Paramedic Care
Principles & Practice
Medicine

Workbook

Fourth Edition

ROBERT S. PORTER

REVISED BY

DEAN C. MEENACH, AAS, RN, BSN, CEN, CCRN, EMT-P
Director of EMS Education
Mineral Area College
Park Hills, Missouri

BRYAN E. BLEDSOE, DO, FACEP, FAAEM, EMT-P
Professor of Emergency Medicine
Director, Prehospital and Disaster Medicine Fellowship
University of Nevada School of Medicine
Attending Emergency Physician
University Medical Center of Southern Nevada
Medical Director, MedicWest Ambulance
Las Vegas, Nevada

ROBERT S. PORTER, MA, EMT-P
Senior Advanced Life Support Educator
Madison County Emergency Medical Services
Canastota, New York

RICHARD A. CHERRY, MS, NREMT-P
Director of Training
Northern Onondaga Volunteer Ambulance
Liverpool, New York

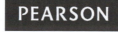

PEARSON

Boston   Columbus   Indianapolis   New York   San Francisco   Upper Saddle River
Amsterdam   Cape Town   Dubai   London   Madrid   Milan   Munich   Paris   Montréal   Toronto
Delhi   Mexico City   São Paulo   Sydney   Hong Kong   Seoul   Singapore   Taipei   Tokyo

Publisher: *Julie Levin Alexander*
Publisher's Assistant: *Regina Bruno*
Editor-in-Chief: *Marlene McHugh Pratt*
Senior Managing Editor for Development: *Lois Berlowitz*
Editorial Project Manager: *Triple SSS Press Media Development, Inc.*
Assistant Editor: *Jonathan Cheung*
Director of Marketing: *David Gesell*
Marketing Manager: *Brian Hoehl*
Marketing Specialist: *Michael Sirinides*
Managing Editor for Production: *Patrick Walsh*
Production Liaison: *Faye Gemmellaro*
Production Editor: *Muralidharan Krishnamurthy/S4Carlisle Publishing Services*
Manufacturing Manager: *Ilene Sanford*
Cover Design: *Kathryn Foot*
Cover Image: © *corepics/Shutterstock*
Composition: *S4Carlisle Publishing Services*
Cover and Interior Printer/Binder: *Edwards Brothers Malloy*

NOTICE ON CPR AND ECC

The national standards for cardiopulmonary resuscitation (CPR) and emergency cardiovascular care (ECC) are reviewed and revised on a regular basis and may change slightly after this manual is printed. It is important that you know the most current procedures for CPR and ECC, both for the classroom and your patients. The most current information may be obtained from the appropriate credentialing agency.

NOTICE ON CARE PROCEDURES

It is the intent of the authors and publisher that this Workbook be used as part of a formal Paramedic program taught by qualified instructors and supervised by a licensed physician. The procedures described in this Workbook are based upon consultation with EMS and medical authorities. The authors and publisher have taken care to make certain that these procedures reflect currently accepted clinical practice; however, they cannot be considered absolute recommendations.

The material in this Workbook contains the most current information available at the time of publication. However, federal, state, and local guidelines concerning clinical practices, including, without limitation, those governing infection control and universal precautions, change rapidly. The reader should note, therefore, that the new regulations may require changes in some procedures.

It is the responsibility of the reader to familiarize himself or herself with the policies and procedures set by federal, state, and local agencies as well as the institution or agency where the reader is employed. The authors and the publisher of this Workbook disclaim any liability, loss, or risk resulting directly or indirectly from the suggested procedures and theory, from any undetected errors, or from the reader's misunderstanding of the text. It is the reader's responsibility to stay informed of any new changes or recommendations made by any federal, state, and local agency as well as by his or her employing institution or agency.

Brady
is an imprint of

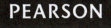

www.bradybooks.com

10 9 8 7 6 5 4 3 2 1

ISBN 10: 0-13-211284-1
ISBN 13: 978-0-13-211284-0

Dedication

*This workbook is dedicated to the important people in your life: your wife/husband,
mother, father, sister, brother . . . and friends who support you and the time and passion
you devote to Emergency Medical Service.
Without them, this endeavor would be lonely and much less rewarding.*

–ROBERT S. PORTER

CONTENTS

INTRODUCTION

Welcome to the self-instructional Workbook for *Paramedic Care: Principles & Practice*. This Workbook is designed to help guide you through an educational program for initial or refresher training that follows the guidelines of the 2009 *National EMS Education Standards*. The Workbook is designed to be used either in conjunction with your instructor or as a self-study guide you use on your own.

This Workbook features many different ways to help you learn the material necessary to become a paramedic, as discussed next.

Features

Review of Chapter Objectives

Each chapter of *Paramedic Care: Principles & Practice* begins with objectives that identify the important information and principles addressed in the chapter reading. To help you identify and learn this material, each Workbook chapter reviews the important content elements addressed by these objectives as presented in the text.

Case Study Review

Each chapter of *Paramedic Care: Principles & Practice* includes a case study, introducing and highlighting important principles presented in the chapter. The Workbook reviews these case studies and points out much of the essential information and many of the applied principles they describe.

Content Self-Evaluation

Each chapter of *Paramedic Care: Principles & Practice* presents an extensive narrative explanation of the principles of paramedic practice. The Workbook chapter (or chapter section) contains between 10 and 50 multiple-choice questions to test your reading comprehension of the textbook material and to give you experience taking typical emergency medical service examinations.

Special Projects

The Workbook contains several projects that are special learning experiences designed to help you remember the information and principles necessary to perform as a paramedic. Special projects include contacting local agencies and services, Internet research, and a variety of other exercises.

Chapter Parts

Several chapters in *Paramedic Care: Principles & Practice* are extensive and contain a great deal of subject matter. To help you to grasp this material more efficiently, the Workbook breaks these chapters into sections with their own objectives, content review, and special projects.

Content Review

The Workbook provides a comprehensive review of the material presented in this volume of *Paramedic Care: Principles & Practice*. After the last text chapter has been covered, the Workbook presents an extensive content self-evaluation component that helps you recall and build upon the knowledge you have gained by reading the text, attending class, and completing the earlier Workbook chapters.

Patient Scenario Flash Cards

This Workbook contains scenario flash cards, each of which presents a patient scenario with signs and symptoms. On the reverse side you will find the appropriate field diagnosis and the care steps you should consider providing for the patient. These cards will help you recognize and remember common serious medical emergencies, their presentation, and the appropriate care that would be given.

HOW TO USE THIS SELF-INSTRUCTIONAL WORKBOOK

The self-instructional Workbook accompanying *Paramedic Care: Principles & Practice* may be used as directed by your instructor or independently by you during your course of instruction. The following recommendations are intended to guide you in using the Workbook independently.

- Examine your course schedule and identify the appropriate text chapter or other assigned reading.

- Read the assigned chapter in *Paramedic Care: Principles & Practice* carefully. Do this in a relaxed environment, free of distractions, and give yourself adequate time to read and digest the material. The information presented in *Paramedic Care: Principles & Practice* is often technically complex and demanding, but it is very important that you comprehend it. Be sure that you read the chapter carefully enough to understand and remember what you have read.

- Carefully read the Review of Chapter Objectives at the beginning of each Workbook chapter (or section). This material includes both the objectives listed in *Paramedic Care: Principles & Practice* and narrative descriptions of their content. If you do not understand or remember what is discussed from your reading, refer to the referenced pages and reread them carefully. If you still do not feel comfortable with your understanding of any objective, consider asking your instructor about it.

- Reread the case study in *Paramedic Care: Principles & Practice*, and then read the Case Study Review in the Workbook. Note the important points regarding assessment and care that the Case Study Review highlights and be sure that you understand and agree with the analysis of the call. If you have any questions or concerns, ask your instructor to clarify the information.

- Take the Content Self-Evaluation at the end of each Workbook chapter (or section), answering each question carefully. Do this in a quiet environment, free from distractions, and allow yourself adequate time to complete the exercise. Correct your self-evaluation by consulting the answers at the back of the Workbook, and determine the percentage you have answered correctly (the number you got right divided by the total number of questions). If you have answered most of the questions correctly (85 to 90 percent), review those that you missed by rereading the material on the pages listed in the answer key and be sure you understand which answer is correct and why. If you have more than a few questions wrong (less than 85 percent correct), look for incorrect answers that are grouped together. This suggests that you did not understand a particular topic in the reading. Reread the text dealing with that topic carefully, and then retest yourself on the questions you got wrong. If incorrect answers are spread throughout the chapter content, reread the chapter and retake the Content Self-Evaluation to ensure that you understand the material. If you don't understand why your answer to a question is incorrect after reviewing the text, consult with your instructor.

- In a similar fashion, complete the exercises in the Special Projects section of the Workbook chapters (or sections). These exercises are specifically designed to help you learn and remember the essential principles and information presented in *Paramedic Care: Principles & Practice*.

- When you have completed this volume of *Paramedic Care: Principles & Practice* and its accompanying Workbook, prepare for a course test by reviewing both the text in its entirety and your class notes. Then take the Content Review examination in the Workbook. Again, review your score and any questions you have answered incorrectly by referring to the text and rereading the page or pages where the material is presented. If you note groupings of wrong answers, review the entire range of pages or the full chapter they represent.

If, during your completion of the Workbook exercises, you have any questions that either the textbook or Workbook doesn't answer, write them down and ask your instructor about them. Prehospital emergency medicine is a complex and complicated subject, and answers are not always black and white. It is also common for different EMS systems to use differing methods of care. The questions you bring up in class, and your instructor's answers to them, will help you expand and complete your knowledge of prehospital emergency medical care.

GUIDELINES TO BETTER TEST-TAKING

The knowledge you will gain from reading the textbook, completing the exercises in the Workbook, listening in your paramedic class, and participating in your clinical and field experience will prepare you to care for patients who are seriously ill or injured. However, before you can practice these skills, you will have to pass several classroom written exams and your state's certification exam. Your performance on these exams will depend not only on your knowledge but also on your ability to answer test questions correctly. The following guidelines are designed to help your performance on tests and to better demonstrate your knowledge of prehospital emergency care.

1. Relax and be calm during the test.

A test is designed to measure what you have learned and to tell you and your instructor how well you are doing. An exam is not designed to intimidate or punish you. Consider it a challenge, and just try to do your best. Get plenty of sleep before the examination. Avoid coffee or other stimulants for a few hours before the exam, and be prepared.

Reread the text chapters, review the objectives in the Workbook, and review your class notes. It might be helpful to work with one or two other students and ask each other questions. This type of practice helps everyone better understand the knowledge presented in your course of study.

2. Read the questions carefully.

Read each word of the question and all the answers slowly. Words such as "except" or "not" may change the entire meaning of the question. If you miss such words, you may answer the question incorrectly even though you know the right answer.

Example:
The art and science of emergency medical services involves all of the following EXCEPT

    A. sincerity and compassion.
    B. respect for human dignity.
    C. placing patient care before personal safety.
    D. delivery of sophisticated emergency medical care.
    E. none of the above.

The correct answer is C, unless you miss the "EXCEPT."

3. Read each answer carefully.

Read each and every answer carefully. Although the first answer may be absolutely correct, so may the rest, and thus the best answer might be "all of the above."

Example:
Indirect medical direction is considered to be

    A. treatment protocols.
    B. training and education.
    C. quality assurance.
    D. chart review.
    E. all of the above.

Although answers A, B, C, and D are each correct, the best and only acceptable answer is "all of the above," E.

4. Delay answering questions you don't understand and look for clues.

When a question seems confusing or you don't know the answer, note it on your answer sheet and come back to it later. This will ensure that you have time to complete the test. You will also find that other questions in the test may give you hints to answer the one you've skipped over. It will also prevent you from being frustrated with an early question and letting it affect your performance.

Example:

Upon successful completion of a course of training as an EMT-P, most states will

- **A.** certify you. (correct)
- **B.** license you.
- **C.** register you.
- **D.** recognize you as a paramedic.
- **E.** issue you a permit.

Another question, later in the exam, may suggest the right answer:

The action of one state in recognizing the certification of another is called:

- **A.** reciprocity. (correct)
- **B.** national registration.
- **C.** licensure.
- **D.** registration.
- **E.** extended practice.

5. Answer all questions.

Even if you do not know the right answer, do not leave a question blank. A blank question is always wrong, whereas a guess might be correct. If you can eliminate some of the answers as wrong, do so. It will increase the chances of a correct guess.

A multiple-choice question with five answers gives a 20 percent chance of a correct guess. If you can eliminate one or more incorrect answers, you increase your odds of a correct guess to 25 percent, 33 percent, and so on. An unanswered question has a 0 percent chance of being correct.

Just before turning in your answer sheet, check to be sure that you have not left any items blank.

Example:

When a paramedic is called by the patient (through the dispatcher) to the scene of a medical emergency, the medical direction physician has established a physician/patient relationship.

- **A.** True
- **B.** False

A true/false question gives you a 50 percent chance of a correct guess.

The hospital health professional(s) responsible for sorting patients as they arrive at the emergency department is (are) usually the

- **A.** emergency physician.
- **B.** ward clerk.
- **C.** emergency nurse.
- **D.** trauma surgeon.
- **E.** both A and C. (correct)

Pulmonology

With each chapter of the workbook, we identify the objectives and the important elements of the text content. You should review these items and refer to the pages listed if any points are not clear.

Because Chapter 1 is lengthy, it has been divided into parts to aid your study. Read the assigned text pages, then progress through the objectives and self-evaluation materials as you would with other chapters. When you feel secure in your grasp of the content, proceed to the next part.

Part 1, p. 1

Review of Chapter Objectives

After reading this part of the chapter, you should be able to:

1. **Define key terms introduced in this chapter.**

    Knowing and being able to apply the key terms in each chapter is critical to understanding chapter concepts. Write the list of key terms. Then write the definition of each one in your own words. Check your understanding by confirming the definitions in the text glossary. Correct any misunderstandings. Create a study aid by writing each key term on the front of an index card and the definition on the back. Use the cards to quiz yourself, or to have someone quiz you.

2. **Adapt the scene size-up, primary assessment, patient history, secondary assessment, and use of monitoring technology to meet the needs of patients with complaints and presentations related to pulmonary disorders.**
    pp. 14–32

    Respiratory emergencies are among the most common EMS calls, and lead to over 200,000 deaths per year. Because of the frequency of such calls, it is critical that you are able to adapt your assessment and treatment priorities to effectively provide care for these patients. When responding to a respiratory emergency, the two monitoring technologies that you will use the most are pulse oximetry and waveform capnography.

    Pulse oximetry is a standard device used to assess the patient's oxygen saturation. A reading of 91 to 94 percent indicates mild hypoxemia. This reading is important in post–cardiac arrest patients. According to the American Heart Association (AHA), post–cardiac arrest care should include maintaining oxygen saturation ≥ 94 percent. Supplemental oxygen should be titrated to the recommended level and hyperoxygenation should be avoided. See Table 1-2 in the text for treatment strategies based on pulse oximetry readings.

    Waveform capnography provides the end-tidal CO_2 ($EtCO_2$) reading and a graphic recording of the ventilatory effort over time. By becoming familiar with waveform capnography readings and waveforms, you can distinguish between many pulmonary conditions. See Table 1-3 in the text for spirometry and peak flow values for adults.

Waveform capnography is also a useful reassessment tool to determine if a treatment is actually improving ventilatory function. Perhaps one of the best uses of waveform capnography is as a tool to guide the rate and depth of assisted ventilations, confirmation of endotracheal tube (ETT) placement, and as an indicator of return of spontaneous circulation (ROSC) during cardiac arrest.

3. **Use a process of clinical reasoning to guide and interpret the patient assessment and management process for patients with pulmonary disorders.** pp. 14–23

As a paramedic, it is vital you develop your clinical reasoning process to quickly recognize and treat acute respiratory conditions to improve patient outcomes. Develop an organized general impression to identify signs of respiratory distress. This will include assessing possible cardiac arrest patients with a CAB assessment instead of the ABC assessment.

4. **Given a variety of scenarios, recognize risk factors for pulmonary disorders.** pp. 3–40

Some risk factors for pulmonary disorders include: the very young and very old; cigarette smoking; alcoholism; exposure to cold temperatures; patients undergoing immune suppressive therapy; conditions of immobility; history of chest trauma; chronic pulmonary disease; inhaled toxic exposure; patients taking corticosteroids; and exposure to communicable disease.

5. **Relate the anatomy and physiology of the respiratory system to the assessment and management of patients with pulmonary disorders.** pp. 4–23

The respiratory system is functionally divided into the upper airway and the lower airway. The upper airway comprises the nasal cavity, pharynx, and larynx. The lower airway comprises the trachea, bronchi, alveoli, and lungs. In pulmonary disorders, these structures function abnormally and a disruption in ventilation, diffusion, or perfusion occurs. Therefore, successful interpretation of your assessment findings will depend upon your understanding of the structure and function of the respiratory system. For example, when secretions, edema, or foreign bodies occlude the upper airway, the process of ventilation is disrupted. When fluid fills the small alveolar sacks, diffusion is impaired. An embolus from a deep vein thrombosis (DVT) may travel to a pulmonary artery and create a pulmonary embolism, halting perfusion (circulation) to lung tissue.

6. **Recognize conditions that lead to disruptions in ventilation.** pp. 12–13

A major function of the respiratory system is the exchange of gases between the person and the environment. Three processes allow the gas exchange to take place: ventilation, diffusion, and perfusion. Ventilation is the movement of air in and out of the lungs. Ventilation may be disrupted by diseases that cause obstruction of any part of the airway, disrupt the normal function of the chest wall, or impair nervous system control of breathing. Conditions that result from disruptions in ventilation include asthma, emphysema, chronic bronchitis, pneumonia, upper respiratory infection, and SARS. Other conditions that cause disruptions in ventilation include tension and spontaneous pneumothorax, hyperventilation syndrome, flail chest, upper airway obstruction, and central nervous system dysfunction.

7. **Recognize conditions that lead to disruptions in diffusion.** pp. 13–14

Diffusion is the movement of gases between the alveoli and the pulmonary capillaries (oxygen from the lungs into the bloodstream; waste carbon dioxide from the bloodstream into the lungs) as well as between the systemic capillaries and the body tissues (oxygen from the bloodstream into the cells; waste carbon dioxide from the cells into the bloodstream). Diffusion can be disrupted by a change in concentration of atmospheric oxygen or carbon dioxide (CO_2), or by any disease that affects the structure or patency of alveoli, the thickness of the respiratory membrane, or the permeability of the capillaries. Conditions that result from disruptions in diffusion include acute respiratory distress syndrome (ARDS), pulmonary edema, emphysema, and atelectasis.

©2013 Pearson Education, Inc.
Paramedic Care: Principles & Practice, Vol. 4, 4th Ed.

8. **Recognize conditions that lead to disruptions in perfusion.** pp. 13–14

Perfusion is the circulation of blood through the capillaries. Adequate perfusion is critical to adequate gas exchange in the lungs and body tissues. Perfusion will be affected by any disease that limits blood flow through the lungs and the body, or reduces the volume of the oxygen-carrying red blood cells or hemoglobin. Conditions that result from disruptions in perfusion include: pulmonary edema, low cardiac output such as in shock states and cardiac arrest, anemia, carbon monoxide poisoning, and cyanide poisoning.

Case Study Review

It is important to review each emergency response you participate in as a paramedic. Similarly, we will review the case study that precedes each chapter. We will address the important points of the response as addressed by the chapter. Often, this will include the scene size-up, patient assessment, patient management, patient packaging, and transport.

Reread the case study on pages 2 and 3 in Paramedic Care: Medicine; *then, read the following discussion.*

This case study demonstrates how paramedics can reach a field diagnosis and choose appropriate emergency treatment in a respiratory emergency. On this call, Tony and Lee gather critical information from the patient history.

Tony and Lee learn that their patient is a 55-year-old male who is having difficultly breathing. He is already being given oxygen.

Once on the scene, they grab the equipment they think they may need, enter the house (checking for safety), and approach the patient, who is seated at the kitchen table, obviously short of breath. They avoid leaping to conclusions and begin their systematic assessment. The primary assessment confirms that the patient has a patent airway, is moving a little air, and has a strong pulse. They replace the nasal cannula the first responder had provided with a nonrebreather mask and continue the assessment.

The physical exam reveals diminished breath sounds, rhonchi, use of accessory muscles of respiration, and cyanosis around the mouth. These findings confirm the original complaint: breathing difficulty. But because this is a medical patient (no mechanism of injury was noted during the scene size-up), Tony and Lee know that the most critical information is likely to come from the history. In fact, they learn that the patient has been diagnosed with emphysema (and has an ongoing 60-pack/year smoking history), and some worsening or exacerbation of this condition is the most likely cause of the patient's current emergency.

Tony and Lee know that emphysema results in bronchoconstriction, alveolar collapse, and a decrease in pulmonary capillaries, which interferes with ventilation and diffusion. The constricted bronchi and destruction of the walls of the small bronchioles make exhalation difficult, causing the rhonchi heard on auscultation of this patient, and also prevent oxygen from reaching the alveoli. The patient no longer has enough healthy alveoli or pulmonary capillaries to provide for adequate oxygen diffusion into the blood-stream. This, they understand, is why the patient's pulse oximetry reading is only 90 percent, even though he is receiving supplemental oxygen.

The two paramedics know that emergency treatment must be aimed at relief of the patient's hypoxia and bronchoconstriction. They continue administration of supplemental oxygen to compensate for the decreased diffusion the patient's diseased alveoli and capillaries are providing. In consultation with medical direction, they start an IV of normal saline, knowing that the fluid may counter any dehydration present and may help to loosen any excess mucus that may be blocking the bronchioles. Additionally, medical direction orders nebulizer administration of levalbuterol (Xopenex) to relieve bronchoconstriction, as well as methyl-prednisolone (Solu-Medrol) by IV push to relieve inflammation.

Monitoring of the patient en route to the hospital shows the effectiveness of these interventions. The patient's respirations slow to a normal rate and his oxygen saturation increases to 96 percent. Waveform capnography shows a plateau phase that is nearly horizontal and an $EtCO_2$ reading of 42 mmHg.

Content Self-Evaluation

Each of the chapters in this workbook includes a short content review. The questions are designed to test your ability to remember what you read. At the end of this workbook, you can find the answers to the questions as well as the pages where the topic of the question was discussed in the text. If you answer the question incorrectly or are unsure of the answer, review the pages listed.

MATCHING—KEY TERMS SECTION A

Match each term with its correct description by writing the letter in the space provided next to the term.

A. characterized by the presence of two diseases—emphysema and chronic bronchitis

B. hemoglobin without oxygen

C. the process by which gases move between the alveoli and pulmonary capillaries

D. absence of breathing

E. chemicals formed due to hyperoxia that can damage body cells and tissues

F. the transport protein that carries oxygen in the blood

G. an above-normal amount of oxygen to the tissues

H. normal level of oxygen in inspired air

I. chest wall injury in which three or more consecutive ribs on the same side of the chest have been fractured in at least two places

J. where the trachea divides into the right and left mainstem bronchus

K. below-normal levels of oxygen in inspired air, resulting in decreased tissue oxygenation

L. a life-threatening condition that affects gas exchange caused by fluid buildup in the interstitial space within the lungs

M. also known as "difficulty breathing"

N. bluish discoloration

O. a respiratory pattern with a rate slower than 12 breaths per minute.

P. right-sided heart failure caused by pulmonary hypertension

Q. coughing up blood

R. compensatory breathing mechanism in which expansion of the nares increases the volume of inspired air

S. molecule formed when hemoglobin and carbon dioxide combine

T. impairment of ventilatory exchange of oxygen and carbon dioxide

U. difficulty breathing while lying flat

V. profuse sweating

W. noise or vibration produced by bones rubbing together

X. toxic chemicals caused by excessive oxygenation

Y. accumulation of blood in the pleural space

©2013 Pearson Education, Inc.
Paramedic Care: Principles & Practice, Vol. 4, 4th Ed.

_____ 1. Acute respiratory distress syndrome (ARDS)

_____ 2. Apnea

_____ 3. Asphyxia

_____ 4. Bradypnea

_____ 5. Carina

_____ 6. Carbaminohemoglobin

_____ 7. Chronic obstructive pulmonary disease (COPD)

_____ 8. Cor pulmonale

_____ 9. Crepitus

_____ 10. Cyanosis

_____ 11. Deoxyhemoglobin

_____ 12. Diaphoresis

_____ 13. Diffusion

_____ 14. Dyspnea

_____ 15. Flail chest

_____ 16. Reactive oxygen species (ROS)

_____ 17. Free radicals

_____ 18. Hemoglobin

_____ 19. Hemoptysis

_____ 20. Hemothorax

_____ 21. Hypoxia

_____ 22. Hyperoxia

_____ 23. Nasal flaring

_____ 24. Normoxia

_____ 25. Orthopnea

MATCHING—KEY TERMS SECTION B

Match each term with its correct description by writing the letter in the space provided next to the term.

A. difficulty breathing at night

B. accumulation of air within the pleural space

C. the presence of air in the subcutaneous tissues

D. a compensatory breathing mechanism in which the accessory muscles of the neck are used to increase negative intrathoracic pressure and increase the volume of inspired air

E. the exchange of gases between a living organism and its environment

F. hemoglobin bound with oxygen

G. an abnormal increase in the number of red blood cells

H. pale skin (paleness) caused by inadequate peripheral circulation

I. a substance that reduces alveolar surface tension so that the alveoli can expand and contract

J. circulation of blood through the capillaries

K. pertaining to the pleura or pleurisy

L. the vibration felt in the chest during vocalization

M. a respiratory rate that exceeds 20 breaths per minute

N. the negative logarithm of the H^+ ion concentration used to measure the acidity or alkalinity of a liquid

O. displacement of the trachea due to mediastinal shifting as a result of increased intrathoracic pressure

P. a process in which cells and tissues are damaged by free radicals (reactive oxygen species)

Q. accumulation of air within the pleural space that occurs in the absence of blunt or penetrating trauma

R. the mechanical process of moving air in and out of the lungs

S. faster-than-normal heart rate

T. intervention used to maintain the patency of the alveoli and adequate oxygenation

_____ **1.** Oxyhemoglobin

_____ **2.** Oxidative stress

_____ **3.** Pallor

_____ **4.** Paroxysmal nocturnal dyspnea

_____ **5.** Perfusion

_____ **6.** PH

_____ **7.** Pleuritic

_____ **8.** Pneumothorax

_____ **9.** Polycythemia

_____ **10.** Positive end-expiratory pressure (PEEP)

_____ **11.** Respiration

_____ **12.** Spontaneous pneumothorax

_____ **13.** Subcutaneous emphysema

_____ **14.** Surfactant

_____ **15.** Tachycardia

_____ **16.** Tachypnea

_____ **17.** Tactile fremitus

_____ **18.** Tracheal deviation

_____ **19.** Tracheal tugging

_____ **20.** Ventilation

©2013 Pearson Education, Inc.
Paramedic Care: Principles & Practice, Vol. 4, 4th Ed.

MULTIPLE CHOICE

_____ 1. Which of the following is considered an intrinsic risk factor for respiratory disease?
  A. Smokestack pollutants
  B. Polluted water
  C. Genetic predisposition
  D. Cigarette smoking
  E. Stress

_____ 2. Which of the following is NOT part of the upper airway?
  A. Nasal cavity
  B. Oropharynx
  C. Laryngopharynx
  D. Trachea
  E. Larynx

_____ 3. Which of the following is part of the lower airway?
  A. Esophagus
  B. Ileum
  C. Tonsils
  D. Hypopharynx
  E. Bronchi

_____ 4. Most of the exchange of oxygen and carbon dioxide takes place in the
  A. trachea.
  B. bronchi.
  C. pulmonary ducts.
  D. bronchioles.
  E. alveoli.

_____ 5. The three processes that allow gas exchange to occur in the lungs and body tissues are
  A. ventilation, diffusion, and perfusion.
  B. inspiration, expiration, and ventilation.
  C. resistance, compliance, and perfusion.
  D. ventilation, inspiration, and expiration.
  E. inspiration, compliance, and diffusion.

_____ 6. The mechanical process of moving air in and out of the lungs is
  A. ventilation.
  B. diffusion.
  C. perfusion.
  D. inspiration.
  E. inhalation.

_____ 7. The process by which gases move between the alveoli and the pulmonary capillaries is
  A. infusion.
  B. perfusion.
  C. respiration.
  D. diffusion.
  E. permeation.

_____ 8. Lung perfusion is dependent on three factors—adequate blood volume, efficient pumping by the heart, and intact
  A. alveoli.
  B. respiratory membrane.
  C. bronchioles.
  D. goblet cells.
  E. pulmonary capillaries.

_____ 9. Any of the following can disrupt ventilation, EXCEPT
  A. obstruction of the upper airway.
  B. obstruction of the lower airway.
  C. blockage of the pulmonary arteries.
  D. impairment of normal function of the chest wall.
  E. abnormalities of the nervous system's control of breathing.

_____ 10. Which of the following abnormal breathing patterns is characterized by long, deep breaths that are stopped during the inspiratory phase and separated by periods of apnea?
  A. Ataxic (Biot's) respirations (seen with increased intracranial pressure)
  B. Central neurogenic hyperventilation (seen with stroke or brainstem injury)
  C. Kussmaul's respirations (seen with metabolic acidosis)
  D. Apneustic respirations (seen with stroke or severe central nervous system disease)
  E. Cheyne-Stokes respirations (seen with terminal illness or brain injury)

11. Which of the following is NOT likely to cause hypoxia (inadequate cellular oxygen supply)?
    A. Ascension to a high altitude
    B. Esophageal ulceration
    C. Black lung disease
    D. Left-sided heart failure
    E. Asbestos inhalation

12. Pulmonary shunting results from
    A. alveolar collapse.
    B. blockage of pulmonary capillaries.
    C. bronchoconstriction.
    D. excess mucus production.
    E. airway obstruction.

13. The most important action when you arrive on the scene and discover that a hazardous material is present is to
    A. have supplemental oxygen available.
    B. assure your own safety.
    C. search for additional patients.
    D. put on self-contained breathing apparatus (SCBA).
    E. call for a hazardous materials team.

14. You are dispatched to a patient with difficulty breathing. Which of the following should be part of the scene size-up?
    A. Establish a patent airway.
    B. Look for clues to the possible cause.
    C. Evaluate AVPU mental status.
    D. Determine respiration rate.
    E. Ready the oxygenation equipment.

15. During the initial assessment, your general impression of the patient's respiratory status should include all of the following elements, EXCEPT
    A. pulse.
    B. position.
    C. color.
    D. mental status.
    E. ability to speak.

16. Which of the following is NOT a classic sign of respiratory distress?
    A. Pursed lips
    B. Tracheal tugging
    C. Diaphoresis
    D. Nasal flaring
    E. Cyanosis

17. Which of the following is TRUE with regard to assessing the airway?
    A. Noisy breathing usually indicates a complete obstruction.
    B. Obstructed breathing is not always noisy breathing.
    C. If the airway is blocked, artificial respiration must be started immediately.
    D. If the airway is blocked, endotracheal intubation must be established.
    E. If the airway is open, the patient is breathing.

18. Which of the following is the MOST ominous sign of possible life-threatening respiratory distress?
    A. Altered mental status
    B. Audible stridor
    C. One- to two-word dyspnea
    D. Tachycardia
    E. Use of accessory muscles

19. Orthopnea is
    A. dizziness when rising from a supine position.
    B. dyspnea that occurs while lying supine.
    C. short attacks of dyspnea that interrupt sleep.
    D. apnea that occurs while in an upright position.
    E. pleuritic pain that occurs during breathing.

©2013 Pearson Education, Inc.
Paramedic Care: Principles & Practice, Vol. 4, 4th Ed.

_____ 20. Which of the following is NOT considered a chronic respiratory disease?
- A. Pneumonia
- B. Emphysema
- C. Chronic bronchitis
- D. Asthma
- E. Lung cancer

_____ 21. Which of the following medications would be of LEAST significance if found in the home of a patient with a respiratory complaint?
- A. Oxygen
- B. Bronchodilator
- C. Vitamin C tablets
- D. Corticosteroid
- E. Antibiotic

_____ 22. Cardiac patients often present with dyspnea.
- A. True
- B. False

_____ 23. Allergic reaction to a medication may be the cause of a respiratory complaint.
- A. True
- B. False

_____ 24. Breathing through pursed lips during respiratory distress helps to
- A. prevent tracheal collapse.
- B. force air past a bronchial obstruction.
- C. bring up excess mucus.
- D. close the epiglottis.
- E. keep the alveoli open.

_____ 25. Pink or bloody sputum is commonly seen with all of the following, EXCEPT
- A. pulmonary edema.
- B. lung cancer.
- C. tuberculosis.
- D. allergic reaction.
- E. bronchial infection.

_____ 26. Asymmetrical chest movement is most likely to be found during
- A. auscultation.
- B. capnometry.
- C. oximetry.
- D. inspection.
- E. percussion.

_____ 27. Subcutaneous emphysema is most likely to be found during
- A. oximetry.
- B. percussion.
- C. capnometry.
- D. palpation.
- E. inspection.

_____ 28. Wheezing is most likely to be detected during
- A. oximetry.
- B. auscultation.
- C. percussion.
- D. capnometry.
- E. palpation.

_____ 29. Rattling sounds in the larger airways associated with excess mucus are called
- A. stridor.
- B. wheezing.
- C. crackles (rales).
- D. snoring.
- E. rhonchi.

_____ 30. A harsh, high-pitched sound heard on inspiration, associated with upper airway obstruction, is called
- A. snoring.
- B. stridor.
- C. crackles (rales).
- D. rhonchi.
- E. rales.

_____ 31. In general, tachycardia is a nonspecific finding seen, for example, with fear, anxiety, or fever. In a patient with a respiratory complaint, however, tachycardia may also indicate
- A. hypothermia.
- B. hypertrophy.
- C. hypotension.
- D. hyperopia.
- E. hypoxia.

32. Drugs that may cause an elevation in both heart rate and blood pressure include
   A. diuretics such as furosemide.
   B. analgesics such as morphine sulfate.
   C. tranquilizers such as diazepam.
   D. sympathomimetics such as albuterol.
   E. beta blockers such as labetalol.

33. An elevated respiratory rate in a patient with dyspnea is most likely caused by
   A. bradycardia.
   B. dysuria.
   C. hypoxia.
   D. anemia.
   E. tachycardia.

34. In a patient with dyspnea, a persistently slow respiratory rate
   A. indicates impending respiratory arrest.
   B. is less critical than a persistently rapid rate.
   C. is a common symptom of asthma.
   D. indicates cardiac involvement.
   E. is commonly associated with pneumonia.

35. Which of the following measures end-expiratory carbon dioxide?
   A. Spirometry
   B. Sphygmomanometry
   C. Capnometry
   D. Oximetry
   E. Tomography

MATCHING

Match each respiratory condition with its identified cause by writing the letter in the space provided next to the respiratory condition. Use the following letters:

V = Abnormal Ventilation   **D = Abnormal Diffusion**   **P = Abnormal Perfusion**

36. Acute respiratory distress syndrome (ARDS)

37. Chronic obstructive pulmonary disease (COPD), either emphysema or chronic bronchitis

38. Asthma

39. Childhood epiglottitis

40. Atelectasis

41. Cardiac-related pulmonary edema

42. Pulmonary embolism

43. Croup

44. Dysfunction of the spinal cord

45. Shock states

46. Cardiac arrest

Label the Diagrams

Supply the missing labels for the drawing of the upper airway by writing the appropriate letters in the spaces provided.

A. cricoid cartilage

B. cricothyroid membrane

©2013 Pearson Education, Inc.
Paramedic Care: Principles & Practice, Vol. 4, 4th Ed.

C. epiglottis

D. esophagus

E. glottic opening

F. thyroid cartilage

G. tongue

H. tonsils and adenoids

I. trachea

J. turbinates

K. laryngopharynx

L. larynx

M. nasal cavity

N. nasopharynx

O. oropharynx

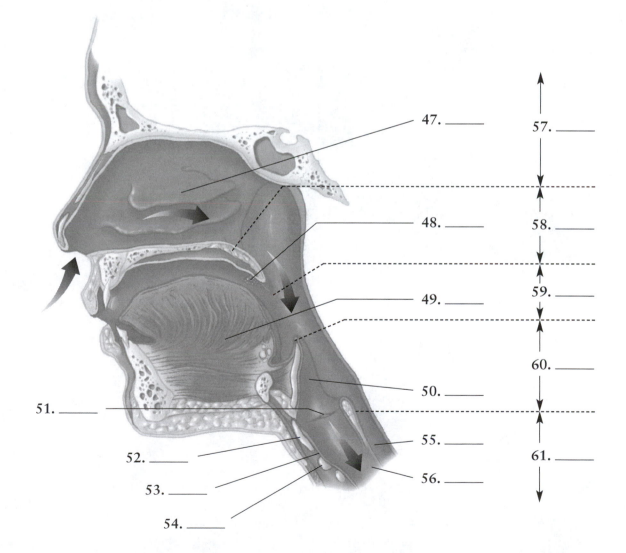

47. _____

48. _____

49. _____

50. _____

51. _____

52. _____

53. _____

54. _____

55. _____

56. _____

57. _____

58. _____

59. _____

60. _____

61. _____

Supply the missing labels for the drawing of the lower airway by writing the appropriate letters in the spaces provided.

A. carina

B. larynx

C. left mainstem bronchus

D. right mainstem bronchus

E. trachea

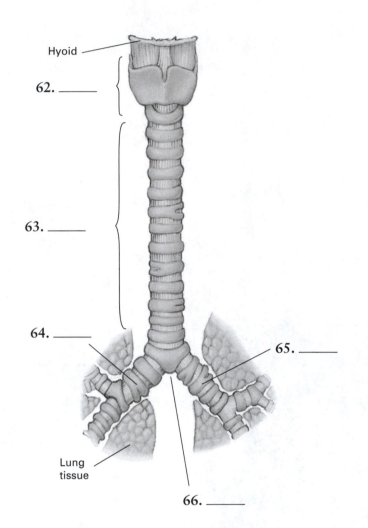

©2013 Pearson Education, Inc.

Paramedic Care: Principles & Practice, Vol. 4, 4th Ed.

Special Project

Evaluating Abnormal Breathing Patterns

Read the following three scenarios about patients who present with abnormal breathing patterns. On the lines—on the basis of the brief information given—write the name of the breathing pattern the patient seems to display and the condition (or conditions, if you think there is more than one possibility) you think is most likely causing the abnormal breathing pattern. Review the text, pages 12–18, for help in completing your answers.

Scenario 1: You are called to the home of an elderly woman who is unresponsive. Her family tells you she had her ninetieth birthday last month but has been bedridden for two weeks and has "not been doing very well." Today, they have not been able to rouse her. On assessment, you find that the patient is breathing in a pattern of progressively increasing tidal volume, followed by progressively declining volume, separated by periods of apnea.

Breathing pattern: _____ **Probable cause:** _____

_____

_____

_____

Scenario 2: You are called to a local fitness center where a middle-aged man who was participating in an exercise class suddenly complained of a terrible headache. He lurched sideways, then sat down hard on the exercise mat. By the time you arrive, he has lost consciousness. When you assess his breathing, you find repeated sets of gasping ventilations separated by periods of apnea.

Breathing pattern: _____ **Probable cause:** _____

_____

_____

_____

Scenario 3: You are dispatched to a downtown office where the billing manager has fallen ill. You find her slumped on a sofa in the women's restroom. She has an altered mental status and is barely coherent. A medical ID bracelet identifies her as a diabetic. A coworker says that she has been diabetic since childhood and takes insulin by injection but has lately been neglecting to take her injections regularly. Her respirations are deep and rapid.

Breathing pattern: _____ **Probable cause:** _____

_____

_____

_____

Review of Chapter Objectives

After reading this part of the chapter, you should be able to:

9. Describe the pathophysiology of specific respiratory disorders, including airway obstruction, acute respiratory distress syndrome, obstructive lung diseases, upper respiratory infection, pneumonia, SARS, lung cancer, toxic inhalation, pulmonary embolism, spontaneous pneumothorax, hyperventilation syndrome, central nervous system dysfunction, dysfunction of the spinal cord, nerves, and muscles.

   a. Upper airway obstruction   pp. 12–24

   Upper airway obstruction is characterized by a partial or complete occlusion of the upper airway structures. Causes may include trauma, infection, allergic reactions, neurologic disorders, endocrine disorders, and drug/alcohol use, just to name a few. Upper airway structures may be obstructed by the tongue (most common), food, secretions, swelling, dentures, or other foreign bodies. Assessment may reveal hoarseness, facial burns, angioedema, choking, stridor, drooling, cyanosis, or even apnea. Prehospital management is based on the nature of the obstruction.

   b. Noncardiac pulmonary edema/acute respiratory distress syndrome   pp. 25–27

   Acute respiratory distress syndrome (ARDS) is characterized by pulmonary edema caused by fluid accumulation in the interstitial spaces in the lungs. The mortality rate is 70 percent. ARDS occurs as a result of increased vascular permeability and decreased fluid removal from the lungs. A variety of lung insults can cause this inability to maintain proper fluid balance, including sepsis, pneumonia, inhalation injuries, emboli, tumors, and others noted in the text chapter. ARDS interferes with diffusion, causing hypoxia. In addition to evaluating the degree of the patient's respiratory distress, assessment is aimed at discovering symptoms and history that point to the underlying condition. Prehospital management is supportive (oxygen supplementation is essential to compensate for diffusion defects); in-hospital care is aimed at treatment of the underlying condition.

   c. Obstructive lung diseases   pp. 27–28

   Obstructive lung disease is a common set of conditions that includes asthma, emphysema, and chronic bronchitis. A condition called chronic obstructive pulmonary disease (COPD) is characterized by the presence of two diseases—emphysema and chronic bronchitis. Each is described in more detail below.

   Emphysema   pp. 28–29

   Like chronic bronchitis, emphysema is classified as a COPD. Alveolar walls are destroyed by exposure to noxious substances such as cigarette smoke or other environmental toxins. The disease also causes destruction of the walls of the small bronchioles, which contributes to a trapping of air in the lungs. The result is a decrease in both ventilation and diffusion. Patients tend to breathe through pursed lips, which creates a positive pressure that helps to prevent alveolar collapse. A developing decrease in PaO_2 leads to a compensatory increase in red blood cell production (polycythemia). Emphysema patients are more susceptible to acute respiratory infections and cardiac dysrhythmias. They become dependent on bronchodilators and corticosteroids and, in the final stages, supplemental oxygen. In contrast to chronic bronchitis sufferers, emphysema patients often lose weight and seldom have a cough except early in the morning. Because of the habit of breathing through pursed lips and the color produced by polycythemia, they are sometimes called "pink puffers." Clubbed fingers are common. Auscultation may reveal diminished breath sounds and, at times, wheezes and rhonchi. There may also be signs of right-sided heart disease. As a result of severe respiratory impairment, COPD patients may exhibit confusion, agitation, somnolence, one- to two-word dyspnea, and use of accessory muscles to assist respiration.

©2013 Pearson Education, Inc.
Paramedic Care: Principles & Practice, Vol. 4, 4th Ed.

Chronic bronchitis
pp. 29–30

Chronic bronchitis is classified, along with emphysema, as a COPD. COPD affects 25 percent of adults, with chronic bronchitis affecting one in five adult males. Chronic bronchitis reduces ventilation as a result of increased mucus production that blocks airway passages. It is often caused by cigarette smoking but also occurs in nonsmokers. There may be a history of frequent respiratory infections. Chronic bronchitis is usually associated with a productive cough and copious sputum. Patients tend to be overweight and often become cyanotic, so they are sometimes called "blue bloaters." Auscultation of the airway often reveals rhonchi as a result of mucus occlusion. The goals of treatment are relief of hypoxia and reversal of bronchoconstriction. Because these patients may be dependent on a hypoxic respiratory drive (low oxygen levels stimulate respiration), respiratory effort may become depressed when oxygen is administered. Needed oxygen should not be withheld, but the patient's respirations must be carefully monitored. IV fluids may help loosen mucous congestion. Medical direction may also order administration of a bronchodilator, such as albuterol, metaproterenol, or ipratropium bromide, and may also recommend corticosteroid administration.

Asthma
pp. 30–34

Asthma is an obstructive lung disease that causes abnormal ventilation. Although deaths from other respiratory diseases are decreasing, deaths from asthma have been on the increase, with 50 percent of those deaths occurring before the patient reaches the hospital. Asthma is thought to be caused by a combination of genetic predisposition and environmental triggers that differ from individual to individual. These include allergens, cold air, exercise, stress, and certain medications. Exposure to a trigger causes release of histamine, which in turn causes both bronchial constriction and capillary leakage that leads to bronchial edema. The result is a significant decrease in expiratory air flow, which is the essence of an "asthma attack." In the early phase of an attack, inhaled bronchodilator medications such as albuterol will help. In the late phase, inflammation sets in and anti-inflammatory drugs are required to alleviate the condition. Assessment must focus first on evaluation and support of the airway and breathing. Most patients will report a history of asthma. The physical exam should focus on the chest and neck to assess breathing effort. The respiratory rate is the most critical of the vital signs. EMS systems should also be able to measure the peak expiratory flow rate. Treatment is aimed at correction of hypoxia (oxygen administration) and relief of bronchospasm and inflammation. A special case is status asthmaticus, a severe, prolonged attack that does not respond to bronchodilators. It is a serious emergency requiring prompt recognition, treatment, and transport. Another special case is asthma in children, which is treated much as for adults but with altered medication dosages and some special medications.

d. Upper respiratory infections (URIs)
pp. 34–35

Infections of the upper airways of the respiratory tract are among the most common infectious conditions for which patients seek medical assistance, and you will see them in the field. Even though these infections are rarely life threatening, they can produce considerable discomfort. At-home management is usually symptomatic, with treatment for pain and fever, as needed, as well as appropriate antibiotic therapy if the infection is bacterial. However, an upper respiratory tract infection in a person with preexisting pulmonary disease can trigger severe problems, and you should pay particularly close attention to airway and ventilation in patients with asthma or COPD. Be sure to monitor the condition with pulse oximetry and electrocardiogram (ECG) during transport to a treatment facility.

e. Pneumonia
pp. 35–36

Pneumonia, or lung infection, is a leading cause of death in the elderly and those with HIV infection and is the fifth leading cause of death in the United States overall. It is an infection most commonly caused by bacterial or viral infection, rarely by fungal and other infections. Risk factors center on conditions that cause a defect in mucus production or ciliary action that weaken the body's natural defenses against invaders of the respiratory system. Common signs and symptoms include an ill appearance, fever and shaking chills, a productive cough, and sputum. Many cases involve pleuritic chest pain. Auscultation usually reveals crackles (rales) in the involved lung segments, or sometimes wheezes or rhonchi, and occasionally egophony (change in spoken "E" sound to "A"). Percussion produces dullness over the affected areas. Some forms of pneumonia do not produce these distinctive symptoms, presenting instead with systemic complaints such as headache, malaise, fatigue, muscle aches, sore throat, nausea, vomiting, and diarrhea. Diagnosis in the field is unlikely and treatment is supportive. Place the patient in a comfortable position and administer high-flow oxygen. In severe cases, ventilatory assistance and possibly endotracheal intubation may be necessary. Medical direction may recommend administration of a beta agonist. Antipyretics may be given to reduce a high fever.

f. Severe acute respiratory syndrome (SARS)   pp. 36–37

Severe acute respiratory syndrome is rapidly progressing respiratory distress caused by a virus similar to that responsible for the common cold. Transmission occurs through droplets as the patient coughs or sneezes and these droplets contact the membranes of the mouth, nose, or eyes. Incubation takes from two to seven days and the patient is considered contagious as long as he displays symptoms. Signs and symptoms associated with SARS include rhinorrhea, chills, muscle aches, headache, diarrhea, and the signs of serious respiratory distress—dyspnea, cough, cyanosis, and hypoxia. Management of the SARS patient includes personal protective equipment (PPE), high-concentration oxygen, pulse oximetry monitoring, and respiratory assistance and endotracheal intubation, as needed. Initiate intravenous fluid administration to ensure adequate hydration and consider a nebulized bronchodilator if wheezing is present.

g. Lung cancer   pp. 37–38

Lung cancer (neoplasms, literally "new growths" or tumors) is the leading cause of cancer-related death in the United States in both men and women. The primary problems are disruption of diffusion and, if the bronchioles are involved, of ventilation as well. The primary risk factor is cigarette smoking. Inhalation of other environmental toxins is also a risk factor. Less commonly, lung cancer can result from the spread of cancer from another part of the body. EMS calls to patients with lung cancer may involve a variety of complaints related to the disease, including cough, hoarseness, chest pain, and bloody sputum. There may be fever, chills, and chest pain if the patient has developed pneumonia. There can be weakness, numbness of the arm, shoulder pain, and difficulty swallowing. The physical exam may reveal weight loss, crackles (rales), wheezes, rhonchi, and diminished breath sounds in the affected lung. There may be venous distention of the arms and neck. Your primary responsibility is to identify and address signs of respiratory distress. Assist ventilation and administer supplemental oxygen as needed. Establish IV access and consult medical direction about possible administration of bronchodilators and corticosteroids. Transport, but be alert for any do not resuscitate (DNR) orders.

h. Toxic inhalation   pp. 38–39

Toxic inhalation may be characterized by history of exposure, pain in the respiratory tract, hypoxemia, dyspnea, abnormal breathing patterns, abnormal lung sounds, chest pain, or airway swelling. Signs and symptoms will depend on the type of exposure, duration of exposure, as well as the patient's age and underlying pulmonary disease. When assessing the patient with possible toxic inhalation exposure, determine the nature of the inhalant. Prehospital management of toxic inhalation will include careful attention to scene safety, supportive measures, and transport to the appropriate specialty care center.

i. Pulmonary embolism   pp. 39–40

A pulmonary embolism is a blood clot (thrombus) that lodges in an artery in the lungs. One in five cases of sudden death is caused by pulmonary thromboembolism. It is a life-threatening condition because it can significantly reduce pulmonary blood flow (perfusion), causing hypoxemia (lack of oxygen in the blood). Immobilization, such as recent surgery, a long bone fracture, or being bedridden, increases the risk of developing an embolism. Other risk factors for clot formation include pregnancy, oral birth control medications, cancer, and sickle cell anemia. The classic symptom of pulmonary embolism is a sudden onset of severe dyspnea, which may or may not be accompanied by pleuritic pain. The physical exam may reveal other signs, including labored breathing, tachypnea, and tachycardia. In severe cases, there may be signs of right-sided heart failure, including jugular vein distention and, possibly, falling blood pressure. Auscultation may reveal no significant findings. In 50 percent of cases, examination of the extremities will reveal signs suggesting deep venous thrombosis (warm, swollen extremity with a thick cord palpated along the medial thigh and pain on palpation or when extending the calf). Because a large embolism may cause cardiac arrest, be prepared to perform resuscitation. Primary care is aimed at support of the airway, breathing, and circulation. As necessary, assist ventilations and provide supplemental oxygen. Endotracheal intubation may be required. Establish IV access, monitor vital signs and cardiac rhythms, and transport expeditiously to a facility that can care for the patient's critical needs.

j. Spontaneous pneumothorax   **pp. 40–41**

Spontaneous pneumothorax, which occurs in the absence of trauma, is a relatively common condition, occurring in roughly 18 persons per 100,000. It is relatively likely to recur as well (with 50 percent recurrence rate at two years). Significant risk factors include male gender, age 20 to 40 years, tall and thin stature, and history of cigarette smoking. Presentation is marked by sudden-onset pleuritic chest or shoulder pain, often precipitated by a bout of coughing or by heavy lifting. The loss of negative pressure in the affected hemithorax prevents proper chest expansion, and the patient may report dyspnea. In individuals who do NOT have significant underlying pulmonary disease, a pneumothorax of up to 15 to 20 percent of the chest cavity can be tolerated fairly well. Monitor symptoms and pulse oximetry readings during transport. Be especially attentive in your ongoing assessment of patients who require positive-pressure ventilation. These patients are at higher risk for development of tension pneumothorax, which is marked by increasing resistance to ventilation, along with hypoxia, cyanosis, and possible hypotension. Exam will reveal tracheal deviation away from the affected side of the chest and distention of the jugular vein. Needle decompression of a tension pneumothorax may be required.

k. Hyperventilation syndrome   **pp. 41–**

Hyperventilation, with rapid breathing, chest pain, and numbness in the extremities, is often associated with anxiety, and it is called hyperventilation syndrome in this setting. However, you should remember that a number of significant and common medical conditions can cause hyperventilation, including cardiovascular and pulmonary conditions such as acute myocardial infarction and pulmonary thromboembolism, sepsis, pregnancy, liver failure, and several metabolic and neurological disorders. Be conservative and consider hyperventilation to be a sign of a serious medical problem until proven otherwise. Management centers on reassurance and assisting the patient to consciously decrease the rate and depth of breathing, maneuvers that will increase PCO_2.

l. Central nervous system dysfunction   **pp. 42–**

Central nervous system dysfunction occurs when the central nervous system (CNS) experiences a temporary or permanent interruption in normal functioning. One role of the CNS is to regulate the rate, pattern, and depth of respirations. When the CNS receives a chemical or physical insult, regulation ceases or becomes abnormal. Causes include brain trauma, stroke, brain tumors, and drugs, to list a few. Assessment findings can include CNS trauma, identified drug ingestion, abnormal respiratory patterns, or apnea. Prehospital management is supportive and may include mechanical ventilation, supplemental oxygenation, suctioning, and transport to a specialty care facility.

m. Dysfunction of the spinal cord, nerves, or respiratory muscles   **pp. 42–**

Several diseases can affect the spinal cord, nerves, and/or respiratory muscles. Assessment findings usually reveal hypoventilation and risk for hypoxemia. Diseases that interfere with respiratory function can include some of the following: spinal cord trauma, polio, amyotrophic lateral sclerosis (ALS), myasthenia gravis, Guillain-Barré syndrome (GBS), multiple sclerosis (MS), and spinal cord tumors. Prehospital management is supportive and may include mechanical ventilation, supplemental oxygenation, suctioning, and transport to a specialty care facility.

10. Demonstrate the steps of assessing the respiratory system.   **pp. 14–23**

The steps of a respiratory assessment include:

- **Complete a scene size-up**—consider scene safety and the patient's appearance.
- **Form a general impression**—consider position, color, mental status, speech, and respiratory effort.
- **Complete a primary assessment**—evaluate ABCs (or use CAB if unresponsive) and identify any life-threatening conditions.
- **Complete a secondary assessment**—obtain a history and physical exam.
- **Complete a physical exam**—inspect, palpate, percuss, and auscultate lung sounds (anterior and posterior).
- **Obtain vital signs**—respiratory rate, pulse rate, blood pressure, pulse oximetry, waveform capnography, work of breathing, temperature, and peak flow (if appropriate).

11. **Recognize signs and symptoms of airway compromise, respiratory distress, and respiratory failure.**   pp. 12–42

Signs and symptoms of *airway compromise* include:

- Stridor
- Noisy breathing
- Apnea
- Signs of choking
- Snoring
- Gurgling
- Speech

Signs and symptoms of *respiratory distress* include:

- Nasal flaring
- Intercostals muscle retractions
- Accessory muscle use
- Cyanosis
- Pursed lips
- Tracheal tugging

Signs and symptoms of *respiratory failure* include:

- Apnea
- Severe tachypnea or decreasing rate and depth of respirations
- Deteriorating pulse oximetry reading
- Increasing $EtCO_2$ readings
- Abnormal waveform capnogram
- Inability to speak
- Unresponsiveness
- Central cyanosis

12. **Apply general principles of management of respiratory disorders in the development and implementation of treatment plans.**   pp. 23–42

General management principles for respiratory conditions include:

- Consider trauma implications and implement spinal immobilization and effective airway positioning to maintain the airway.
- Provide supplemental oxygen for hypoxia.
- Avoid hypoxia and hyperoxia.
- Support the patient's respiratory effort with proper positioning.
- Suction the patient as needed.
- Consider pharmacologic interventions as appropriate.
- Use appropriate monitoring devices.
- Consider age-related changes and chronic pulmonary disease in developing and implementing any treatment plan.

13. **Apply a process of clinical reasoning to evaluate patients for specific respiratory disorders, including the following:**   pp. 12–42

- **a.** Upper airway obstruction.
- **b.** Noncardiogenic pulmonary edema/acute respiratory distress syndrome.
- **c.** Obstructive lung diseases, including emphysema, chronic bronchitis, and asthma.
- **d.** Upper respiratory infection
- **e.** Pneumonia
- **f.** Severe acute respiratory syndrome (SARS)
- **g.** Lung cancer
- **h.** Toxic inhalation
- **i.** Pulmonary embolism

©2013 Pearson Education, Inc.
Paramedic Care: Principles & Practice, Vol. 4, 4th Ed.

j. Spontaneous pneumothorax
k. Hyperventilation syndrome
l. Central nervous system dysfunction
m. Dysfunction of the spinal cord, nerves, and muscles

As a paramedic, you will evaluate objective and subjective data from your scene size-up, general impression, patient interview and history, and assessments to determine an appropriate clinical path. Your understanding of common clinical presentations (signs and symptoms), pathophysiology, risk factors, and epidemiology will assist you in forming a presumptive conclusion. Your treatment plan will be formed from considering common practice, standards of care, evidence-based practice, treatment guidelines, local protocols, empirical experience, and your patient's wishes. Implementation of prehospital care can be influenced by the stability of your patient's condition, availability of resources, scene location, and access to specialty care centers. Your reassessment is ongoing and can evolve the clinical decision-making process as you evaluate the effectiveness of treatments and changing patient condition.

14. **Given a variety of scenarios, develop treatment plans for patients with respiratory disorders.**
pp. 12–24

During your training as a paramedic, you will participate in many classroom sessions involving simulated patients. You will also spend some time in the emergency departments of local hospitals as well as in advanced-level ambulances gaining clinical experience. During these times, use your knowledge of pulmonary disease to help you assess and care for the simulated or real patients you attend.

Content Self-Evaluation

MULTIPLE CHOICE

_____ 1. Supplemental oxygen may induce respiratory depression due to hypoxic drive in
   A. asthma and pneumonia.
   B. spontaneous pneumothorax and pneumonia.
   C. asthma and emphysema.
   D. asthma and acute respiratory distress syndrome.
   E. chronic bronchitis and emphysema.

_____ 2. The pulmonary edema characteristic of acute respiratory distress syndrome (ARDS) is caused by
   A. left-sided cardiac ventricular failure.
   B. right-sided cardiac ventricular failure.
   C. accumulation of fluid in the pulmonary interstitial spaces.
   D. obstruction of pulmonary capillaries by thrombi.
   E. chronic constriction of terminal airways and alveoli.

_____ 3. Factors that commonly cause acute aggravation of symptoms due to chronic obstructive pulmonary disease (COPD) include all of the following, EXCEPT
   A. progression of lung cancer.
   B. exertion, including heavy lifting and exercise.
   C. allergens such as foods and dust.
   D. tobacco smoke.
   E. occupational airborne pollutants such as chemical fumes.

_____ 4. Common physical attributes of a person with emphysema include all of the following, EXCEPT
   A. chronic cough.
   B. barrel chest.
   C. clubbing of the fingers.
   D. pinkish tone to skin.
   E. thin build.

5. Common physical attributes of a person with chronic bronchitis include all of the following, EXCEPT
   A. chronic cough.
   B. thin build.
   C. bluish, cyanotic tone to skin.
   D. cough producing large amounts of sputum.
   E. ankle edema.

6. Which of the following is NOT part of the epidemiology of asthma?
   A. There has been an increase in the mortality rate over the past decade.
   B. The death rate in whites is roughly twice that in blacks.
   C. It is a common disorder in both males and females.
   D. The mortality change is seen mostly in persons over age 45 years.
   E. Half of asthma deaths occur in the prehospital setting.

7. Medications commonly used by persons with asthma include all of the following, EXCEPT
   A. beta agonists administered via inhaler.
   B. oral doses of aspirin.
   C. anticholinergic administered via inhaler.
   D. oral doses of corticosteroid.
   E. cromolyn sodium administered via inhaler.

8. The chief management goals for an acute asthma attack involve improvement in
   A. blood pH (acidosis), hypoxia, and wheezing.
   B. hypoxia, bronchospasm, and wheezing.
   C. blood pH (acidosis), hypoxia, and local inflammation.
   D. hypoxia, bronchospasm, and local inflammation.
   E. hypoxia, wheezing, and local inflammation.

9. Be prepared for which of the following when caring for a patient with status asthmaticus?
   A. Respiratory acidosis with electrolyte imbalance
   B. Dehydration with early signs of renal failure
   C. Respiratory depression when administered supplemental oxygen
   D. Respiratory arrest requiring endotracheal intubation
   E. Tracheal inflammation causing airway obstruction

10. Upper respiratory infections can affect all of the following, EXCEPT the
    A. sinuses.
    B. lungs.
    C. middle ear.
    D. nose.
    E. pharynx.

11. Pleuritic chest pain associated with pneumonia is
    A. dull and aching in character.
    B. sharp or tearing in character.
    C. cramplike and hard to localize.
    D. likely to radiate to the jaw or left arm.
    E. only present on deep inspiration.

12. The patient with SARS is considered contagious during which time period?
    A. While the patient displays signs and symptoms
    B. For 2 to 7 days after contact
    C. For 10 to 14 days after contact
    D. For 2 to 7 days after symptoms first appear
    E. For 10 to 14 days after symptoms first appear

13. Standard management of lung cancer includes all of the following, EXCEPT
    A. checking for instructions such as do not resuscitate (DNR) orders.
    B. placement of electrocardiogram (ECG) leads for cardiac monitoring.
    C. administration of supplemental oxygen.
    D. airway and ventilatory support as needed.
    E. emotional support of patient and family.

_____ 14. Roughly one in five cases of sudden death is due to pulmonary emboli.
   A. True
   B. False

_____ 15. The mortality rate for pulmonary emboli is greater than 50 percent.
   A. True
   B. False

_____ 16. Risk factors for pulmonary emboli include all of the following, EXCEPT
   A. obesity.
   B. pregnancy.
   C. prolonged immobilization.
   D. deep vein thrombophlebitis.
   E. use of oral contraceptives, especially in smokers.

_____ 17. The ventilation-perfusion mismatch characteristic of pulmonary embolism is due to loss of blood flow to a ventilated segment of lung tissue.
   A. True
   B. False

_____ 18. Common physical findings in pulmonary embolism include all of the following, EXCEPT
   A. evidence suggestive of deep venous thrombosis.
   B. labored, painful breathing.
   C. tachypnea and tachycardia.
   D. cardiac dysrythmias.
   E. normal chest auscultation.

_____ 19. Which of the following statements about spontaneous pneumothorax is FALSE?
   A. Most patients have acute-onset pain in the chest or shoulder region.
   B. Onset of pain often follows coughing or heavy lifting.
   C. Spontaneous pneumothorax is much more common in women than in men.
   D. Spontaneous pneumothorax is more common among smokers and persons with COPD.
   E. Supplemental oxygen is sufficient therapy for the majority of patients with spontaneous pneumothorax.

_____ 20. The respiratory alkalosis of hyperventilation syndrome often results in
   A. cramping of the muscles of the hands and feet.
   B. slowing of cardiac electrical conduction, causing bradycardia.
   C. cramping of facial muscles, causing characteristic grimace.
   D. one of several cardiac dysrhythmias.
   E. altered mental status, specifically, lethargy and depression.

_____ 21. Respiratory emergencies due to central nervous system (CNS) dysfunction are relatively rare.
   A. True
   B. False

_____ 22. Numerous peripheral nervous system conditions can cause respiratory compromise, including the diseases of polio and amyotrophic lateral sclerosis, as well as Guillian-Barré syndrome.
   A. True
   B. False

_____ 23. The processes of ventilation, diffusion, and perfusion allow gas exchange to occur efficiently in the lungs and other body tissues. The derangement in pulmonary embolism is principally of
   A. ventilation.
   B. diffusion.
   C. perfusion.
   D. a combination of ventilation and diffusion.
   E. a combination of diffusion and perfusion.

24. Carbon monoxide exposure is potentially life threatening because carbon monoxide displaces oxygen from hemoglobin in red blood cells.
    A. True
    B. False

25. The most common auscultation finding in a patient with pneumonia is
    A. stridor over the involved segment.
    B. decreased or absent breath sounds over the involved segment.
    C. expiratory wheezing over the involved segment.
    D. crackles (rales) over the involved segment.
    E. pleural friction rub over the involved segment.

26. Common causes of central nervous system dysfunction include
    A. Rous sarcoma virus.
    B. positional asphyxiation.
    C. tension pneumothorax.
    D. traumatic brain injury.
    E. hyperoxia.

27. Dysfunction of the spinal cord, nerves, or respiratory muscles can lead to
    A. hyperventilation.
    B. hypoventilation.
    C. hyperoxia.
    D. PEEP.
    E. hypocarbia.

28. Management of suspected carbon monoxide exposure includes
    A. evacuation of the care team and patient from the environment.
    B. performing immediate rapid-sequence intubation and providing PEEP.
    C. decontaminating the patient by removing contaminated clothing.
    D. administration of bronchodilators and intravenous corticosteroids.
    E. measuring the patient's oxyhemoglobin by using CO-oximetry.

29. Central nervous system dysfunction is a common cause of respiratory emergencies.
    A. True
    B. False

30. All patients suffering from carbon monoxide exposure should be emergently transported to a specialty care facility with a hyperbaric oxygen chamber.
    A. True
    B. False

MATCHING

Match each respiratory emergency with its key prehospital management steps by writing the letter of the steps in the space provided next to the emergency.

A. correct hypoxia, reverse bronchospasm, and reduce inflammation

B. ensure safety of rescue personnel, remove patient for transport, maintain open airway, and deliver humidified, high-concentration oxygen

C. maintain airway and ventilation as needed; deliver oxygen; establish IV access, cardiac monitoring, and pulse oximetry; and transport to facility for care of underlying condition

D. maintain airway, ventilation, and circulation as needed; deliver oxygen; establish IV access, cardiac monitoring, and pulse oximetry; and check extremities during transport to appropriate facility

E. maintain airway and ventilation as needed, with the exception that examination of the throat should be avoided

©2013 Pearson Education, Inc.
Paramedic Care: Principles & Practice, Vol. 4, 4th Ed.

F. relieve hypoxia, reverse bronchoconstriction, assist ventilations as needed

G. deliver oxygen, support ventilation as allowed by orders or advance directive, correct hypoxia as possible, and provide emotional support

_____ **31.** Acute respiratory distress syndrome (ARDS)

_____ **32.** Chronic obstructive pulmonary disease (COPD), either emphysema or chronic bronchitis

_____ **33.** Asthma

_____ **34.** Childhood epiglottitis

_____ **35.** Lung cancer

_____ **36.** Inhalation of a toxic substance

_____ **37.** Pulmonary embolism

Special Project

Assessing Respiratory Emergencies

Read the assessment written for each of the three patients evaluated in a prehospital setting and identify the probable cause for each emergency. Check the Assessment section of the textbook for each disorder to refamiliarize yourself with characteristic findings in the history and physical examination.

Scenario 1: You are called to an elementary school where a student has become "suddenly ill" during a class birthday party. You find a distressed 7-year-old child who is breathing rapidly and shallowly and whose skin tone is becoming dusky. The use of accessory muscles to breathe is evident. The school nurse offers you a box containing an inhaler that she says the child uses on an "as-needed" basis and states she isn't sure what ingredients were in the cupcakes brought for the party. She adds that the boy has several severe food allergies.

Probable cause: _____

Scenario 2: You are called to a home where an elderly man is "short of breath." On arrival, you find a thin, elderly man with a broad chest whose breathing is labored despite use of a home supplemental oxygen setup. His daughter tells you that he has had a cold recently, and he suddenly became "shorter of breath" this morning. On exam, the man has a fever of 101°F, is somewhat confused in answering your questions, and can say only two or three words before needing to breathe again. Breath sounds are diminished bilaterally and crackles (rales) are present at the right base.

Probable cause for acute emergency: _____

Probable underlying disorder: _____

Scenario 3: You are called to a home where a visitor has fallen ill. The man's son tells you that his father had just arrived after a two-day car trip to visit the family and had seemed fine until after dinner. Then the older man complained of a sudden inability "to catch his breath" and "awful pain in the shoulder like a knife." The patient is standing over a couch, breathing rapidly and shallowly. Tachycardia is present but rhythm is even. Blood pressure is normal and chest auscultation is within normal limits.

Probable cause: _____

Cardiology

Because Chapter 2 is lengthy, it has been divided into three parts to aid in your study. Read the assigned text pages, then progress through the objectives and self-evaluation materials as you would with other chapters. When you feel secure in your grasp of the content, proceed to the next part.

Part 1, p. 45

Review of Chapter Objectives

After reading this part of the chapter, you should be able to:

1. Define key terms introduced in this chapter.

Knowing and being able to apply the key terms in each chapter is critical to understanding chapter concepts. Write the list of key terms. Then write the definition of each one in your own words. Check your understanding by confirming the definitions in the text glossary. Correct any misunderstandings. Create a study aid by writing each key term on the front of an index card and the definition on the back. Use the cards to quiz yourself, or to have someone quiz you.

2. Describe the significance of the prevalence of cardiovascular disease (CVD) in the United States. **pp. 48–49**

It is important that paramedics understand epidemiology of CVD. Every year almost 466,000 people die of cardiovascular disease. Almost half (225,000) die in the prehospital environment. In the United States, a person suffers from a nonfatal heart attack every 29 seconds. About once every minute, an American will die from coronary artery disease (CAD).

Knowing these statistics, paramedics must be competent to manage a wide range of cardiovascular emergencies. These emergencies range from sudden death to acute coronary syndrome. As patient advocates, paramedics must seek opportunities to educate the public about CVD risk factors, prevention, and cardiovascular health strategies while empowering themselves with the latest evidence-based treatment guidelines.

3. Describe risk factors for cardiovascular disease. **p. 49**

Risk factors that have been *proven* to increase the risk of cardiovascular disease include:

- Smoking
- Older age
- Family history of cardiac disease
- Hypertension (high blood pressure)
- Hypercholesterolemia (excessive cholesterol in the blood)
- Carbohydrate intolerance (diabetes mellitus)

- Cocaine use
- Male gender
- Lack of exercise

Risk factors that are *believed* to increase the risk of cardiovascular disease include:

- Diet
- Obesity
- Oral contraceptives (birth control pills)
- Type A personality (competitive, aggressive, hostile)
- Psychosocial tensions (stress)

4. Relate the anatomy and physiology of the cardiovascular system to cardiac rhythm generation and to pathophysiology and assessment of patients with cardiac disorders.   **pp. 49–102**

The heart is regulated by two divisions of the autonomic nervous system: the parasympathetic and sympathetic divisions. The sympathetic nervous system innervates the atria and the ventricles through the cardiac plexus. Parasympathetic control affects the atria and upper ventricles of the heart and occurs through the vagus nerve (10th cranial nerve). Both nervous systems affect the sinoatrial (SA) node in the right atrium and the atrioventricular (AV) node just above the bundle of His. Stimulation from the sympathetic division increases heart rate and cardiac contractile force. Stimulation from the parasympathetic decreases heart rate and atrioventricular conduction.

Heart rhythms that are too slow (bradycardic) may be a result of not enough sympathetic stimulation or too much parasympathetic stimulation. In contrast, rhythms that are too fast (tachycardic) may be a result of too much sympathetic stimulation or decreased parasympathetic stimulation. Certain types of atrioventricular heart blocks, such as second-degree type 1 AV block, can be caused by an increase in parasympathetic tone.

Adequate heart function depends on adequate venous return and other vascular factors, as well as the intrinsic factors of myocardial health and function and adequacy of the electrical conduction system. Hypertension, atherosclerosis, and diabetes are risk factors for cardiac disease because they damage blood vessels, including the coronary arteries. Impaired perfusion of the myocardium (particularly the left ventricle responsible for cardiac output to the body) can lead to ischemia or myocardial infarction (MI). If infarction occurs, the amount of functional myocardium decreases, and this can ultimately lead to a decrease in cardiac output dependent on the area involved and the amount of myocardium lost.

There are innate disorders of the electrical conduction system, including developmental variants in the accessory pathways, that can make arrhythmias more likely (such as Wolff-Parkinson-White syndrome). In addition, ischemia or infarction of the fibers of the conduction system can also make development of arrhythmias more likely, including some (such as the tachycardias and the ventricular arrhythmias) that can impair cardiac output to some degree or be directly life threatening by precluding the adequacy of cardiac output (namely, ventricular fibrillation).

External agents that can harm cardiac function and possibly damage cardiac tissue include drugs. In some cases, drugs used to treat cardiac dysfunction can cause different cardiac problems.

5. Describe the purpose and process of electrocardiographic monitoring.   **pp. 61–69**

The purpose of electrocardiographic monitoring is to maintain a real-time assessment and ongoing trend of the heart's electrical activity. This becomes very important in patients who are experiencing an acute coronary syndrome (ACS) because these patients are at risk for sudden death and immediate intervention is vital for survival. In addition, many arrhythmias are treated in the prehospital setting and electrocardiogram (ECG) monitoring provides a method for reevaluation of interventions. For example, stable patients experiencing supraventricular tachycardia (SVT) can receive Adenocard to slow down the heart rate and even convert the arrhythmia. In this case, ECG monitoring while the medication is being administered is very important in determining the effectiveness of the drug. Patients experiencing symptomatic bradycardia in third-degree AV heart block most likely will require transcutaneous pacing. During this intervention, the continuous monitoring of the ECG will allow the paramedic to recognize electrical capture during pacing.

©2013 Pearson Education, Inc.
Paramedic Care: Principles & Practice, Vol. 4, 4th Ed.

6. **Relate the waves and intervals of an ECG tracing to the electrical events in the heart.** pp. 61–69

- *P wave.* The first component of the ECG, the P wave, corresponds to atrial depolarization. On lead II, it is a positive, rounded wave before the QRS complex.
- *QRS complex.* The QRS complex reflects ventricular depolarization. The *Q wave* is the first negative deflection after the P wave; the *R wave* is the first positive deflection after the P wave; and the *S wave* is the first negative deflection after the R wave. Not all three waves are always present, and the shape of the QRS complex can vary among individuals.
- *T wave.* The T wave reflects repolarization of the ventricles. Normally positive in lead II, it is rounded and usually moves in the same direction as the QRS complex.
- *U wave.* Occasionally, a U wave appears. U waves follow T waves and are usually positive. U waves may be associated with electrolyte abnormalities, or they may be a normal finding.
- *PR interval (PRI) or P-Q interval (PQI).* The PR interval is the distance from the beginning of the P wave to the beginning of the QRS complex. It represents the time the impulse takes to travel from the atria to the ventricles. Occasionally, the R wave is absent, in which case this interval is called the P-Q interval. The terms *PR interval* and *P-Q* interval may be used interchangeably.
- *QRS interval.* The QRS interval is the distance from the first deflection of the QRS complex to the last. It represents the time necessary for ventricular depolarization.
- *ST segment.* The ST segment is the distance from the S wave to the beginning of the T wave. Usually it is an isoelectric line; however, it may be elevated or depressed in certain disease states, such as ischemia.

7. **Describe the significance of changes in ECG tracings from expected normal findings.** pp. 61–102

Understanding the normal ECG tracings is the foundation for recognizing abnormal findings. P waves are expected to be upright and occur before the QRS complex in lead II. P waves that are absent indicate that the atria depolarized at the same time as the ventricles depolarized. P waves that are inverted in the bipolar limb leads indicate that atrial depolarization occurred in a retrograde fashion instead of from a superior-to-inferior direction. If P waves appear inverted and after the QRS complex, it indicates that atrial depolarization occurred retrograde and after ventricular depolarization. These variations are often observed in junctional rhythms.

The PR interval is usually less than 0.20 seconds. When the PR interval is observed longer than 0.20 seconds, it indicates that conduction through the atria and AV junction was delayed. This is often seen in first-degree AV heart block.

The QRS complex usually is no more than 0.12 seconds in duration. However, when the QRS is wide (> 0.12 seconds), it indicates that there was a delay in conduction through the interventricular septum, ventricles, or Purkinje system. This is often seen in high-degree AV heart blocks such as second-degree type II AV block and third-degree AV heart block.

The QT interval is normally between 0.33 and 0.42 seconds and represents complete ventricular activity. QT intervals and heart rate have an inverse relationship: Increases in heart rate usually decrease the QT interval, whereas decreases in heart rate usually prolong it. A prolonged QT interval is thought to be related to an increased risk of certain ventricular arrhythmias and sudden death. Numerous medications, particularly some of the antipsychotic medications, have been associated with prolongation of the QT interval. A prolonged QT interval is significant because it also prolongs the relative refractory period. This places the patient at increased risk for R-on-T phenomena, V-tach, and V-fib.

The ST segment is usually an isoelectric line. Myocardial infarctions, which are caused by lack of blood flow to a part of the heart, produce changes in this line. The affected area is then electrically dead and cannot conduct electrical impulses. Ischemia causes ST segment depression or an inverted T wave. The inversion is usually symmetrical. Injury elevates the ST segment, most often in the early phases of a myocardial infarction. As the tissue dies, a significant Q wave appears. A significant Q wave is at least one small square wide, lasting 0.04 second, or is more than one-third the height of the QRS complex. Q waves may also indicate extensive transient ischemia.

8. **Explain general mechanisms of cardiac arrhythmias.** pp. 63–102

The general causes of cardiac arrhythmias include:

- **Disturbed Automaticity:** This may involve a speeding up or slowing down of areas of automaticity such as the SA node, AV node, or the myocardium. Abnormal beats (more appropriately called *depolarizations* rather than *beats* or *contractions*) may arise through this mechanism from the atria, AV junction, or the ventricles. Abnormal rhythms, such as atrial or ventricular tachycardia, may also occur.
- **Disturbed Conduction:** Conduction may be either too rapid (as in Wolf-Parkinson-White syndrome) or too slow (as in atrioventricular block).
- **Combination of Disturbed Automaticity and Disturbed Conduction:**
  - A premature atrial contraction (disturbed automaticity) plus first-degree AV block (disturbed conduction).
  - Atrial flutter (disturbed automaticity) with 3:1 or higher grades of AV block (disturbed conduction).

9. **Use systematic analysis and apply knowledge of criteria for specific arrhythmias to interpret the ECG tracings of normal sinus rhythm and specific arrhythmias.** pp. 63–102

It is very important to use a systematic approach when interpreting arrhythmias. Use the following approach and compare your findings with the established criteria for each arrhythmia. When analyzing the P waves, ask yourself the following questions:

- Are P waves present?
- Are the P waves regular?
- Is there one P wave for each QRS complex?
- Are the P waves upright or inverted (compared to the QRS complex)?
- Do all the P waves look alike?

10. **Identify potential causes of cardiac arrhythmias.** pp. 67–102

Causes of cardiac arrhythmias may differ. The causes of arrhythmias include:

- Myocardial ischemia, necrosis, or infarction
- Autonomic nervous system imbalance
- Distention of the chambers of the heart (especially in the atria, secondary to congestive heart failure)
- Blood gas abnormalities, including hypoxia and abnormal pH
- Electrolyte imbalances (Ca^{++}, K^+, Mg^{++})
- Trauma to the myocardium (cardiac contusion)
- Drug effects and drug toxicity
- Electrocution
- Hypothermia
- CNS damage
- Idiopathic events
- Normal occurrences

Case Study Review

The Case Study Review for this chapter is found in Part 2.

©2013 Pearson Education, Inc.
Paramedic Care: Principles & Practice, Vol. 4, 4th Ed.

Content Self-Evaluation

MULTIPLE CHOICE

C 1. Each year, how many people in the United States die from coronary heart disease (CHD)?
   A. 144,000
   B. 225,000
   C. 466,000
   D. 1 million
   E. 1.3 million

E 2. Which of the following is (are) a risk factor(s) for cardiovascular and coronary heart disease?
   A. Obesity
   B. Oral contraceptive use
   C. Cocaine use
   D. Family history
   E. All of the above

D 3. From innermost to outermost, the three tissue layers of the heart are
   A. the endocardium, the pericardium, and the myocardium.
   B. the endocardium, the myocardium, and the syncytium.
   C. the endocardium, the myocardium, and the pericardium.
   D. the myocardium, the epicardium, and the pericardium.
   E. the epicardium, the myocardium, and the endocardium.

B 4. The apex of the heart is the location where the great vessels connect to the heart.
   A. True
   B. False

B 5. The heart valve located between the right atrium and ventricle is the
   A. mitral.
   B. tricuspid.
   C. aortic.
   D. pulmonic.
   E. semilunar.

E 6. Which of the following blood vessels carries oxygenated blood?
   A. Pulmonary vein
   B. Superior vena cava
   C. Aorta
   D. Pulmonary artery
   E. Both A and C

A 7. The blood supply to the left ventricle, interventricular septum, part of the right ventricle, and the heart's conduction system comes from the two branches of the left coronary artery, which are the
   A. anterior descending artery and the circumflex artery.
   B. anterior descending artery and the posterior descending artery.
   C. circumflex artery and the posterior descending artery.
   D. circumflex artery and the marginal artery.
   E. marginal artery and the posterior descending artery.

C 8. The tunica adventicia is which layer of the artery?
   A. The inner endothelial layer
   B. The muscle middle layer
   C. The fibrous covering layer
   D. A ligamentous intermediate layer
   E. None of the above

D 9. The normal cardiac output is approximately what volume?
   A. 500 mL
   B. 1,200 mL
   C. 2,400 mL
   D. 5,000 mL
   E. 6,000 mL

_____D_____ 10. Stimulation of the heart by the sympathetic nervous system results in
    A. negative inotropic and chronotropic effects.
    B. negative chronotropic and dromotropic effects.
    C. positive chronotropic and dromotropic effects.
    D. positive inotropic and chronotropic effects. *chrono-*
    E. positive inotropic and dromotropic effects. *HR*

_____ 11. The hormones released by the heart during hemodynamic stress provide which of the following actions?
    A. Loss of water (diuresis)   D. Vasodilation
    B. Reduced automaticity   E. All of the above except B
    C. Loss of sodium (natriuresis)

_____ 12. Specialized myocardial structures called intercalated discs enable the atria to act as an electrophysiological syncytium and the ventricles to act as another one.
    A. True
    B. False

_____ 13. Which of the following is an important property of cardiac tissue?
    A. Automaticity   D. Contractility
    B. Conductivity   E. All of the above
    C. Excitability

_____ 14. All of the following can cause an artifact on the ECG, EXCEPT
    A. a diaphoretic patient.   D. shivering by the patient.
    B. an enlarged heart.   E. loose electrodes.
    C. movement by the patient.

_____ 15. Which of the following is NOT an electrode location used for the bipolar leads?
    A. Right leg   D. Left arm
    B. Left leg   E. All of the above are used.
    C. Right arm

_____ 16. A single monitoring lead CANNOT identify which of the following?
    A. Presence of an infarct   D. Quality of pumping actions
    B. Location of an infarct   E. All of the above
    C. Axis deviation information

_____ 17. The smallest box on the ECG paper represents what period of time?
    A. 0.02 seconds   D. 0.20 seconds
    B. 0.04 seconds   E. 0.25 seconds
    C. 0.10 seconds

_____ 18. Which of the following represents the first (generally) positive deflection (on lead II) of the ECG?
    A. P wave   D. U wave
    B. QRS complex   E. P-R interval
    C. T wave

_____ 19. Which element of the ECG is normally between 0.8 and 0.12 seconds in duration?
    A. P wave   D. ST segment
    B. PR interval   E. T wave
    C. QRS interval

_____ 20. A prolonged QT interval is longer than 0.38 second.
    A. True
    B. False

©2013 Pearson Education, Inc.
Paramedic Care: Principles & Practice, Vol. 4, 4th Ed.

21. Which of the following is NOT part of the criteria for ECG rhythm strip analysis?
    A. Memorize the rules for each rhythm.
    B. Always be consistent and analytical.
    C. Identify the dysrhythmia by its similarity to established rules.
    D. Use the eyeball approach for the initial analysis.
    E. Analyze a given rhythm strip according to a specific formula.

22. In your analysis of a dysrhythmia, you determine there is no relationship among R-R intervals. You would classify this dysrhythmia as
    A. regular.
    B. occasionally irregular.
    C. irregularly irregular.
    D. regularly irregular.
    E. reciprocating.

23. Common causes of dysrhythmias include all of the following, EXCEPT
    A. myocardial ischemia or infarction.
    B. electrolyte and pH disturbances.
    C. CNS or autonomic nervous system damage.
    D. drug effects.
    E. hyperthermia.

24. In the bradycardia algorithm, the first drug in the intervention sequence is
    A. procainamide.
    B. epinephrine.
    C. atropine.
    D. isoproterenol.
    E. dopamine.

25. Which of the following dysrhythmias has an R-R interval that often varies with respiration?
    A. Sinus arrest
    B. Paroxsysmal supraventricular tachycardia
    C. Sinus dysrhythmia
    D. Sinus bradycardia
    E. Sinus tachycardia

26. Of the following atrial dysrhythmias, which is often an indication of serious underlying medical disease?
    A. Atrial tachycardia
    B. Atrial flutter
    C. Premature atrial contractions (PACs)
    D. Multifocal atrial tachycardia (MAT)
    E. Paroxysmal supraventricular tachycardia (PSVT)

27. Which of the following dysrhythmias has a characteristic sawtooth-shaped P wave?
    A. Atrial flutter
    B. Atrial fibrillation
    C. Ventricular fibrillation
    D. Mobitz I second-degree block
    E. Mobitz II second-degree block

28. Which of the following dysrhythmias is rhythm irregularly irregular?
    A. Atrial flutter
    B. Atrial fibrillation
    C. Paroxysmal supraventricular tachycardia
    D. Sinus dysrhythmia
    E. All of the above

29. The diagnostic finding for first-degree AV block on an ECG is
    A. the presence of some QRS complexes not preceded by a P wave.
    B. a P-R interval longer than 0.20 second.
    C. a QRS complex widened to longer than 0.12 second.
    D. an R-T interval widened for those beats with an initial P wave.
    E. the presence of some P waves without following QRS complexes.

30. The chief difference between type I and type II second-degree AV block is the pattern of lengthening P-R interval before the blocked impulse in type I second-degree AV block.
    A. True
    B. False

31. The type of heart block where two P waves precede each QRS complex is called which of the following?
    A. First degree
    B. Second degree, type I
    C. Second degree type II
    D. 2:1 AV block
    E. Third degree

32. All of the following statements about third-degree AV block are true, EXCEPT
    A. the atrial rate is unaffected, and ventricular rate depends on site of ventricular pacemaker.
    B. P waves are normal but show no relationship to the QRS complex.
    C. there is an absence of conduction between the atria and the ventricles.
    D. both atrial and ventricular rhythms are usually regular.
    E. QRS complexes are normal in length.

33. Lidocaine is contraindicated with frequent PVCs when the underlying rhythm is third-degree block.
    A. True
    B. False

34. All of the following statements about ECG findings for dysrhythmias originating in the AV junction are true, EXCEPT
    A. P-R interval is less than 0.12 second.
    B. P waves are inverted in lead II.
    C. T waves are blunted and widened.
    D. QRS complexes are normal in duration.
    E. P waves are masked if atrial depolarization occurs during ventricular depolarization.

35. A junctional bradycardia is defined as a junctional rhythm with a rate below ___ beats per minute.
    A. 20
    B. 30
    C. 40
    D. 50
    E. 60

36. Accelerated junctional rhythm is usually well tolerated; however, because it is often caused by underlying ischemia, you must carefully watch for the development of other dysrhythmias.
    A. True
    B. False

37. All of the following statements about dysrhythmias originating in the ventricles are true, EXCEPT
    A. ischemia, hypoxia, and drug effects are common causes.
    B. T waves are blunted and widened.
    C. P waves are absent.
    D. the pacemaker site determines QRS morphology.
    E. QRS complexes are 0.12 second or longer in duration.

38. The treatment of choice for symptomatic bradydysrhythmias is
    A. lidocaine.
    B. atropine.
    C. vagal maneuvers.
    D. synchronized cardioversion.
    E. all but A.

39. The treatment of choice for ventricular escape rhythms is lidocaine.
    A. True
    B. False

©2013 Pearson Education, Inc.
Paramedic Care: Principles & Practice, Vol. 4, 4th Ed.

40. Possible characteristics of malignant PVCs include all of the following, EXCEPT
   A. R on T phenomenon.
   B. couplets or longer runs of ventricular tachycardia.
   C. four PVCs per minute.
   D. multifocal origin within the ventricles.
   E. accompanying chest pain.

41. Torsades de pointes varies in both cause and ECG appearance from other forms of
   A. ventricular escape rhythm.
   B. accelerated idioventricular rhythm.
   C. ventricular fibrillation.
   D. premature ventricular contraction.
   E. ventricular tachycardia.

42. Nonperfusing ventricular tachycardia and ventricular fibrillation are treated identically, including an immediate countershock and cardiopulmonary resuscitation (CPR) followed by
   A. epinephrine 1:10,000 IV bolus.
   B. adenosine IV bolus.
   C. transcutaneous cardiac pacing (TCP).
   D. glucagon IV bolus.
   E. atropine IV bolus.

43. The usual dose for amiodarone in perfusing ventricular tachycardia is which of the following dosages?
   A. 100 mg
   B. 150 mg
   C. 200 mg
   D. 3 mg
   E. Amiodarone is not indicated.

44. You are attending a patient and apply ECG electrodes and note a rhythm with a dramatic spike preceding each bizarre but regular QRS complex (at a rate of 70 bpm). What is the likely cause of this rhythm?
   A. Monitor failure
   B. A low battery
   C. Monitor is set on cardioversion mode
   D. Patient has a pacemaker
   E. Wandering atrial pacemaker

45. Causes of asystole include all of the following, EXCEPT
   A. preexisting alkalosis (respiratory or metabolic).
   B. hyperkalemia.
   C. hypokalemia.
   D. drug overdose.
   E. hypothermia.

46. Which of the following is a possible cause of PEA?
   A. Hypovolemia
   B. Tension pneumothorax
   C. Massive pulmonary embolism
   D. Cardiac tamponade
   E. All of the above

47. Which of the following is most likely to cause a tall, pointed T wave?
   A. Hypokalemia
   B. Hyperkalemia
   C. Hypocalcemia
   D. Hypercalcemia
   E. Hypothermia

48. Which of the following is most likely to cause a shortened ST segment?
   A. Hypokalemia
   B. Hyperkalemia
   C. Hypocalcemia
   D. Hypercalcemia
   E. Hypothermia

49. Which of the following is most likely to cause a prominent U wave to appear on the ECG?
   A. Hypokalemia
   B. Hyperkalemia
   C. Hypocalcemia
   D. Hypercalcemia
   E. Hypothermia

50. Which of the following is an ECG disturbance you might expect with a patient who is experiencing hypothermia?

    A. J or Osborn wave   **D.** Atrial flutter

    B. T wave inversion   **E.** All of the above

    C. PR interval prolongation

MATCHING

Write the letter of the definition or description regarding cardiac function in the space provided next to the term to which it applies. The same description or definition may be used more than once or not at all.

A. the ratio of blood pumped from the ventricle compared with the amount contained at the end of diastole

B. the series of events between the end of a cardiac contraction to the end of the next

C. the resistance against which the heart must pump

D. the phase of the cardiac cycle during which the heart contracts

E. the amount of blood pumped by the ventricle during one cardiac contraction

F. the amount of blood pumped by the ventricle during 1 minute

G. the phase of the cardiac cycle during which the heart muscle is relaxed

H. the end-diastolic volume in the ventricle

I. the phase of the cardiac cycle during which blood enters the coronary arteries

_____ **51.** Cardiac cycle

_____ **52.** Diastole

_____ **53.** Systole

_____ **54.** Ejection fraction

_____ **55.** Preload

_____ **56.** Afterload

_____ **57.** Cardiac output

_____ **58.** Stroke volume

Write the letter of innate rate of impulse discharge in beats per minute (bpm) in the space provided next to the part of the cardiac conduction system to which it applies.

A. 60 to 100 bpm

B. 15 to 40 bpm

C. 40 to 60 bpm

_____ **59.** Purkinje system

_____ **60.** AV node

_____ **61.** SA node

Label the Diagrams

Supply the missing labels for the drawing showing the chambers of the heart by writing the appropriate letters in the spaces provided.

A. right ventricle

B. interatrial septum

C. left atrium

©2013 Pearson Education, Inc.
Paramedic Care: Principles & Practice, Vol. 4, 4th Ed.

D. right atrium

E. interventricular septum

F. left ventricle

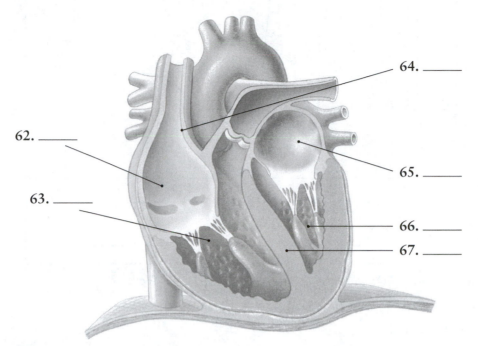

Supply the missing labels for the drawing showing the cardiac conductive system by writing the appropriate letters in the spaces provided for Figure 2.

A. Purkinje system

B. left bundle branch

C. SA node

D. AV node

E. bundle of His

F. internodal atrial pathway

G. AV junction

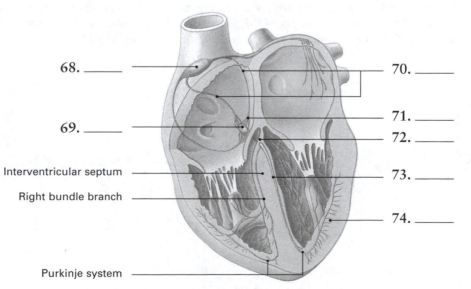

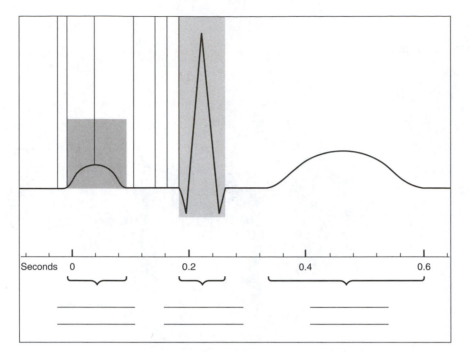

Use the following terms to fill in the missing labels in the spaces provided.

A. QRS complex

B. ventricular depolarization

C. atrial depolarization

D. T wave

E. ventricular repolarization

F. P wave

Special Project

ECG Interpretation

The chapter introduces a five-step procedure for analyzing ECG strips: (1) analysis of rate; (2) analysis of rhythm; (3) analysis of P waves; (4) analysis of P-R interval; and (5) analysis of QRS complexes.

Look at each of the five ECG tracings shown and complete the information grid asked for below each tracing.

ECG 1

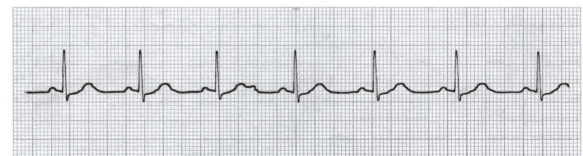

Rate: _____

Rhythm: _____

P waves: _____

P-R interval: _____

QRS complexes: _____

Overall rhythm (or dysrhythmia): _____

ECG 2

Rate: _____

Rhythm: _____

P waves: _____

P-R interval: _____

QRS complexes: _____

Overall rhythm (or dysrhythmia): _____

ECG 3

Rate: _____

Rhythm: _____

P waves: _____

P-R interval: _____

QRS complexes: _____

Overall rhythm (or dysrhythmia): _____

ECG 4

Rate: _____

Rhythm: _____

P waves: _____

P-R interval: _____

QRS complexes: _____

Overall rhythm (or dysrhythmia): _____

ECG 5

Rate: _____

Rhythm: _____

P waves: _____

P-R interval: _____

QRS complexes: _____

Overall rhythm (or dysrhythmia): _____

ECG 6

©2013 Pearson Education, Inc.
Paramedic Care: Principles & Practice, Vol. 4, 4th Ed.

Rate: _____

Rhythm: _____

P waves: _____

P-R interval: _____

QRS complexes: _____

Overall rhythm (or dysrhythmia): _____

ECG 7

Rate: _____

Rhythm: _____

P waves: _____

P-R interval: _____

QRS complexes: _____

Overall rhythm (or dysrhythmia): _____

ECG 8

Rate: _____

Rhythm: _____

P waves: _____

P-R interval: _____

QRS complexes: _____

Overall rhythm (or dysrhythmia): _____

ECG 9

Rate: _____

Rhythm: _____

P waves: _____

P-R interval: _____

QRS complexes: _____

Overall rhythm (or dysrhythmia): _____

ECG 10

Rate: _____

Rhythm: _____

P waves: _____

P-R interval: _____

QRS complexes: _____

Overall rhythm (or dysrhythmia): _____

ECG 11

Rate: _____

Rhythm: _____

P waves: _____

P-R interval: _____

QRS complexes: _____

Overall rhythm (or dysrhythmia): _____

ECG 12

Rate: _____

Rhythm: _____

P waves: _____

P-R interval: _____

QRS complexes: _____

Overall rhythm (or dysrhythmia): _____

ECG 13

Rate: _____

Rhythm: _____

P waves: _____

P-R interval: _____

QRS complexes: _____

Overall rhythm (or dysrhythmia): _____

ECG 14

Rate: _____

Rhythm: _____

P waves: _____

P-R interval: _____

QRS complexes: _____

Overall rhythm (or dysrhythmia): _____

ECG 15

Rate: _____

Rhythm: _____

P waves: _____

P-R interval: _____

QRS complexes: _____

Overall rhythm (or dysrhythmia): _____

ECG 16

©2013 Pearson Education, Inc.
Paramedic Care: Principles & Practice, Vol. 4, 4th Ed.

Rate: _____

Rhythm: _____

P waves: _____

P-R interval: _____

QRS complexes: _____

Overall rhythm (or dysrhythmia): _____

ECG 17

Rate: _____

Rhythm: _____

P waves: _____

P-R interval: _____

QRS complexes: _____

Overall rhythm (or dysrhythmia): _____

ECG 18

Rate: _____

Rhythm: _____

P waves: _____

P-R interval: _____

QRS complexes: _____

Overall rhythm (or dysrhythmia): _____

ECG 19

Rate: _____

Rhythm: _____

P waves: _____

P-R interval: _____

QRS complexes: _____

Overall rhythm (or dysrhythmia): _____

ECG 20

Rate: _____

Rhythm: _____

P waves: _____

P-R interval: _____

QRS complexes: _____

Overall rhythm (or dysrhythmia): _____

Part 1 continued, Part 2

Review of Chapter Objectives

After reading this part of the chapter, you should be able to:

11. Describe the clinical significance of specific cardiac arrhythmias.   **pp. 69–102**

Sinus bradycardia occurs when the sinus rate is less than 60 bpm. The decreased heart rate can cause decreased cardiac output, hypotension, angina, or CNS symptoms. This is especially true for rates slower than 50 beats per minute. The slow heart rate may also lead to atrial ectopic or ventricular ectopic rhythms. In a healthy athlete, sinus bradycardia may be normal and have no clinical significance.

Sinus tachycardia occurs when the sinus rate is greater than 100 bpm. Sinus tachycardia is often benign. In some cases, it is a compensatory mechanism for decreased stroke volume. If the rate is greater than 140 beats per minute, cardiac output may fall because ventricular filling time is inadequate. Very rapid heart rates increase myocardial oxygen demand and can precipitate ischemia or infarct in diseased hearts. Prolonged sinus tachycardia accompanying acute myocardial infarction (AMI) is often an ominous finding suggesting cardiogenic shock.

Sinus arrhythmia often results from a variation of the RR interval. Sinus arrhythmia is a normal variant, particularly in the young and the aged.

Sinus arrest occurs when the sinus node fails to discharge for a brief period, resulting in short periods of cardiac standstill. Frequent or prolonged episodes may compromise cardiac output, resulting in syncope (fainting) and other problems. There is always the danger of complete cessation of SA node activity. Usually, an escape rhythm develops; however, cardiac standstill occasionally can result.

Sinus block, also called *sinus exit block*, occurs when the sinus node fires on time but the impulse is blocked before it exits the sinus node. Frequent or prolonged episodes may compromise cardiac output, resulting in syncope (fainting) and other problems. There is always the danger of complete cessation of SA node activity. Usually, an escape rhythm develops; however, cardiac standstill occasionally can result.

A *sinus pause* occurs when the sinus node fails to discharge for a brief period, resulting in missing a single PQRST complex. Frequent or prolonged episodes may compromise cardiac output, resulting in syncope (fainting) and other problems. There is always the danger of complete cessation of SA node activity. Usually, an escape rhythm develops; however, cardiac standstill occasionally can result.

Sick sinus syndrome is not an arrhythmia per se, but a combination of arrhythmias. Sick sinus syndrome occurs when the sinus node is diseased or ischemic. It is characterized by wild swings in the heart rate—often moving rapidly from a profound bradycardia to a severe tachycardia and back. Frequent or prolonged episodes may compromise cardiac output, resulting in syncope (fainting) and other problems. There is always the danger of complete cessation of SA node activity. Usually, an escape rhythm develops; however, cardiac standstill occasionally can result.

Wandering atrial pacemaker (also called *ectopic tachycardia*) is the passive transfer of pacemaker sites from the sinus node to other latent pacemaker sites in the atria and AV junction. Wandering atrial pacemaker usually has no detrimental effects. Occasionally, it can be a precursor of other atrial arrhythmias such as atrial fibrillation. It sometimes indicates digitalis toxicity.

Multifocal atrial tachycardia (MAT) is usually seen in acutely ill patients. Basically, multifocal atrial tachycardia is a wandering pacemaker rhythm with a rate greater than 100. Frequently these patients are acutely ill; this arrhythmia may indicate a serious underlying medical illness.

Premature atrial contractions (PACs) result from a single electrical impulse originating in the atria outside the SA node, which in turn causes a premature depolarization of the heart before the next expected sinus beat. Isolated PACs are of minimal significance. Frequent PACs may indicate organic heart disease and may precede other atrial arrhythmias.

Paroxysmal supraventricular tachycardia (PSVT) occurs when rapid atrial depolarization overrides the SA node. It often occurs in paroxysm with sudden onset, may last minutes to hours, and terminates abruptly. It may be caused by increased automaticity of a single atrial focus or by reentry phenomenon at the AV node. *Note:* "Paroxysmal" means that it starts and stops. Young patients with good cardiac reserves may tolerate PSVT well for short periods. Patients often sense PSVT as palpitations. However, rapid rates can cause a marked reduction in cardiac output because of inadequate ventricular filling time. The reduced diastolic phase of the cardiac cycle can also compromise coronary artery perfusion. PSVT can precipitate angina, hypotension, or congestive heart failure.

Supraventricular tachycardia (SVT) refers to tachycardias that originate above the ventricles. The pacemaker site is often difficult to determine because of the heart rate. A rapid heart rate often makes the P waves indiscernible. The pacemaker site can be in the SA node, the atria, or the AV junction. Young patients with good cardiac reserves may tolerate SVT well for short periods. Patients often sense SVT as palpitations. However, rapid rates can cause a marked reduction in cardiac output because of inadequate ventricular filling time. The reduced diastolic phase of the cardiac cycle can also compromise coronary artery perfusion. SVT can precipitate angina, hypotension, or congestive heart failure.

Atrial flutter results from a rapid atrial reentry circuit and an AV node that physiologically cannot conduct all impulses through to the ventricles. Atrial flutter with normal ventricular rates is generally well tolerated. Rapid ventricular rates may compromise cardiac output and result in symptoms. Atrial flutter often occurs in conjunction with atrial fibrillation and is referred to as "atrial fib-flutter."

Atrial fibrillation results from multiple areas of reentry within the atria or from multiple ectopic foci bombarding an AV node that physiologically cannot handle all of the incoming impulses. In atrial fibrillation, the atria fail to contract and the so-called atrial kick is lost, thus reducing cardiac output 20 to 25 percent. There is frequently a *pulse deficit* (a difference between the apical and peripheral pulse rates). If the rate of ventricular response is normal, as often occurs in patients on digitalis, the rhythm is usually well tolerated. If the ventricular rate is less than 60, cardiac output can fall. Suspect digitalis toxicity in patients taking digitalis with atrial fibrillation and a ventricular rate less than 60. If the ventricular response is rapid, coupled with the loss of atrial kick, cardiovascular decompensation may occur, resulting in hypotension, angina, infarct, congestive heart failure, or shock.

A *first-degree AV block* is a delay in conduction at the level of the AV node rather than an actual block. First-degree block is usually no danger in itself. However, a newly developed first-degree block may precede a more advanced block.

A *type I second-degree AV block* (also called *second-degree Mobitz I*, or *Wenckebach*) is an intermittent block at the level of the AV node. If beats are frequently dropped, second-degree block can compromise cardiac output by causing problems such as syncope and angina. This block is often a transient phenomenon that occurs immediately after an inferior wall myocardial infarction.

A *type II second-degree AV block* (also called *second-degree Mobitz II,* or *infranodal*) is an intermittent block characterized by P waves that are not conducted to the ventricles, but without associated lengthening of the PR interval before the dropped beats. A Mobitz II block can compromise cardiac output, causing problems such as syncope and angina if beats are frequently dropped. Because this block is often associated with cell necrosis resulting from myocardial infarction, it is considered much more serious than Mobitz I. Many Mobitz II blocks develop into full AV blocks.

A *2:1 AV block* is a type of second-degree AV block where there are two P waves for each QRS complex. A 2:1 AV block can compromise cardiac output, causing problems such as syncope and angina if beats are frequently dropped. This block is often associated with cell necrosis resulting from myocardial infarction. A 2:1 AV block can develop into full AV block (third-degree AV block).

A *third-degree AV block,* or *complete block,* is the absence of conduction between the atria and the ventricles resulting from complete electrical block at or below the AV node. Third-degree block can severely compromise cardiac output because of decreased heart rate and loss of coordinated atrial kick.

A *junctional escape beat,* or *junctional escape rhythm,* is an arrhythmia that results when the rate of the primary pacemaker, usually the SA node, is slower than that of the AV node. The slow heart rate can decrease cardiac output, possibly precipitating angina and other problems. If the rate is fairly rapid, the rhythm can be well tolerated.

A *junctional bradycardia* is a junctional arrhythmia with a heart rate less than the intrinsic rate of the AV node (< 40 beats per minute). A slow rate can significantly compromise cardiac output. The slow heart rate can decrease cardiac output, possibly precipitating angina and other problems.

An *accelerated junctional rhythm* results from increased automaticity in the AV junction, causing the AV junction to discharge faster than its intrinsic rate. An accelerated junctional rhythm is usually well tolerated. However, because ischemia is often the etiology, the patient should be monitored for other arrhythmias.

A *ventricular escape beat* (*ventricular escape rhythm* or *idioventricular rhythm*) results either when impulses from higher pacemakers fail to reach the ventricles or when the discharge rate of higher pacemakers becomes less than that of the ventricles (normally 15–40 beats per minute). The slow heart rate can significantly decrease cardiac output, possibly to life-threatening levels. The ventricular escape rhythm is a safety mechanism that you should not suppress. Escape rhythms can be perfusing or nonperfusing.

Accelerated idioventricular rhythm is an abnormally wide ventricular arrhythmia that usually occurs during an acute myocardial infarction. The principal action should be aggressive treatment of the underlying myocardial infarction as indicated, including appropriate prehospital care.

Ventricular tachycardia (VT) consists of three or more ventricular complexes in succession at a rate of 100 beats per minute or more. Ventricular tachycardia usually results in poor stroke volume, which, coupled with the rapid ventricular rate, may severely compromise cardiac output and coronary

©2013 Pearson Education, Inc.
Paramedic Care: Principles & Practice, Vol. 4, 4th Ed.

artery perfusion. Whether ventricular tachycardia is perfusing or nonperfusing dictates the type of treatment. Ventricular tachycardia may eventually deteriorate into ventricular fibrillation.

Torsades de pointes (TDP) is a polymorphic ventricular tachycardia that differs in appearance and cause from ventricular tachycardia in general. It is more common in women than men. Because TDP produces poor cardiac output, patients with TDP typically are unstable and require immediate intervention.

Ventricular fibrillation is a chaotic ventricular rhythm usually resulting from the presence of many reentry circuits within the ventricles. There is no ventricular depolarization or contraction. Ventricular fibrillation is a lethal arrhythmia. The absence of cardiac output or an organized electrical pattern results in cardiac arrest.

Asystole (cardiac standstill) is the absence of all cardiac electrical activity. Asystole results in cardiac arrest. The prognosis for resuscitation is very poor.

12. Describe the treatments generally indicated for specific cardiac arrhythmias.
pp. 69–102

Treatment for sinus bradycardia is generally unnecessary unless signs of poor perfusion (e.g., acute altered mental status, ongoing chest pain, hypotension, or other signs of shock) are present. If there are signs of poor perfusion, prepare for transcutaneous pacing. Consider administering a 0.5-mg bolus of atropine sulfate. Repeat every 3–5 minutes until you have obtained a satisfactory rate or have given 3.0 mg of the drug. If atropine fails, consider transcutaneous cardiac pacing (TCP) or a dopamine or epinephrine infusion.

The treatment for sinus tachycardia is directed at the underlying cause. For example, hypovolemia, fever, hypoxia, or other causes should be corrected. When treating a patient for sinus arrhythmia, you usually are just supportive in nature.

If the patient in sinus arrest, sinus block, or sinus pause is asymptomatic, observation is all that is required unless there are signs of poor perfusion (e.g., acute altered mental status, ongoing chest pain, hypotension, or other signs of shock) are present. If there are signs of poor perfusion, prepare for transcutaneous pacing. Consider administering a 0.5-mg bolus of atropine sulfate. Repeat every 3–5 minutes until you have obtained a satisfactory rate or have given 3.0 mg of the drug. If atropine fails, consider TCP or a dopamine or epinephrine infusion.

If the patient with sick sinus syndrome is asymptomatic, observation is all that is required unless there are signs of poor perfusion (e.g., acute altered mental status, ongoing chest pain, hypotension, or other signs of shock) are present. If there are signs of poor perfusion, begin TCP or consider a dopamine or epinephrine infusion. Also, if the patient with wandering atrial pacemaker is asymptomatic, observation is all that is required. If the patient is symptomatic, consider adenosine.

The treatment of SVT and PSVT starts with considering whether the patient is stable or unstable. If the patient is stable, obtain a 12-lead ECG and establish IV access.

1. *Vagal maneuvers.* Ask the patient to perform a Valsalva maneuver. This is a forced expiration against a closed glottis, or the act of "bearing down" as if to move the bowels. This results in vagal stimulation, which may slow the heart. If this is unsuccessful, attempt carotid artery massage, if the patient is eligible. Do not attempt carotid artery massage in patients with carotid bruits or known cerebrovascular or carotid artery disease.

2. *Pharmacological therapy.* Adenosine (Adenocard) is safe and highly effective in terminating PSVT, especially if its etiology is reentry. Administer 6 mg of adenosine by rapid IV bolus over 1–3 sec through the medication port closest to the patient's heart or central circulation. (Adenosine has a very short half-life, and you must immediately follow administration with a bolus of normal saline to allow the medication to reach its site of action while it is still effective.) If the patient does not convert after 1–2 minutes, administer a second bolus of 12 mg over 1–3 sec in the medication port closest to the patient's heart or central circulation. If this fails and the patient has a normal blood pressure, then look again at the width of the cardiac QRS. Discerning narrow-complex tachycardia from wide-complex tachycardia can be difficult. It is sometimes helpful to look at lead V_1 (or MCL_1) to determine whether the arrhythmia is actually a narrow- or wide-complex tachycardia. In many instances, a narrow-complex tachycardia will be complicated by a bundle branch block, which can be more apparent in these leads. This determination is important, as the treatments are considerably different for the two arrhythmias. If the patient has a narrow-complex tachycardia and is stable, then provide supportive care. If the patient becomes unstable, it is prudent to proceed with synchronized cardioversion.

If the patient in SVT or PSVT is unstable (e.g., altered mental status, ongoing chest pain, hypotension, or other signs of shock) then consider:

1. *Electrical therapy.* Use synchronized cardioversion if the rate is greater than 150 beats per minute. If time allows, sedate the patient and apply synchronized DC countershock of 50 to 100 joules (or biphasic equivalent). If this is unsuccessful, repeat the countershock at increased energy (200 joules monophasic, 120 joules biphasic) as ordered by medical direction. DC countershock is contraindicated if you suspect digitalis toxicity as the PSVT's cause.

   If the patient in A-fib or A-flutter with rapid heart rate is stable, obtain a 12-lead ECG and establish IV access.

2. *Pharmacologic therapy.* Consider rate control with diltiazem or beta blockers if the patient is unstable (e.g., altered mental status, ongoing chest pain, hypotension, or other signs of shock).

   Generally, no treatment is required for first-degree AV block except observation, unless the heart rate drops significantly. If possible, avoid drugs that slow AV conduction, such as lidocaine and procainamide. The same is done for type I second-degree AV block. If the heart rate falls and the patient becomes symptomatic, administer 0.5 mg of atropine IV. Repeat every 3–5 minutes until you have obtained a satisfactory rate or have given 3.0 mg of the drug. If atropine fails, consider TCP or a dopamine or epinephrine infusion.

   Treatment is generally unnecessary for type II second-degree AV block, third-degree AV block, junctional escape rhythm, junctional bradycardia, and ventricular escape rhythm unless there are signs of poor perfusion (e.g., acute altered mental status, ongoing chest pain, hypotension, or other signs of shock). If there are signs of poor perfusion, prepare for TCP. Consider administering a 0.5-mg bolus of atropine sulfate. Repeat every 3–5 minutes until you have obtained a satisfactory rate or have given 3.0 mg of the drug. If atropine fails, consider TCP or a dopamine or epinephrine infusion.

   The treatment of perfusing ventricular tachycardia has changed dramatically in recent years. Perfusing ventricular tachycardia that is causing hypotension, acutely altered mental status, signs of shock, ischemic chest pain, and/or acute heart failure should be treated with synchronized cardioversion. Perfusing ventricular tachycardia that is not accompanied by the findings detailed above should be treated with adenosine (if regular and monomorphic) and/or an antiarrhythmic infusion (e.g., procainamide, amiodarone, sotalol). If the patient is nonperfusing, follow the protocol for ventricular fibrillation. Treatment includes defibrillation, epinephrine, and amiodarone.

   Treatment for torsades de pointes (TDP) focuses on rapid recognition. Treatment is 1–2 g of magnesium sulfate placed in 10 mL of D_5W and administered over 1–2 minutes. This can be repeated every 4 hours with close monitoring of the deep tendon reflexes. Ultimately, overdrive pacing may be required. Correct any underlying electrolyte problems, especially hyperkalemia.

   Ventricular fibrillation and nonperfusing ventricular tachycardia are treated identically. Follow the cardiac arrest algorithm found in the American Heart Association (AHA) guidelines. In addition, uninterrupted chest compressions are extremely important.

13. **Adapt the scene size-up, primary assessment, patient history, secondary assessment, and use of monitoring technology to meet the needs of patients with complaints and presentations related to cardiac disorders.**   pp. 102–174

Your scene size-up will focus on making sure that you have the appropriate equipment and resources available. For instance, a cardiac patient with dyspnea may require continuous positive airway pressure (CPAP) or capnography. This may require you to carry extra equipment into the scene.

The primary assessment will focus on rapid recognition of high-risk patients and patients currently experiencing conditions that require time-sensitive treatments or transport to a specialty care center. For example, a patient complaining of chest pain will require a 12-lead ECG within the first several minutes and will likely require transport to an accredited chest pain center with cath-lab capabilities.

The patient history will include rapid completion of the OPQRST components, SAMPLE history, and a thorough consideration of the past medical history. The recent history provides many alarm clues for your field diagnosis. For instance, a patient who is complaining of chest pain and is 2 days post–coronary artery stent placement is at a much higher risk for another acute myocardial infarction (AMI) than a patient with no remarkable cardiac history at all.

The secondary assessment will include a cardiac focused exam. Important exam findings include some of the following: jugular venous distension (JVD), peripheral edema, crackles (rales), nail clubbing, cyanosis, frothy cough, presence of pace maker, sternal scars, and presence of S3 or S4 heart sounds. Important monitoring devices include automatic blood pressure devices, capnography, pulse oximetry, multi-lead cardiac monitoring, and frequent 12-lead ECGs.

Your assessment of the patient with a cardiovascular emergency should vary according to the acuity of the situation. Patients with serious illnesses should have a limited, yet focused exam. Patients who are less seriously ill should receive a more comprehensive assessment. It is important to remember that the cardiovascular system affects virtually every other body system. Signs of cardiac disease may initially be evident only in the respiratory system as dyspnea. A comprehensive exam, however, will often reveal subtle findings that point to cardiovascular disease as the cause.

14. Use a process of clinical reasoning to guide and interpret the patient assessment and management process for patients with cardiac and vascular disorders. pp. 102–174

As a paramedic, you will evaluate objective and subjective data from your scene size-up, general impression, patient interview and history, and assessments to determine an appropriate clinical path. Your understanding of common clinical presentations (signs and symptoms), pathophysiology, risk factors, and epidemiology will assist you in forming a presumptive conclusion. Your treatment plan will be formed by considering common practice, standards of care, evidence-based practice, treatment guidelines, local protocols, empirical experience, and your patient's wishes. Implementation of prehospital care can be influenced by the stability of your patient's condition, availability of resources, scene location, and access to specialty care centers. Your reassessment is ongoing and can evolve the clinical decision-making process as you evaluate the effectiveness of treatments and changing patient condition. Your transport decision will be based on current scientific evidence as it applies to your patient's clinical condition. For instance, the patient's outcome when experiencing an acute coronary syndrome such as an AMI depends upon a time-critical diagnosis and management. Therefore, such patients should be transported to an appropriate cardiac catheterization facility.

15. Describe the therapeutic roles of pharmacological, electrical, and other basic life support and advanced life support interventions in the management of patients with cardiac disorders. pp. 102–174

There is a multitude of pharmacologic and electrical therapies used in coordination with BLS and ALS interventions for patients with cardiac disorders.

Nitroglycerin is used to treat ischemic chest pain and congestive heart failure (CHF). Aspirin is used to inhibit platelet aggregation and to prevent arterial occlusion from developing further. Narcotic analgesics are used when nitrates fail to relieve chest pain. Benzodiazepines and/or narcotics are used to sedate patients for painful electrical procedures such as pacing and synchronized cardioversion. Sodium channel blockers are used to treat ventricular tachyarrhythmias. Calcium channel blockers and beta blockers are used to treat narrow-complex tachyarrhythmias and hypertension. Vasopressors such as dopamine and norepinephrine can be used to treat hypotension in cardiogenic shock.

Transcutaneous pacing (TCP) and the parasympatholytic drug atropine are used to treat symptomatic bradycardia. TCP is effective when electrical capture and physiologic capture occur. Electrical capture occurs when pacer spikes are followed by ventricular complexes on the monitor. Physiologic capture occurs when a pulse is felt with each electrical capture. Adjusting the pacer rate can be performed once if hemodynamic status has not improved with the initial rate of pacing. If hemodynamic status has not improved, epinephrine or dopamine IV infusions should be initiated and titrated.

Reperfusion therapy using fibrinolytic or percutaneous coronary intervention (PCI) can reopen occluded coronary arteries and restore blood supply to damaged areas of the heart.

Continuous positive airway pressure (CPAP) has proven to be an effective therapy for acute congestive heart failure. CPAP, if applied in time, can often prevent the need for endotracheal intubation and mechanical ventilation. CPAP maintains a constant pressure within the airway throughout the respiratory cycle via a tight-fitting mask that is applied to the mouth and nose. Nitrates (either sublingual or IV) that decrease preload and afterload and ACE inhibitors that decrease afterload can be used along with CPAP to treat acute CHF.

Electrical cardioversion (synchronized cardioversion) is used to emergently treat patients experiencing an unstable tachycardia. Defibrillation is used to emergently treat patients who are pulseless in V-tach, V-fib, and torsades de pointes (TDP). Basic life support with uninterrupted, high-quality CPR is the cornerstone of treating all pulseless patients, regardless of associated arrhythmia.

16. Demonstrate the steps in basic life support and advanced life support interventions used in the management of cardiac disorders. pp. 107–120

Basic life support with uninterrupted, high-quality CPR is the cornerstone of treating all pulseless patients, regardless of associated arrhythmia. These include the basic airway maneuvers as well as CPR. Review basic life support techniques frequently to keep your skills at their peak.

Most of the procedures that paramedics employ to manage cardiovascular emergencies are considered advanced life support. The number of skills will vary from system to system. Advanced prehospital skills used in managing cardiovascular emergencies include:

- ECG monitoring (3-lead and 12-lead)
- Vagal maneuvers (carotid sinus massage)
- Pharmacological therapy
- Defibrillation
- Synchronized cardioversion
- Transcutaneous cardiac pacing
- Diagnostic (12-lead) ECG

17. List causes of chest pain. p. 120–135

It is important to remember that there are other causes of chest pain. Although cardiac ischemia is one of its major causes, chest pain can arise from problems in the cardiovascular, respiratory, gastrointestinal, and musculoskeletal systems. Causes of chest pain include:

- Cardiovascular causes
  - Cardiac ischemia
  - Pericarditis (viral or autoimmune)
  - Thoracic dissection of the aorta
- Respiratory causes
  - Pulmonary embolism
  - Pneumothorax
  - Pneumonia
  - Pleural irritation (pleurisy)
- Gastrointestinal causes
  - Cholecystitis
  - Pancreatitis
  - Hiatal hernia
  - Esophageal disease
  - Gastroesophageal reflux disease (GERD)
  - Peptic ulcer disease
  - Dyspepsia
- Musculoskeletal causes
  - Chest wall syndrome
  - Costochondritis
  - Acromioclavicular disease
  - Herpes zoster (shingles)
  - Chest wall trauma
  - Chest wall tumors

©2013 Pearson Education, Inc.
Paramedic Care: Principles & Practice, Vol. 4, 4th Ed.

18. **Describe the pathophysiology of specific cardiac and vascular disorders, including the following:**

a. **Acute coronary syndrome**   p. 120

Coronary artery disease involves progressive narrowing of the lumen of the coronary arteries (atherosclerosis) caused by the development of thick, hard plaques (atheromas). As the narrowing of the coronary arteries progresses, it leads to the clinical spectrum of myocardial ischemia, injury, and infarction. This spectrum of coronary occlusive disease is known as acute ischemic coronary syndrome.

Myocardial ischemia is caused by an imbalance of oxygen supply and demand—either a decreased oxygen supply or increased oxygen demand. Impairment of oxygen delivery is the primary contributor to decreased oxygen supply. Impaired oxygen delivery is caused by occlusion of the coronary arteries either by spasm, stenosis, thrombus, or a combination of these. Other factors that might contribute to the decreased oxygen supply to the coronary arteries are any factors that produce low blood pressure, such as volume loss, drug effects, or infection. Physical exertion and emotional stress are factors that increase myocardial oxygen demand.

Thrombus formation is considered an integral factor in coronary artery disease. The process is usually initiated by endothelial damage, usually from disruption of an atherosclerotic plaque, which leads to platelet aggregation and thrombus formation. The resulting thrombus can occlude the vessel lumen, leading to myocardial ischemia, injury, and infarction. The consequences of coronary artery occlusion depend on the preexisting atherosclerotic plaque, the extent of occlusion by the thrombus formation, and the rate of development of the occlusion. Occlusions that occur more slowly give the body time to develop collateral circulation in an attempt to compensate for the decrease in blood flow to the area involved.

b. **Heart failure**   p. 128

Heart failure is generally divided into left ventricle or right ventricle failure. Left ventricular failure occurs when the left ventricle fails as an effective forward pump, causing back pressure of blood into the pulmonary circulation, which often results in pulmonary edema. Its causes include various types of heart disease, such as myocardial infarction (MI), valvular disease, chronic hypertension, and arrhythmias. In left ventricular failure, the left ventricle cannot eject all of the blood that the right heart delivers to it via the lungs. Left atrial pressure rises and is subsequently transmitted to the pulmonary veins and capillaries. When pulmonary capillary pressure becomes too high, it forces the blood plasma into the alveoli, resulting in pulmonary edema. Progressive fluid accumulation in the alveoli decreases the lungs' oxygenation capacity and can cause death from hypoxia. Because MI is a common cause of left ventricular failure, consider that all patients with pulmonary edema may have had an MI.

In right ventricular failure, the right ventricle fails as an effective forward pump, resulting in back pressure of blood into the systemic venous circulation and venous congestion. The most common cause of right ventricular failure is left ventricular failure, because myocardial infarction is more common in the left ventricle than in the right and because chronic hypertension affects the left ventricle more adversely than the right. Right ventricular failure is also caused by systemic hypertension, which can affect both sides of the heart and can cause pure right ventricular failure. Pulmonary hypertension and *cor pulmonale* (heart failure due to pulmonary disease) result from the effects of chronic obstructive pulmonary disease (COPD). These problems are related to increased pressure in the pulmonary arteries, which results in right ventricular enlargement, right atrial enlargement, and, if untreated, right-heart failure.

c. **Cardiac tamponade**   p. 131

In cardiac tamponade, excess fluid accumulates inside the pericardium. (The normal amount of fluid between the visceral pericardium and the parietal pericardium is approximately 25 cc.) This excess fluid causes an increase in intrapericardial pressure that impairs diastolic filling and drastically decreases the amount of blood the ventricles can expel with each contraction. Chest pain or dyspnea is the chief complaint; depending on the underlying cause, the chest pain may be dull or sharp and severe.

d. Hypertensive emergencies   p. 133

Hypertension is a chronic disease. However, in some patients, the disease is not well controlled and will sometimes result in a life-threatening elevation in blood pressure. These elevations are usually classified as a hypertensive emergency. A hypertensive emergency is a life-threatening elevation of blood pressure and is quite rare—occurring in 1 percent or less of patients with hypertension, usually when the hypertension is poorly controlled or untreated. The different types of hypertensive problems are detailed in Table 2-6 in the text. A hypertensive emergency is characterized by an increase in blood pressure accompanied by end- or target-organ changes. It often occurs with hypertensive encephalopathy, a condition of acute or subacute consequence of severe hypertension characterized by altered mental status, vomiting, visual disturbances (including transient blindness), paralysis, seizures, stupor, and coma. On occasion, this condition may cause left ventricular failure, pulmonary edema, or stroke.

e. Cardiogenic shock   p. 135

Cardiogenic shock, the most severe form of pump failure, is shock that remains after existing arrhythmias, hypovolemia, or altered vascular tone have been corrected. It occurs when left ventricular function is so compromised that the heart cannot meet the body's metabolic demands and the compensatory mechanisms are exhausted. This usually happens after extensive myocardial infarction, often involving more than 40 percent of the left ventricle, or with diffuse ischemia.

f. Cardiac arrest   p. 136

Cardiac arrest with sudden death accounts for 60 percent of all deaths from coronary artery disease. Cardiac arrest is the absence of ventricular contraction that immediately results in systemic circulatory failure. Sudden death is any death that occurs within 1 hour of symptom onset. At autopsy, actual infarction often is not present. Because severe atherosclerotic disease is common, authorities usually believe that a lethal arrhythmia is the mechanism of death. The risk factors for sudden death are basically the same as those for atherosclerotic heart disease (ASHD) and coronary artery disease (CAD). In a large number of patients, cardiac arrest is the first manifestation of heart disease.

g. Aortic aneurysm and dissecting aortic aneurysm   p. 142

Aneurysm is a nonspecific term meaning "dilation of a vessel." Abdominal aortic aneurysm commonly results from atherosclerosis and occurs most frequently in the aorta, below the renal arteries and above the bifurcation of the common iliac arteries. It is 10 times more common in men than in women and most prevalent between ages 60 and 70. Degenerative changes in the smooth muscle and elastic tissue of the aortic media cause most dissecting aortic aneurysms. This can result in a hematoma and, subsequently, aneurysm. The original tear often results from cystic medial necrosis, a degenerative disease of connective tissue often associated with hypertension and, to a certain extent, aging. Predisposing factors include hypertension, which is present in 75–85 percent of cases. It occurs more frequently in patients older than 40–50, although it can occur in younger individuals, especially pregnant women. A tendency for this disease also runs in families.

h. Pulmonary embolism   p. 142

Acute pulmonary embolism occurs when a blood clot or other particle lodges in a pulmonary artery and blocks blood flow through that vessel. Pulmonary emboli may be composed of air, fat, amniotic fluid, or blood clots. Factors that predispose a patient to blood clots include prolonged immobilization, *thrombophlebitis* (inflammation and clots in a vein), use of certain medications, and atrial fibrillation.

i. Acute arterial occlusion   p. 142

An acute arterial occlusion is the sudden occlusion of arterial blood flow due to trauma, thrombosis, tumor, embolus, or idiopathic means. Emboli are probably the most common cause. They can arise from within the chamber (*mural emboli*), from a thrombus in the left ventricle, from an atrial thrombus secondary to atrial fibrillation, or from a thrombus caused by abdominal aortic atherosclerosis. Arterial occlusions most commonly involve vessels in the abdomen or extremities.

j. Vasculitis   p. 142

Vasculitis is an inflammation of the blood vessels. Most vasculitis stems from a variety of rheumatic diseases and syndromes. The inflammatory process is usually segmental, and inflammation within the media of a muscular artery tends to destroy the internal elastic lamina. Necrosis and hypertrophy (enlarging) of the vessel occur, and the vessel wall has a high likelihood of breaching, leaking fibrin and red blood cells into the surrounding tissue. This potentially can lead to partial or total vascular occlusion and subsequent necrosis.

©2013 Pearson Education, Inc.
Paramedic Care: Principles & Practice, Vol. 4, 4th Ed.

k. Peripheral arterial disease

p. 143

Peripheral arterial (atherosclerotic) disease is a progressive degenerative disease of the midsize and large arteries. It affects the aorta and its branches, the brachial and femoral peripheral arteries, and the cerebral arteries. For reasons unknown, it does not affect coronary arteries. It is a gradual, progressive disease, often associated with diabetes mellitus. In extreme cases, significant arterial insufficiency may lead to ulcers and gangrene. Occlusion of the peripheral arteries causes chronic and acute ischemia.

l. Deep vein thrombosis

p. 143

Deep vein (venous) thrombosis (DVT) is a blood clot in a vein. It most commonly occurs in the larger veins of the thigh and calf. Predisposing factors include a recent history of trauma, inactivity, pregnancy, and varicose veins.

m. Varicose veins

p. 143

Varicose veins are dilated superficial veins, usually in the lower extremities. Predisposing factors include pregnancy, obesity, and genetics. Signs and symptoms include the visible distention of the leg veins, lower leg swelling and discomfort (especially at the end of the day), and skin color and texture changes in the legs and ankles. If the condition is chronic, venous stasis ulcers, a noncritical condition, can develop. Venous stasis ulcers can rupture, but direct pressure usually can control the bleeding, which occasionally is significant.

19. Demonstrate the steps of assessing patients with cardiac complaints and presentations.

pp. 102–107

Your assessment of the patient with a cardiovascular emergency should vary according to the acuity of the situation. Patients with serious illnesses should have a limited, yet focused exam. Patients who are less seriously ill should receive a more comprehensive assessment. It is important to remember that the cardiovascular system affects virtually every other body system. Signs of cardiac disease may initially be evident only in the respiratory system as dyspnea. A comprehensive exam, however, will often reveal subtle findings that point to cardiovascular disease as the cause.

Always do visual inspection first. (1) Look for tracheal position. If it isn't in its normal midline position but is toward one side, there may be a pneumothorax. (2) Check neck veins for signs of jugular distention (have the patient elevated about 45° and with head turned to the side). Jugular venous distention (JVD) is evidence of back pressure from causes such as heart (pump) failure or cardiac tamponade. (3) Thorax and chest movement while breathing should be observed with proper exposure so you can see chest shape (barrel chests may indicate COPD) and effort during respiration, such as retractions of the soft tissues between the ribs. Accessory muscles are used when breathing is difficult and may include those of the neck, back, and abdomen. Always look for surgical scars; a scar over the sternum may indicate prior cardiac surgery. (4) Evaluate the epigastrium while the chest wall is exposed, looking for distention and visible pulsations. Pulsations may signal an aortic aneurysm dissection or rupture. (5) Position-dependent edema may be found in the ankles or sacral area, depending on whether the patient has been sitting or lying in bed. Pitting edema (a depression that persists after you stop applying firm pressure) is significant. (6) Skin changes associated with cardiovascular disease include pallor and diaphoresis (indicating increased sympathetic tone and peripheral vasoconstriction) or a mottled appearance (often an indicator of chronic cardiac failure). (7) Subtle changes associated with cardiovascular disease include not only surgical scars but subcutaneous batteries for a pacemaker or nitroglycerin skin patches.

Auscultation includes listening to the lungs, to the heart, and over the carotid arteries. (1) Assess the lung fields for equality and for sounds such as crackles (rales), rhonchi (whistling or snoring-like sounds), or wheezes, which may signal pulmonary edema or primary pulmonary disease. Note that patients with pulmonary edema may have foamy, blood-tinged sputum evident at the mouth and nose. In advanced cases, you may even hear a gurgling-like sound as the patient breathes. (2) It is difficult to auscultate the heart well in the field because of the number and intensity of background noises. Ideally, you want to listen for heart sounds at four classic sites: aortic, pulmonic, mitral (left AV valve), and tricuspid (right AV valve). The point on the chest wall where the heartbeat is the loudest or is best felt is called the point of maximum impulse (PMI). (3) Auscultation over the carotid arteries may reveal bruits, murmur sounds due to turbulent flow. A bruit over any artery indicates partial obstruction due to atherosclerosis. Never attempt carotid sinus massage in a patient with a bruit because you might dislodge atherosclerotic material that could lodge in a cerebral artery, causing a stroke or other mishap.

Palpation should cover three areas: peripheral pulse, thorax, and epigastrium. (1) Determine rate and regularity of the pulse as well as equality. A pulse deficit (intensity less than expected) may indicate underlying peripheral vascular disease and should be reported to medical direction. (2) Thoracic palpation is extremely important and may reveal crepitus, akin to "bubble wrap" crackling under your fingers, which suggests subcutaneous emphysema. Check for tenderness or possible rib fracture. Remember that at least 15 percent of MI patients have some associated chest wall tenderness. (3) Abdominal exam may reveal distention or pulsations.

20. Describe the roles of diagnostic procedures in the evaluation of myocardial infarction, including 12-lead ECGs and laboratory tests.   **pp. 107–128**

Physical exam findings, ECG findings, and other diagnostic testing (e.g., stress tests, coronary angiography) should always be used together to complete the evaluation of patients with suspected myocardial infarction.

Myocardial ischemia occurs almost immediately following loss of blood supply. The ischemic tissue is deprived of oxygen and other nutrients. Ischemic tissue can still depolarize, but ischemia tends to affect repolarization. Myocardial ischemia can cause depression of the ST segment and inversion of the T wave on the ECG. Both of these findings are due to abnormalities of repolarization. If blood supply is restored promptly to ischemic tissue, then permanent myocardial injury often can be avoided.

If myocardial ischemia is allowed to progress untreated, *myocardial injury* will occur. Myocardial injury reflects actual injury to the myocardium. The degree of injury depends on how quickly blood supply is restored. Injured myocardium tends to be partially or completely depolarized. This tissue, often called stunned myocardium, does not contract and does not contribute to the heart's pumping ability. In addition, injured myocardium can be very irritable and a source of serious and potentially life-threatening arrhythmias. With myocardial injury, current flows between the pathologically depolarized area and the normally depolarized areas. Thus, with myocardial injury, the injured tissue remains depolarized. It effectively emits a negative electrical charge into the surrounding fluids when the surrounding normal myocardium is positively charged. This current of injury can sometimes be seen on the ECG as elevation of the ST segment (STEMI).

Cardiac enzymes are certain chemicals that are released by the heart when myocardial cells are damaged. Thus, an increase in these specific cardiac enzymes is an indicator of myocardial damage. For the most part, measurement of cardiac enzymes has been limited to in-hospital settings. However, with the advent of rapid enzyme assays, it is possible to quickly measure some cardiac enzymes in the prehospital setting. Cardiac enzymes routinely monitored include:

- *Creatine kinase (CK) or creatine phosphokinase (CPK).* This enzyme (CK is the newer term; CPK the older term) can be found in the heart muscle, skeletal muscle, and the brain. However, each specific form (isoenzyme) is different and can be measured separately. For example, CK from the brain is called CK-BB, CK from skeletal muscle is called CK-MM, and CK from the heart is called CK-MB. Thus, an elevation in total CK tells you nothing about the heart. But when CK is fractionated, any elevation in the MB isoenzyme fraction indicates myocardial damage. An elevated CK-MB is seen in about 90 percent of myocardial infarctions. The CK begins to rise 4–6 hours postinfarction, peaks at 24 hours, and returns to near normal levels in 3–4 days. The CK-MB fraction rises and returns to normal faster than the total CK. It typically begins to rise within 3–4 hours postinfarction and returns to normal within 2 days.
- *Lactic dehydrogenase (LDH).* Also called *lactate dehydrogenase*, LDH can be found in heart muscle, skeletal muscle, the liver, erythrocytes, the kidneys, and some types of tumors. It is increased in over 90 percent of myocardial infarctions. However, increases in LDH can also be seen in other disease processes. The LDH will tend to rise within 24 hours after a myocardial infarction, reach a peak level in 3 days, and return to normal in 8–9 days. Isoenzyme forms of LDH can be assayed separately. They are as follows:
  - LD_1 = heart, erythrocytes, renal cortex
  - LD_2 = reticuloendothelial system
  - LD_3 = lung tissue
  - LD_4 = placenta, kidney, liver
  - LD_5 = skeletal muscle, liver

Paramedic Care: Principles & Practice, Vol. 4, 4th Ed.

A reversal of the LD_1/LD_2 ratio suggests myocardial infarction with a sensitivity of 80–85 percent.

- *Myoglobin.* Myoglobin is chemically similar to hemoglobin, but it is found exclusively within striated (skeletal and cardiac) muscle. It is released into the circulation when skeletal or cardiac muscle is damaged. Myoglobin levels begin to rise within 2 hours after myocardial infarction, peak at 6–8 hours, and return to normal within 20–36 hours. False positive myoglobin levels can be associated with skeletal muscle injury and renal failure.
- *Troponin.* Troponins are proteins within the contractile regions of the cardiac fibers. There are three isoforms of troponin: troponin I (TnI), troponin T (TnT), and troponin C (TnC). Troponin I is the form most frequently assessed. It is very specific for cardiac injury and is not found in the serum of healthy people. TnI begins to rise within 4–6 hours after injury, peaks in 12–16 hours, and stays elevated for up to 10 days.

21. Describe the roles of fibrinolytic therapy, percutaneous coronary interventions, coronary artery bypass grafts, and pharmacological treatments in the management of myocardial infarction. pp. 110–126

Definitive treatment of myocardial ischemia with fibrinolytic (also called thrombolytic) agents is one of the most important recent advances in medicine. In some instances, fibrinolytic therapy may be beneficial in the field. This is especially true in areas that have a long transport time to a definitive care facility. Fibrinolytic agents are very expensive, and their use requires a diagnostic 12-lead ECG.

The increased availability of cardiac catheterization labs and the development of STEMI teams now allow MI patients to be immediately taken to the lab for diagnosis and treatment via percutaneous coronary intervention (PCI). A catheter is placed into an artery (usually the femoral) and advanced to the heart. Radiographic contrast dye is administered into the coronary arteries and their anatomy is visualized. This process, called a coronary arteriogram (or coronary angiogram), will detail any blockages or lesions that might be causing the patient's problem. If the lesions can be treated in the lab, they are immediately treated with angioplasty (properly referred to as percutaneous transluminal coronary angioplasty [PTCA]). A balloon is advanced into the affected coronary artery to the point of the lesion. The balloon is inflated and the artery dilated. Often the artery will remain dilated after angioplasty. Sometimes it does not. When it does not, a stent is placed to keep the artery open. This procedure, called primary coronary stenting, is commonly employed.

Coronary artery bypass grafting (CABG), also referred to as aortocoronary grafting, is used when the patient has disease that is extensive or not amenable to PCI techniques. This procedure is rarely done emergently.

Medications that are indicated for the treatment of suspected AMI focus on improving perfusion, decreasing oxygen demand and workload, pain relief, and preventing further occlusion. Medications typically indicated for the patient suspected of MI include the following:

- Aspirin
- Nitroglycerin
- Morphine sulfate
- Fentanyl
- Medications that might be indicated include:
- Clopidogrel (Plavix)
- Heparin (or low-molecular weight heparin)
- Beta blockers
- Glycoprotein IIb/IIIa inhibitors (tirofiban [Aggrastat], eptifibatide [Integrilin])

22. Describe considerations in post-resuscitation care of cardiac arrest patients with return of spontaneous circulation. pp. 139–140

Management of the successful post–cardiac arrest patient generally presents an unusual situation. The patient's blood pressure can return at low, normal, or high readings because of the drugs used in resuscitation. In addition, the pulse can return at bradycardic, normal, or tachycardic rates. The blood pressure may return at low readings. The ideal range of the blood pressure is 80–100 mmHg in the postarrest patient. Do not be concerned if the postarrest patient does not show any signs of response. He has endured a very harsh environment, and recovery, if any, can be slow. The postarrest setting can be unnerving, with the patient's vitals and ECG changing every minute. Approach problems one at a time, and do not be fooled by a return in pulse that fades away while the monitor still has a rhythm (pulseless electrical activity [PEA]).

It has now become common practice to cool survivors of cardiac arrest in the immediate post-resuscitation period. This procedure, called induced therapeutic hypothermia (ITH), has been shown to improve survival and neurological outcome in cardiac arrest survivors. The cooling process helps to slow metabolism and minimize the effects of hypoxic injury and oxidative stress (reperfusion injury), thus providing some degree of neuroprotection. The patient is typically cooled with chilled IV fluids and ice packs to a temperature of $32°–34°C$ $(90°–92°F)$. Once cooled, the patient is usually maintained in the hypothermic state for at least 24 to 48 hours. Problems detected (e.g., STEMI) can be addressed during the hypothermic interval.

23. Describe considerations in withholding resuscitation in cardiac arrest and in terminating resuscitative efforts in the field. pp. 140–141

In some situations, the certainty that the patient will not survive indicates not initiating resuscitation efforts. Rigor mortis, fixed dependent lividity (pooling of the blood), decapitation, decomposition, and incineration are all situations in which you should withhold resuscitation. In addition, withhold resuscitation efforts if the patient has an out-of-hospital advance directive. A physician must sign and date the advance directive, and it must state conditions that apply to the patient at the time of the arrest. For example, the directive may state that resuscitation should be withheld if the patient has an end-stage terminal illness. Each state and many local regions treat advance directives differently. Review local protocol and medical direction before you might have to decide whether to honor an advance directive.

In some instances, poor prognosis and survivability of many nontraumatic cardiac arrest patients makes termination of resuscitation in the field a consideration. Some of the inclusion criteria for termination of resuscitation are:

- 18 years or older
- Arrest is presumed to be nontraumatic in origin and not associated with a treatable cause such as hypothermia, overdose, or hypovolemia
- Successful definitive airway management and ventilation
- ACLS standards have been applied throughout the arrest
- On-scene ALS efforts have been sustained for 25 minutes, or the patient remains in asystole through four rounds of ALS drugs
- Patient's rhythm is asystolic or agonal when the decision to terminate is made, and this rhythm persists until the resuscitation efforts are actually terminated

Depending on local protocol, the exclusion criteria for termination of resuscitation may include:

- Under 18 years old
- Etiology that could benefit from in-hospital treatment (such as hypothermia)
- Transient return of a pulse
- Signs of neurological viability

Criteria that should not be considered as either inclusionary or exclusionary:

- The patient's age if 18 or over (for example, geriatric)
- Downtime before EMS arrival
- Presence of a nonofficial do not resuscitate (DNR) order
- Quality-of-life evaluations by EMS

Review local protocols and medical direction before attempting termination of resuscitation. Most systems use documented protocols and direct communication with an on-line medical director or physician to approve or deny termination of resuscitation. The medical director or physician may base his or her decision on the following information:

- Medical condition of the patient
- Known etiological factors
- Therapy rendered
- Family's presence and appraisal of the situation

- Communication of any resistance or uncertainty on the part of the family
- Continuous documentation, including the ECG

The family should receive grief support. This requires EMS personnel or a community agency to be in place soon after termination of resuscitation. EMS personnel deal not only with the living or viable but also with the families of lost loved ones, especially when they have witnessed the death. Many systems employ assigned personnel to support the family after termination of resuscitation. In other systems, paramedics on the scene provide support until a predetermined person from another local agency can arrive. Although this supportive role can be uncomfortable, it will be part of your job.

24. **Apply a process of clinical reasoning to evaluate patients for specific cardiac and vascular disorders, including the following (see objective 14):**   pp. 102–143

   a. Acute coronary syndrome
   b. Heart failure
   c. Cardiac tamponade
   d. Hypertensive emergencies
   e. Cardiogenic shock
   f. Cardiac arrest
   g. Aortic aneurysm and dissecting aortic aneurysm
   h. Pulmonary embolism
   i. Acute arterial occlusion
   j. Vasculitis
   k. Peripheral arterial disease
   l. Deep vein thrombosis
   m. Varicose veins

As a paramedic, you will evaluate objective and subjective data from your scene size-up, general impression, patient interview and history, and assessments to determine an appropriate clinical path. Your understanding of common clinical presentations (signs and symptoms), pathophysiology, risk factors, and epidemiology will assist you in forming a presumptive conclusion. Your treatment plan will be formed by considering common practice, standards of care, evidence-based practice, treatment guidelines, local protocols, empirical experience, and your patient's wishes. Implementation of prehospital care can be influenced by the stability of your patient's condition, availability of resources, scene location, and access to specialty care centers. Your reassessment is ongoing and can evolve the clinical decision-making process as you evaluate effectiveness of treatments and changing patient condition.

Case Study Review

Reread the case study on pages 47–48 in Paramedic Care: Medicine; *then, read the following discussion.*

Chris and Kim are dispatched to a "difficulty breathing" call. On arrival, they find just that, a patient breathing 34 times per minute and in distress. However, Chris and Kim know that sometimes respiratory signs and symptoms in elderly patients are due to causes other than respiratory problems. During their assessment they will do much to assure there are no other reasons for the dyspnea. Sure enough, Mr. Williams's history reveals congestive heart failure and hypertension. Chris and Kim will provide an assessment to rule out a heart attack or an exacerbation of the congestive heart failure.

The initial assessment identifies the patient is in severe distress but denies chest pain, an important pertinent negative. His advanced age would suggest he is more likely to experience the MI without chest pain. Mr. Williams has one-word-dyspnea, loud crackles (rales), and an oximetry reading of only 83 percent, even with supplemental oxygen. The distended jugular veins (while the patient is seated) and pitting edema support a diagnosis of congestive heart failure. His blood pressure of 140/98 may be low for a patient with reported hypertension. Chris and Kim should investigate this during their focused assessment. Their patient's ECG demonstrates atrial fibrillation, further supporting a diagnosis of CHF.

Continuous positive airway pressure (CPAP) increases the pressure within the alveoli, which does two things to help the patient. It increases the partial pressure of oxygen, assuring better movement across the alveolar and capillary walls. It also helps to push the fluid back into the capillary (vascular) space, permitting better oxygen and carbon dioxide exchange. Nitroglycerin also eases some of the congestion by reducing afterload and providing better circulation through the coronary arteries and to the heart muscle. The reduced afterload means the left heart can better move blood out of the pulmonary circulation. The patient improves markedly, as demonstrated by the reduced respiratory rate and the increasing SpO_2. Increasing the PEEP value to 15 continues that trend.

Preparing the intubation equipment and placing a saline lock identify that both Kim and Chris are looking ahead. Often, patients with congestive heart failure are difficult to treat and become more symptomatic during care. These actions assure the team is prepared for the worst. Fortunately, their care is very effective and Mr. Williams arrives at the hospital in a condition much better than when they found him.

Content Self-Evaluation

MULTIPLE CHOICE

_____ 1. Chest pain is the most common chief complaint among patients with cardiac disease, but not all patients with cardiac disease will have chest pain.
  A. True
  B. False

_____ 2. Which element of the OPQRST acronym represents those activities that either increase or decrease the severity of a symptom or complaint?
  A. "O"
  B. "P"
  C. "Q"
  D. "R"
  E. "S"

_____ 3. Which patient might you expect NOT to have chest pain while experiencing an MI?
  A. Young male
  B. Middle-aged female
  C. Athlete
  D. Diabetic
  E. Patient with no recent exertion

_____ 4. A family cardiac history is significant unless the family member had heart problems before the age of 40.
  A. True
  B. False

_____ 5. Ascultation of the carotid artery reveals a murmur. This finding is
  A. normal.
  B. suggestive of the need for carotid massage.
  C. called a bruit.
  D. indicative of hypertension.
  E. a contraindication for thrombolytic therapy.

_____ 6. Which of the following is likely to cause a poor ECG signal?
  A. Excessive body hair
  B. Dried conductive gel
  C. Poor electrode placement
  D. Diaphoresis
  E. All of the above

_____ 7. Atropine, lidocaine, and adenosine are in which group of drugs?
  A. Sympathomimetics
  B. Sympatholytics
  C. Fibrinolytics
  D. Antidysrhythmics
  E. Drugs used for myocardial ischemia and its pain

8. Dopamine, dobutamine, and epinephrine are in which group of drugs?
   A. Sympatholytics
   B. Drugs used for myocardial ischemia and its pain
   C. Antidysrhythmics
   D. Parasympathomimetics
   E. Sympathomimetics

9. Nitrous oxide, nitroglycerin, fentanyl, and morphine are in which group of drugs?
   A. Sympathomimetics
   B. Drugs used for myocardial ischemia and its pain
   C. Antidysrhythmics
   D. Antiatherosclerotics
   E. Sympatholytics

10. A potent loop diuretic used to relax the venous system and decrease intravascular fluid volume is
    A. promethazine.
    B. alteplase.
    C. furosemide.
    D. sodium nitroprusside.
    E. isoproterenol.

11. Digitalis (digoxin) has all of the following effects, EXCEPT that it
    A. increases the force of cardiac contractions.
    B. suppresses atrial ectopy as an antidysrhythmic.
    C. increases cardiac output.
    D. decreases ventricular response to certain supraventricular dysrhythmias.
    E. decreases conduction through the AV node.

12. The alkalizing agents such as sodium bicarbonate are first-line drugs in the treatment of asystole.
    A. True
    B. False

13. A smaller paddle size decreases the transthoracic resistance and allows the delivery of more energy to the heart.
    A. True
    B. False

14. Indications for synchronized cardioversion in an unstable patient include all of the following, EXCEPT
    A. rapid atrial fibrillation.
    B. nonperfusing ventricular tachycardia.
    C. paroxysmal supraventricular tachycardia.
    D. perfusing ventricular tachycardia.
    E. 2:1 atrial flutter.

15. When using the transthoracic pacer, you should set the rate
    A. between 60 and 80.
    B. between 40 and 60.
    C. between 80 and 100.
    D. never lower than 75.
    E. at the patient's current heart rate.

16. To ensure the defibrillator delivers the electrical energy at the right time during the heart's electrical sequence, you must be sure the defibrillator is in the synchronized cardioversion mode and that
    A. the patient is premedicated.
    B. the energy is set to 100 joules.
    C. there is R wave capture.
    D. the defibrillator is fully energized.
    E. all of the above.

_____ **17.** If initial carotid massage does not slow the heart rate, massage both arteries simultaneously.
- **A.** True
- **B.** False

_____ **18.** Potentially urgent noncardiac causes of chest pain include all of the following, EXCEPT
- **A.** stroke.
- **B.** peptic ulcer disease.
- **C.** pneumothorax.
- **D.** pulmonary embolism.
- **E.** esophageal disease.

_____ **19.** The type of myocardial infarction where the injury affects the full thickness of the myocardium is termed
- **A.** non–Q wave infarction.
- **B.** angina.
- **C.** angina pectoris.
- **D.** transmural infarction.
- **E.** subendocardial infarction.

_____ **20.** The greatest threat to the patient's life secondary to the myocardial infarction is
- **A.** hypoxia.
- **B.** dysrhythmias.
- **C.** cardiac enzyme release.
- **D.** pulmonary emboli.
- **E.** nerve injury.

_____ **21.** Always consider the possibility of cardiac tamponade when you encounter a patient
- **A.** with a chest wall tumor.
- **B.** with muffled or distant heart and lung sounds.
- **C.** with a gallop rhythm (S_1, S_2, S_3, S_4 heart sounds).
- **D.** who has just entered ventricular fibrillation.
- **E.** who received CPR and later deteriorated.

_____ **22.** Causes of cardiogenic shock include all of the following, EXCEPT
- **A.** subendocardial MI.
- **B.** tension pneumothorax.
- **C.** pulmonary embolism.
- **D.** diffuse myocardial ischemia.
- **E.** prosthetic valve malfunction.

_____ **23.** Return of spontaneous circulation occurs when resuscitation results in resumption of a pulse; spontaneous breathing may or may not return.
- **A.** True
- **B.** False

_____ **24.** Which of the following is NOT a possible criterion for termination of resuscitation efforts?
- **A.** Successful airway and ventilation
- **B.** A patient 48 years of age
- **C.** On-scene ALS efforts have been sustained for 25 minutes
- **D.** Arrest is associated with a pediatric patient or hypothermia
- **E.** ACLS standards have been applied throughout the arrest

_____ **25.** Which of the following is NOT a sign or symptom of abdominal aortic aneurysm?
- **A.** Hypotension
- **B.** Back pain
- **C.** Blood in the urine
- **D.** Urge to defecate
- **E.** Abdominal pain

MATCHING

Write the letter of the definition in the space provided next to the term to which it applies.

- **A.** inflammation and clots within a vein

- **B.** relief of dyspnea on sitting upright

- **C.** alternation of weak and strong pulse over time

- **D.** pain in the calf muscles secondary to local ischemia

©2013 Pearson Education, Inc.
Paramedic Care: Principles & Practice, Vol. 4, 4th Ed.

E. episodes of being awakened at night by shortness of breath

F. murmur heard over an artery due to turbulent blood flow

G. drop of more than 10 mmHg in systolic blood pressure with inspiration

_____ 26. Orthopnea

_____ 27. Bruit

_____ 28. Paroxysmal nocturnal dyspnea

_____ 29. Pulsus paradoxus

_____ 30. Pulsus alternans

_____ 31. Intermittent claudication

_____ 32. Thrombophlebitis

Write the letter of the definition in the space provided next to the procedure to which it applies.

A. effort made immediately after onset of ventricular fibrillation or pulseless ventricular tachycardia that may cause conversion to organized rhythm

B. passage of electrical current through the heart during a specific part of the cardiac cycle to terminate certain dysrhythmias

C. manipulation of an arterial baroreceptor in an effort to increase parasympathetic tone

D. electrical pacing of the heart with the use of special skin electrodes

E. passage of electrical current through a fibrillating heart to depolarize a critical mass of myocardium, resulting in conversion to an organized rhythm

_____ 33. Defibrillation

_____ 34. Transcutaneous cardiac pacing

_____ 35. Precordial thump

_____ 36. Synchronized cardioversion

_____ 37. Carotid sinus massage

Write the letter of the probable diagnosis in the space provided next to the appropriate description of the condition. A letter response may be used more than once or not at all.

A. pulmonary edema

B. heart failure

C. acute MI

D. left ventricular failure

E. right ventricular failure

F. cardiac arrest

G. cardiac tamponade

H. hypertensive encephalopathy

_____ 38. Constant chest pain that is not relieved by rest or nitroglycerin and lasts longer than 30 minutes

_____ 39. Progressive fluid accumulation in the lungs

_____ 40. Syndrome in which the heart's pumping ability does not meet the body's needs

_____ 41. Unresponsiveness with apnea and pulselessness

_____ **42.** Jugular venous distension, engorged liver, edema, tachycardia

_____ **43.** Electrical paradoxus and pulsus alternans

_____ **44.** Dyspnea, orthopnea, decreased systolic blood pressure (BP) with narrowing pulse pressures

_____ **45.** Severe headache, visual disturbance, seizures, stupor, diagnostic vital signs

Part 3, p. 102

Review of Chapter Objectives

After reading this part of the chapter, you should be able to:

25. Given a variety of scenarios, develop treatment plans for patients with cardiac disorders. pp. 102–144

During your training as a paramedic, you will participate in many classroom sessions involving simulated patients. You will also spend some time in the emergency departments of local hospitals as well as in advanced-level ambulances gaining clinical experience. During these times, use your knowledge of cardiac disease to help you assess and care for the simulated or real patients you attend.

26. Describe the process and purpose of 12-lead ECG interpretation. pp. 144–175

The 12-lead ECG records the same series of electrical events within the heart from 12 different perspectives. This allows for examination of the heart in two planes. Many abnormalities can be detected with the 12-lead ECG. It is important to point out that the ECG records only the electrical events that occur. It does not provide any information about the heart's pumping efficiency. The ECG, like other pieces of medical information, must be used in association with a good history and physical examination, vital sign determination, and other ancillary testing and diagnostic equipment available for advanced prehospital care.

The 12-lead ECG can be performed several ways, depending on the machine being used. The most common 12-lead presentation is a three-channel machine that provides short strips of each lead. The most common format is to place the bipolar limb leads on the left with lead I at the top, lead II in the middle, and lead III at the bottom. To the right of this, in the second column, are the augmented limb leads with aVR at the top, aVL in the middle, and aVF at the bottom. To the right of the augmented limb leads are the precordial leads. Leads V_1 through V_3 are placed in the third column, and leads V_4 through V_6 in the fourth column. This system functionally groups the leads based on their view of the heart.

27. Identify findings associated with ACS in a variety of 12-lead ECGs. pp. 144–175

Each ECG lead is designed to visualize a particular part of the heart. The bipolar and augmented limb leads evaluate the heart from the frontal plane, whereas the precordial leads look at the heart from a horizontal plane.

Various ECG leads look at a specific part of the myocardium. Abnormalities of the ECG in certain leads, with a few exceptions, indicate problems in the part of the heart those leads visualize. The following is a generalized description of the various ECG lead groupings associated with various locations of acute myocardial infarction. These descriptions are generalized and some overlapping may occur:

- _Anterior._ Leads I, V_2, V_3, and V_4 are immediately over the anterior surface of the heart. ST segment elevation, T wave inversion, and the development of significant Q waves in these leads indicate myocardial infarction involving the anterior surface of the heart. Leads V_2 and V_3 overlie the ventricular septum. Ischemic changes in these leads, and possibly in the adjoining precordial leads, are often referred to as septal infarctions.

- *Anterolateral.* Leads I, aVL, V_5, and V_6 examine the anterior and lateral surface of the heart. ST segment elevation, T wave inversion, and the development of significant Q waves in these leads indicate myocardial infarction involving the anterolateral surface of the heart.
- *Lateral.* Leads V_5 and V_6 visualize the lateral surface of the heart. ST segment elevation, T wave inversion, and the development of significant Q waves in these leads indicate myocardial infarction involving the lateral surface of the heart.
- *High lateral.* Leads I and aVL visualize the high lateral surface of the heart. Changes in these leads can often be seen in the other lateral leads (V_5 and V_6). ST segment elevation, T wave inversion, and the development of significant Q waves in these leads indicate myocardial infarction involving the high lateral surface of the heart.
- *Inferior.* Leads II, III, and aVF visualize the inferior (diaphragmatic) surface of the heart. ST segment elevation, T wave inversion, and the development of significant Q waves in these leads indicate myocardial infarction involving the inferior surface of the heart. Inferior infarcts can sometimes primarily affect the right ventricle, causing right ventricular failure and elevated right ventricular filling pressures. These occur despite relatively normal left ventricular filling pressures. The classic clinical triad of right ventricular infarction includes distended neck veins, clear lung fields, and hypotension. All patients with inferior-wall myocardial infarction should have a right-sided ECG performed. ST segment elevation in lead V_4R is the single most powerful predictor of right ventricular infarction. Patients with this finding (right ventricular infarction) are a high-risk group of patients in the setting of inferior-wall myocardial infarction.
- *Inferolateral.* Leads II, III, aVF, and V_6 visualize the inferolateral portion of the heart. ST segment elevation, T wave inversion, and the development of significant Q waves in these leads indicate myocardial infarction involving the inferolateral surface of the heart.
- *True posterior.* There are no ECG leads over the posterior surface of the heart. True posterior infarctions, although rare, can be diagnosed by looking for reciprocal changes in the anterior leads (V_1 and V_2). Normally, the R wave in leads V_1 and V_2 is principally negative. An unusually large R wave in lead V_1 and V_2 can actually be a reciprocal of a posterior Q wave. Likewise, an upright T wave in these leads would be a reciprocal of posterior T wave inversion. These findings are subtle and require practice to learn. Alternatively, posterior leads (V_7 through V_{12}) can be applied to the back to confirm the presence of a true posterior myocardial infarction.

28. Describe the use of 15-lead and 18-lead ECGs in posterior-wall myocardial infarctions.   **pp. 159–175**

The classic 12-lead ECG is designed to detect the most common types of cardiac problems—usually those involving the left side of the heart and the left anterior descending coronary artery. However, problems that arise in the right ventricle and the posterior wall of the left ventricle may not be readily visible on the standard 12 leads. Because of this, some clinicians recommend the use of a 15-lead or 18-lead ECG to increase the sensitivity of the test. These supplemental leads specifically look at the right ventricle and the posterior wall of the left ventricle.

To the standard 12 leads (I, II, III, aVR, aVL, aVF, and V_1 through V_6), the 18-lead ECG adds three right-sided chest leads (V_4R, V_5R, and V_6R) and three posterior leads (V_7, V_8, and V_9). The 15-lead ECG is a subset of the 18-lead ECG, using V_4R, V_8, and V_9 as additional leads to the standard 12-lead ECG. Placement of the right chest electrodes mirrors left chest placement. The V_4R electrode is placed in the fifth intercostal space at the right midclavicular line. V_5R is placed level with V_4R at the right anterior axillary line. V_6R is placed level with V_5R at the right midaxillary line. The V_7 to V_9 electrodes extend in a horizontal line from V_6. V_7 is placed lateral to V_6 at the posterior axillary line. V_8 is placed at the level of V_7 at the midscapular line. V_9 is placed at the level of V_8 at the paravertebral line.

29. Use a 12-lead ECG to indentify cardiac conduction disorders and chamber enlargement.   **pp. 144–167**

Conduction disorders in the bundle branches can be described as affecting the right bundle branch, the left bundle branch, or even one fascicle of the thicker left bundle branch. Note that although AV blocks can be diagnosed from a single-lead rhythm strip, you need a 12-lead ECG to diagnose bundle branch blocks. In a bundle branch block, ventricular depolarization will be abnormal. The impulse will be passed properly through the AV node into the bundle of His and then into the right and left bundles, but the block will occur at some distal point. If the right bundle branch is blocked, the impulse will travel properly through the left bundle branch. The impulse will then eventually pass through the interventricular septum to depolarize the right ventricle. Likewise, if a blockage is in the left bundle branch, the impulse will pass properly through the right bundle branch, the interventricular septum, and eventually the left ventricle. Because of the circuitous passage of the depolarizing impulse toward the ventricle whose bundle branch bears the block, depolarization of that ventricle will be delayed. You can see this prolongation of ventricular depolarization as a QRS complex of 0.12 second or longer. In addition, the same delay can result in an abnormal QRS complex shape.

Right bundle branch block

Right bundle branch block results from an electrical obstruction at some point in that bundle branch. The right ventricle is the one affected by the delay in the depolarizing impulse. The right ventricle is also the lower pressure pump, and it has a thinner myocardium than the left ventricle. Thus, under normal circumstances the electrical forces in the right ventricular myocardium are overshadowed by those in the more massive left ventricle. In the case of right bundle branch block, the delayed right ventricular depolarization is anterior and to the right compared with the vector for left ventricular depolarization. A complete right bundle branch block is detected as a prolonged QRS complex (at least 0.12 second in length) and as an abnormal, later portion of the QRS that is directed toward the right ventricle (and away from the left ventricle).

Look at lead I and you will see a broad S wave. You will also see a characteristic RSR (R-S-R prime) complex in lead V_1. The RSR reflects the abnormal septal depolarization and the subsequent right ventricular depolarization. Lead V_1 overlies the right ventricle and is useful not only for detecting right bundle branch block but also other right ventricular abnormalities.

Clinically, right bundle branch block is a relatively common finding. It is a relatively thin bundle of fibers compared to the left bundle branch and thus it is more vulnerable to injury. Right bundle branch block can result from acute MI, drugs, electrolyte abnormalities, and general age-related deterioration of the cardiac conduction system.

Left bundle branch block

Left bundle branch block is derived from an obstruction at the level of the bundle of His, which divides into the anterior and posterior fascicles of the left bundle branch before terminating in the Purkinje system of the left ventricle. The left ventricle is the one affected by the delay in the depolarizing impulse. The left ventricle is also the higher-pressure pump, and it has a thicker myocardium than the right ventricle. Unlike the case of right bundle branch block, the direction of depolarization in left bundle branch block is still right to left, and thus nearly the same as in a normal heart. The QRS complexes in the heart with left bundle branch block are prolonged (at least 0.12 second in length) and bizarre in appearance. Typically, wide, notched QRS complexes are seen in leads I, aVL, V_5, and V_6. The changes are most pronounced in these leads because they visualize the lateral surface of the heart, which is principally the left ventricle. You may also see deep S waves in lead V_1, V_2, or V_3 or tall R waves in leads I, aVL, V_5, and V_6.

Left bundle branch block usually indicates significant and widespread myocardial disease. Like right bundle branch block, it can be caused by MI, drugs, electrolyte abnormalities, and age-related degenerative disease. Most MIs affect the left ventricle, and the presence of a left bundle branch block may mask new-onset ischemic changes associated with an acute MI. Thus, a patient may have a significant acute MI and the "characteristic" ECG changes will not be seen because of the presence of the left bundle branch block. In fact, the presence of left bundle branch block negates any possibility of localizing an MI with use of a 12-lead ECG.

Detection of bundle branch blocks, especially left bundle branch blocks, is important in the field for two reasons: (1) The block can mask ischemic changes associated with an acute MI and (2) some ST segment elevation usually appears in the precordial leads (V_1 to V_6) with left bundle branch blocks, which can make 12-lead tracings useless in the field.

The left bundle branch (which feeds the far thicker left ventricular myocardium) divides into anterior and posterior fascicles. Blocks (termed *hemiblocks*) can occur in either of these fascicles, and such hemiblocks are a fairly common finding.

©2013 Pearson Education, Inc.
Paramedic Care: Principles & Practice, Vol. 4, 4th Ed.

Hemiblocks

- Left posterior hemiblock results from blockage of the posterior fascicle and consequent delayed depolarization of the region of the left ventricle that it innervates. Note that a left posterior hemiblock does NOT typically result in a prolonged QRS interval or abnormally shaped QRS complex. Instead, the chief ECG finding is a rightward shift in QRS axis (right QRS deviation). This is often difficult to confirm, especially in the presence of right ventricular or pulmonary disease. Generally, the QRS axis must be equal to or greater than 120° to consider a left posterior hemiblock likely. This form of hemiblock is usually due to degenerative disease of the conductive system or to ischemic heart disease.
- Left anterior hemiblock results from blockage of the anterior fascicle. Anterior hemiblock does NOT result in a delay in ventricular depolarization, and so the QRS complex is of normal duration and is usually of normal shape (without the notching characteristic of bundle branch blocks). Instead, the chief ECG finding is a far leftward shift in QRS axis (typically more negative than 230°), which is manifest as a negative QRS complex in leads II, III, and aVF. A left anterior hemiblock is usually caused by degenerative disease of the conduction system or ischemic heart disease; it is usually a benign finding.

Chamber enlargement

Enlargement of any of the heart's four chambers rarely affects care in the field; however, you should understand the basic pathophysiology because it can cause changes in the ECG that might mislead you into consideration of ischemia. Any disease process that causes a prolonged increase in pressure in a chamber can lead to chamber enlargement. Right atrial enlargement (RAE) is often due to pulmonary disease such as emphysema or chronic bronchitis (COPD) or to pulmonary emboli. In these cases, the problem of origin produces pulmonary hypertension, which causes the increased pressure in the right atrium. Right ventricular hypertrophy (RVH, thickening of the right ventricle due to enlargement by stretching of the individual muscle cells) typically follows. In a similar fashion, left atrial enlargement (LAE), which is often due to long-term systemic hypertension, is a precursor to left ventricular hypertrophy (LVH).

- Atrial enlargement—Because the P wave represents atrial depolarization, atrial enlargement affects its formation. The first half of the P wave, which represents right atrial depolarization, is normally rounded like a quarter-circle. The second half of the P wave, which represents left atrial depolarization, has the same quarter-circle shape. RAE appears on a 12-lead tracing as a tall, spiked first half of the P wave (taller than 2 mm, two small boxes). LAE appears as a biphasic (two-part), widened P wave of 2.5 mm. Leads II, aVL, V_1, and V_2 offer the best views of RAE and LAE.
- Ventricular enlargement—Because the QRS complex represents ventricular depolarization, ventricular enlargement affects it. Abnormally deep S waves or tall waves in the precordial leads suggest RVH or LVH. RVH generally appears as an R wave taller than 7 mm with a right axis deviation. You need to look at the S wave of V_1 or V_2 and the R wave of V_5 or V_6 to detect LVH. Add the amplitude of the deeper S wave (of V_1 or V_2) to the amplitude of the taller R wave (of V_5 or V_6). A sum equal to or greater than 35 mm indicates LVH. Clinically, it is important for you to be able to detect LVH because its ST pattern often mimics the ST segment elevation expected with myocardial injury.

Echocardiography is the usual diagnostic test for chamber enlargement, but 12-lead monitors with programmed interpretative capability may detect the condition. Even if you have one of the most advanced monitors with computerized interpretation, you should remember that they can detect only about 50 percent of these cases.

Case Study Review

The Case Study Review for this chapter is found in Part 2.

Content Self-Evaluation

MULTIPLE CHOICE

1. A positive deflection on the tracing for a certain lead means that the electrical current is flowing toward the positive electrode for that lead, whereas a negative deflection for the same lead signifies a flow of electrical current away from the positive electrode.
   A. True
   B. False

2. If current is flowing directly toward the positive lead, the deflection will be less than it would be if the current were flowing obliquely toward the positive lead.
   A. True
   B. False

3. When the flow of current is exactly perpendicular to the line of the negative and positive electrode for a certain lead, the tracing will show no deflection at all.
   A. True
   B. False

4. The leads that examine heart activity in the horizontal plane are
   A. I, II, and III.
   B. aVR, aVL, and aVF.
   C. I, II, III, aVR, aVL, and aVF.
   D. V_1, V_2, V_3, V_4, V_5, and V_6.
   E. all 12 leads.

5. The normal cardiac axis orientation is between
   A. 29° and +105°.
   B. 0° and 190°.
   C. +90° and +180°.
   D. 0° and 90°.
   E. 90° and 180°.

6. Left axis deviation exists when the QRS axis lies between
   A. 29° and 105°.
   B. 0° and +90°.
   C. +90° and +180°.
   D. 0° and −90°.
   E. 90° and 180°.

7. Myocardial injury is shown on an ECG as
   A. an isoelectric ST segment.
   B. ST segment depression.
   C. ST segment elevation.
   D. a lengthened QRS complex.
   E. ST segment prolongation.

8. Myocardial tissue will die if the blood supply is not restored after how many hours?
   A. 1
   B. 2
   C. 4
   D. 6
   E. 12

9. Which of the 12 ECG lead groupings will give you a direct look at the posterior myocardial wall?
   A. V_5 and V_6
   B. I, II, and III
   C. I, II, and aVF
   D. I, V_2, V_3, and V_4
   E. None of the above

10. Which of the 12 ECG lead groupings will give you a direct look at the lateral myocardial wall?
    A. V_5 and V_6
    B. I, II, and III
    C. I, II, and aVF
    D. I, V_2, V_3, and V_4
    E. None of the above

11. The right ventricle is perfused during both systole and diastole.
    A. True
    B. False

©2013 Pearson Education, Inc.
Paramedic Care: Principles & Practice, Vol. 4, 4th Ed.

_____ 12. Which of the following is NOT commonly associated with a right ventricular infarction?
  A. Increased pulmonary arterial pressure
  B. Distended neck veins
  C. Clear lung fields
  D. Hypotension
  E. Preload-reducing drug sensitivity

_____ 13. On very hot days or with a patient who is diaphoretic, you may wish to apply which substance to the skin in order to achieve a good skin–electrode interface for an ECG?
  A. Betadine   D. Soap and water
  B. Normal saline   E. Tincture of Benzoin
  C. Rubbing alcohol

_____ 14. Which of the following represents the proper placement of the V_1 lead?
  A. Left of the sternum, 4th intercostal space
  B. Right of the sternum, 4th intercostal space
  C. Midclavicular line, 5th intercostal space
  D. Anterior axillary line, same level as V_4
  E. Midaxillary line, same level as V_4

_____ 15. Which of the following represents the proper placement of the V_6 lead?
  A. Left of the sternum, 4th intercostal space
  B. Right of the sternum, 4th intercostal space
  C. Midclavicular line, 5th intercostal space
  D. Anterior axillary line, same level as V_4
  E. Midaxillary line, same level as V_4

MATCHING

Write the letter of the ECG leads in the space provided next to the type of leads they are.

A. I, II, III

B. V_1, V_2, V_3, V_4, V_5, V_6

C. aVR, aVL, aVF

_____ 16. Unipolar (augmented)

_____ 17. Bipolar

_____ 18. Precordial

Localization of myocardial ischemia, injury, or infarction is done by examining the ECG tracings among leads reflecting different regions of the heart. Write the letter of the myocardial region in the space provided next to the leads that examine it.

A. inferior

B. lateral

C. anterolateral

D. high lateral

E. true posterior

F. inferolateral

G. anterior

_____ 19. II, III, and aVF

_____ 20. I, V_2, V_3, and V_4

_____ 21. II, III, aVF, and V_6

_____ **22.** I, aVL, V$_5$, and V$_6$

_____ **23.** V$_5$ and V$_6$

_____ **24.** I and aVL (sometimes with V$_5$ and V$_6$)

_____ **25.** V$_1$ and V$_2$ (looking for reciprocal changes)

Write the letter of the description of the conduction disturbance in the space provided next to the name of the disturbance.

A. prolonged QRS complex with bizarre, notched complexes in leads I, aVL, V$_5$, and V$_6$, along with deep S waves in lead V$_1$, V$_2$, or V$_3$ or tall R waves in leads I, aVL, V$_5$, and V$_6$

B. R wave 7 mm tall and presence of right axis deviation

C. prolonged QRS complex with broad S wave in lead I and RSR complex in lead V$_1$

D. normal QRS length and appearance; right deviation in QRS axis ($\geq 120°$)

E. biphasic, widened P wave

F. sum of deeper S wave (in V$_1$ or V$_2$) and taller R wave (in V$_5$ or V$_6$) ≥ 35 mm; possible ST segment elevation

G. Normal QRS length and appearance; left deviation in QRS axis with negative QRS complexes in leads II, III, and aVF

_____ **26.** right bundle branch block

_____ **27.** left bundle branch block

_____ **28.** left posterior hemiblock

_____ **29.** left anterior hemiblock

_____ **30.** left atrial enlargement (LAE)

_____ **31.** right ventricular hypertrophy (RVH)

_____ **32.** left ventricular hypertrophy (LVH)

Special Project

Interpreting an ECG

You receive a call to check out the medical status of an elderly man who has been seen wandering along the side of a local highway. As you drive down the road, you pass an empty car and note its license plate in case it belongs to the man you are to check out. About 0.4 mile farther down the road, you spot the man walking unsteadily and slowly along the shoulder and pull in behind him.

The patient is a thin, elderly man who seems out of breath but aware of you and your partner as you approach. When you draw near, you explain that you are paramedics who are there to see if he is all right or needs help. He replies that his name is Adam Benon, that he is 81 years old, and that he has lost his car. You notice that he is tachypneic and breathing with great effort, and you ask him how he feels as you gently take his shoulder and turn him toward the ambulance.

Within a few minutes you learn that Mr. Benon felt dizzy and nauseated while driving and pulled over to the side of the road. The patient cannot remember getting out of the car, but he does remember walking toward the next exit looking for help. He notes that his chest hurts more now than it did a while ago and he feels that he cannot take a deep breath.

Mr. Benon has a regular pulse of 90, and his ECG is shown on the next page.

1. What preexisting cardiac problem is strongly suggested by the ECG tracing?

2. What, if any, significance does this hold for your current attempt to determine whether Mr. Benon is having an acute cardiac problem such as ischemia or acute MI?

©2013 Pearson Education, Inc.
Paramedic Care: Principles & Practice, Vol. 4, 4th Ed.

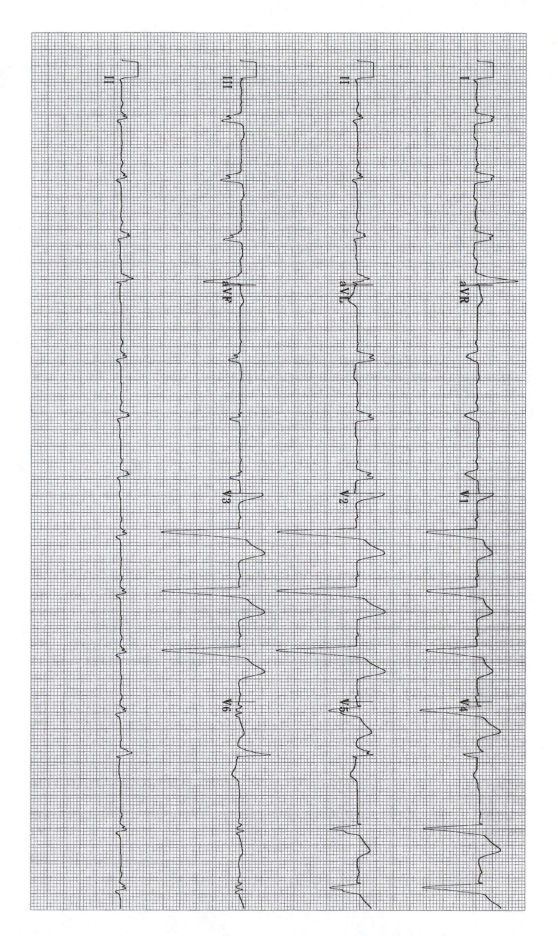

3

Neurology

Review of Chapter Objectives

After reading this chapter, you should be able to:

1. Define key terms introduced in this chapter.

Knowing and being able to apply the key terms in each chapter is critical to understanding chapter concepts. Write the list of key terms. Then write the definition of each one in your own words. Check your understanding by confirming the definitions in the text glossary. Correct any misunderstandings. Create a study aid by writing each key term on the front of an index card and the definition on the back. Use the cards to quiz yourself, or to have someone quiz you.

2. Describe the significance of the prevalence of neurologic disorders in the United States

p. 181

Diseases and conditions of the nervous system affect millions of Americans. You will see neurological emergencies in the field, and you will also see patients who present with another complaint but who have coexisting neurological conditions. Epilepsy affects about 2.5 million persons, who may present with a neurological emergency or have another condition complicated by their seizure disorder. Strokes are medical emergencies, and they affect about 500,000 people annually, of whom about 150,000 die. Strokes are also a frequent source of considerable morbidity. Recent studies have shown that early recognition and intervention in certain strokes due to thromboembolism may decrease their morbidity and mortality. Neoplasms affecting the central nervous system (CNS) occur in about 40,000 persons annually; morbidity and mortality depend on variables including tumor type and location. The miscellaneous group termed the degenerative disorders account for considerable morbidity for many Americans, and they often account for premature death, as well. Multiple sclerosis affects about 300,000 to 400,000 Americans, and typical first presentation is at the age range of 20 to 40 years. Parkinson's disease affects more than 500,000 Americans, who are typically 60 years or older.

Other neurological conditions are extremely common and of variable cause and morbidity/ mortality. For instance, nearly half of all Americans will have a syncopal episode in their lifetime, and syncope accounts for roughly 3 percent of all emergency department visits. Headaches of various causes are extremely common, with nearly 45 million persons affected by chronic headaches. Low back pain can be either acute or chronic, and roughly 60 to 90 percent of Americans will experience some type of lower back pain in their lifetime.

3. Relate the anatomy and physiology of the nervous system to the pathophysiology and assessment of patients with neurologic disorders.

pp. 181–196

The nervous system is the body's chief control for virtually every major function. It is divided physically into the central nervous system (CNS) and peripheral nervous system (PNS). The CNS consists of the brain and spinal cord.

Messages within the CNS, as well as those that connect it with the rest of the body, travel as nerve impulses. The complex network of nerves outside the CNS makes up the peripheral nervous system.

The messages that carry information regarding critical body functions such as respiration pass through a part of the PNS called the autonomic nervous system; these functions do not require any conscious effort to maintain them. In contrast, messages that involve voluntary, or conscious, actions and thoughts travel through the other part of the PNS, the somatic nervous system. Both the autonomic and somatic nervous systems have two parallel tracks: one of nerves that carry messages to the brain, and a second that carries messages from the brain. In terms of the computer analogy, the PNS carries the various input and output messages that run between the brain and spinal cord and the rest of the body. The autonomic nervous system is also structurally and functionally broken into two parts: the sympathetic and parasympathetic nervous systems. These two parts work together to make sure the net balance of stimulatory and inhibitory messages from the brain keep body functions such as blood pressure within normal limits.

The basic structural and functional unit is the neuron, or nerve cell. Nerve cells have a body that contains the essential cell machinery of the nucleus, mitochondria, and so on. Nerve processes (usually there are many) that are capable of receiving impulses from other neurons or body cells are called dendrites. An impulse that is picked up by a dendrite travels toward the cell body. Another process, the axon, carries the impulse away from the cell body. Axons may have multiple tips, which means a neuron has the capacity to send the impulse onward to more than one other nerve or other cell. Dendrites associated with neurons of the major sense organs (such as the eye or ear) convert an environmental stimulus into a nerve impulse that can be forwarded via the axon to other nerves, and eventually the brain. Dendrites associated with neurons that monitor internal conditions such as PaO_2 also convert that information into an impulse and send it to the brain. Eventually all such information is analyzed by neurons in the brain and response impulses travel back through the PNS. These impulses eventually affect a motor neuron, causing a muscle cell to contract, or affect another type of cell such as one in a gland. Messages cannot pass directly from an axon to a dendrite because there is a tiny physical gap, called a synapse, between each pair of neurons. As the wave of electrical depolarization (due to ion fluxes of potassium rapidly leaving the neuron and sodium rapidly entering) reaches the axon tip, it causes a chemical called a neurotransmitter to be released into the synapse. (There are multiple neurotransmitters within the body. Either acetylcholine or norepinephrine is found in the neurons of the PNS. Neurotransmitters within the CNS include dopamine and serotonin.) When the neurotransmitter crosses the synapse and is taken up by the dendrite on the other side, a wave of depolarization is started in that dendrite and the nerve impulse is then carried toward the cell body.

Most of the CNS is protected by the bones of the cranium and spine. The spinal column is made up of 33 vertebrae running from the neck to the junction with the pelvis. There is also an inner shock-absorbing, cushioning protection system. The cells of the brain and spinal cord are bathed in cerebrospinal fluid, and there are three layers of protective membranes between the neural surface and the outer, protective bone. These meninges are called the dura mater, arachnoid membrane, and pia mater (in outer-to-inner sequence).

The human brain has six obvious structural regions: the cerebrum, the diencephalon, the mesencephalon (or midbrain), the pons, the medulla oblongata, and the cerebellum. Sometimes, this is simplified into the terminology of the forebrain (cerebrum and diencephalon), the midbrain, and the hindbrain (the brain stem—pons, medulla oblongata—and the cerebellum). The largest part of the brain, with its characteristic folded outer surfaces, is the cerebrum. The cerebrum has left and right sides, or hemispheres, which are connected physically and functionally by tissue called the corpus callosum. The cerebrum is responsible for intelligence, learning, memory, and language, as well as analysis and response to sensory and motor activities. The diencephalon is covered by the cerebrum, and it is made up of several vital structures: the thalamus, hypothalamus, and the limbic system. This primal part of the brain is responsible for many involuntary functions such as temperature regulation, sleep, water balance, stress response, and emotion. It also has an important role in regulating the autonomic nervous system. The brain stem consists of the mesencephalon, pons, and medulla oblongata. The mesencephalon is located between the diencephalon and the pons, and it plays a role in motor coordination. It is the major region controlling eye movement. The pons is a major connection point between the upper portions of the brain and the medulla and cerebellum. The medulla oblongata itself marks the division between the brain and the spinal cord. The major centers for control of respiration, cardiac activity, and vasomotor activity are located here. The cerebellum is located in the posterior fossa of the cranium, and it also has two hemispheres, which are closely coordinated to the brain stem and higher centers. The cerebellum coordinates fine motor movement, posture, equilibrium, and muscle tone.

©2013 Pearson Education, Inc.
Paramedic Care: Principles & Practice, Vol. 4, 4th Ed.

The hemispheres of the cerebrum do not contain identical centers. Rather, the functional responsibilities of the cerebrum have been mapped as a whole. Important centers with clinical implications for you in cases such as stroke or trauma include the following: (1) speech, which is located in the temporal lobe; (2) vision, which is located in the occipital lobe; (3) personality, which is located in the frontal lobes; (4) sensory, which is located in the parietal lobes; and (5) motor, which is located in the frontal lobes. As noted previously, balance and coordination are located in the cerebellum. Another important center is called the reticular activating system (RAS), which operates in the lateral portion of the medulla, pons, and especially the mesencephalon. The RAS sends impulses to and receives messages from the cerebral cortex (the outer portion of the cerebrum). This diffuse system of interlaced cells is responsible for maintaining consciousness and the ability to respond to external stimuli. Dysfunction or interruption in the RAS results in altered level of consciousness.

The brain receives about 20 percent of the body's total blood flow per minute. Vascular supply to the brain is provided by two systems, a physical arrangement that provides secondary supply if one system is occluded or severed. The anterior system is the carotid, and the posterior system is the vertebrobasilar. They join at the circle of Willis before entering the structures of the brain itself. Venous drainage is via the venous sinuses and the internal jugular veins. As previously noted, there is also cerebrospinal fluid (CSF) bathing the tissues of the brain and spinal cord. Most of the intracranial CSF is found in the ventricles. When CSF becomes infected, it causes the meninges to become infected in a condition called meningitis.

The spinal cord is 17 to 18 inches long on average in adults. It leaves the brain at the medulla and passes through an opening in the skull called the foramen magnum to enter the spinal canal. The spinal cord, which ends near the level of the first lumbar vertebra (the reason why spinal taps are done below that level), conducts impulses to and from the peripheral nervous system and locally for motor reflexes. Thirty-one pairs of nerves exit the spinal cord between adjacent vertebrae. The dorsal nerve roots carry afferent fibers, which carry impulses to the brain. The ventral roots carry efferent fibers, which carry impulses from the brain to the periphery. Each nerve root has a corresponding area of skin called a dermatome, to which it supplies sensation. In the field, you may be able to correlate sensory deficits to the level of a spinal cord problem. The reason why our protective motor reflexes are so fast and effective lies in the fact that the afferent and efferent impulses are coordinated in the spinal cord—they do not travel the whole way to the brain before coming back. However, because they are mediated in the spinal cord, they lack fine motor control.

The peripheral nervous system (PNS) contains 12 pairs of cranial nerves, which extend directly from the lower surface of the brain and exit through small holes in the skull, and the peripheral nerves, which exit from the spinal cord as noted previously. The nerves of the PNS control both voluntary and involuntary activities. The cranial nerves supply nervous control for the head, neck, and certain thoracic and abdominal organs. The peripheral nerves can be divided into four classes: (1) somatic sensory, afferent nerves that carry impulses concerned with touch, pressure, pain, temperature, and position; (2) somatic motor, efferent nerves that carry impulses to the skeletal (voluntary) muscles; (3) visceral (autonomic) sensory, afferent nerves that carry impulses of sensation from the visceral organs (examples being fullness in the bladder or distension of the rectum); and (4) visceral (autonomic) motor, efferent nerves that serve the involuntary cardiac muscle and the smooth muscle of the viscera and the glands. Peripheral neuropathy occurs when there is a malfunction in or damage to the peripheral nerves. This can affect muscle activity, sensation, reflexes, or internal organ function.

The involuntary division of the PNS is called the autonomic nervous system, and it has two components: the sympathetic nervous system and the parasympathetic nervous system. The sympathetic system is associated with the primitive "fight-or-flight" response to sensory stimuli. Its major nerve roots are located near the thoracic and lumbar parts of the spinal cord. Stimulation causes increased heart rate and blood pressure, pupillary dilation, rise in blood glucose, as well as bronchodilation, all responses that ready the body for stress. The neurotransmitters norepinephrine and epinephrine mediate its actions, and sympathetic activity is also closely correlated to activity in the adrenal gland, tissue that is of nervous system origin and that also relies on norepinephrine and epinephrine. The parasympathetic nervous system is responsible for controlling vegetative functions such as normal heart rate and blood pressure. It is associated with the cranial nerves and the sacral plexus of nerves, and it is mediated by the neurotransmitter acetylcholine. When stimulated, it causes a decrease in heart rate, an increase in digestive activity, pupillary constriction, and a reduction in blood glucose. In patients experiencing neurogenic shock, there is a disruption in the sympathetic nervous system. Complete transection of the spinal cord at or above T-6 results in suspending central nervous system communication to the adrenal glands. Without this communication the adrenal glands fail to release epinephrine and norepinephrine. Consequently, the expected sympathetic compensatory responses to shock are not seen in neurogenic shock.

Because many signs and symptoms of neurological dysfunction are subtle, you should use the observations made during the scene size-up and formation of general impressions to look for evidence suggesting focus on the neurological system. Environmental clues may include medical equipment, medication bottles, Medic-Alert identification, alcohol bottles, and so on. Note, for instance, whether the patient is conscious, and, if so, whether he is confused or lucid. Are his posture and gait normal? Speech can give many clues, particularly if either the patient or a bystander can tell you if the speech you hear is normal for the patient. Skin color, temperature, and moisture are valuable, as is any evidence of facial drooping or muscle spasm. Mental status can then be quickly ascertained through the AVPU method. Assessment of higher cerebral functioning includes assessment of emotional status. Try to evaluate the patient's affect, thought patterns, perceptions, judgments, and memory and attention. Any alteration from the patient's normal mental status or mood is considered significant and warrants further assessment. After that level of assessment is done, evaluate for the ABCs, including respiration pattern, effort of breathing, heart rate, rhythm, and electrocardiogram (ECG) pattern. An unresponsive patient can be evaluated further with use of the Glasgow Coma Scale (GCS). Be aware that a midlevel GCS score (such as 5, 6, or 7) that drops on reevaluation has grim implications.

Respiratory derangements are common with CNS illness or injury. Five abnormal breathing patterns may be commonly observed in this setting: Cheyne-Stokes respiration is a pattern marked by apnea lasting 10 to 60 seconds followed by gradually increasing depth and frequency of respiration. It can be seen with brain damage due to trauma or cerebral hemorrhage and with chronic hypoxia. Kussmaul's respirations are deep, rapid breaths caused by severe metabolic or CNS problems. Central neurogenic hyperventilation is caused by a lesion in the CNS and is marked by rapid, deep, noisy respirations. Ataxic respirations are poor breaths due to CNS damage causing ineffective thoracic muscular coordination. Apneustic respiration is breathing marked by prolonged inspiration unrelieved by expiration attempts and it is due to damage in the upper pons. Always remember that carbon dioxide (CO_2) has a critical effect on cerebral vessels: Increased levels cause vascular dilation, whereas low levels cause vasoconstriction. This is the basis for controlled hyperventilation in settings where some degree of vasoconstriction might minimize brain swelling.

4. **Adapt the scene size-up, primary assessment, patient history, secondary assessment, and use of monitoring technology to meet the needs of patients with complaints and presentations related to neurologic disorders.** pp. 190–214

During the scene size-up, your general impression will be very important, as you will be looking for clues that can indicate the patient's condition. Because diagnosis and treatment with many neurologic emergencies is time sensitive, it will be your goal to develop your assessment process to recognize neurologic disorders rapidly. The causes of altered mental status and abnormal neurologic signs and symptoms are numerous. One of the first questions you will answer will be if there is a history of trauma or toxic exposure. These may also present scene safety considerations for you and your crew. Evaluate the patient's level of consciousness using the AVPU method, speech, skin appearance, and posture. The patient's emotional status may also provide clues to the patient's cerebral function. Complete your primary ABCD assessment and recognize any findings that would indicate a neurologic emergency. Your secondary assessment should include a detailed neurologic exam, accurate history, and physical exam with a full set of vital signs. Initiate all appropriate monitoring devices. For example, alterations in ventilatory function may be observed in a patient experiencing a neurologic emergency. Capnography measures exhaled or end-tidal CO_2 and can assist the paramedic in evaluating the ventilation rate and quality in such a patient. Pulse oximetry is used to monitor a patient's general state of perfusion. Patients with abnormal neurologic function are at risk for vomiting and aspiration, so frequent assessment of the airway, breathing, and circulation is vital. Because hypoglycemia can result in neurologic focal deficits, every patient with an abnormal neurologic exam should have his blood glucose measured.

©2013 Pearson Education, Inc.
Paramedic Care: Principles & Practice, Vol. 4, 4th Ed.

5. **Use a process of clinical reasoning to guide and interpret the patient assessment and management process for patients with neurologic disorders.** pp. 190–214

As a paramedic, it is vital that you develop your clinical reasoning process to quickly recognize and treat acute neurologic conditions to improve patient outcome. This is because diagnosis and treatment with many neurologic emergencies is time sensitive. Develop an organized general impression to rapidly identify signs and symptoms of neurologic emergencies. This will include assessing possible acute neurologic changes using standardized scoring systems such as the Cincinnati Prehospital Stroke Scale (CPSS) or Los Angeles Prehospital Stroke Screen (LAPSS). In addition, you must also consider transport decisions early, as patients with traumatic brain injury and stroke have better outcomes when treated at specialty care centers.

The primary treatment for nervous system emergencies in the field is supportive. Make a strong effort to make the patient comfortable, keep NPO, prevent aspiration, and be prepared for seizures. Consider the following:

- *Airway and breathing.* Properly position any patient that you suspect has a neurological emergency and protect the airway. If there is known or possible trauma, maintain C-spine immobilization. Administer supplemental oxygen if the patient is hypoxic—but only enough to correct hypoxia. Avoid hyperoxia. If the patient is breathing inadequately or is apneic, initiate ventilatory assistance. If an airway problem is detected, first apply basic airway maneuvers such as head positioning or the modified jaw-thrust maneuver. Intubate, if indicated.
- *Circulatory support.* Establish a saline lock. It is important to have an accessible route for medications.
- *Pharmacological interventions.* Medications are available to alleviate signs and symptoms in patients with neurological emergencies. Medications include aspirin, dextrose, thiamine, naloxone, and diazepam.
- *Psychological support.* Patients suffering from a nervous system emergency, acute or chronic, are likely also to suffer anxiety. Neurological deficits of any kind are frightening experiences. Provide the patient with emotional support and explain the treatment regimen. In most cases, it is appropriate to explain to the patient what is occurring and why. Careful explanation and emotional support will help allay anxiety and apprehension.
- *Transport considerations.* Assess, provide emergency care, and package the patient as quickly and safely as possible. Rapidly transport any patient with a neurological deficit or altered mental status to an appropriate emergency department, equipped with a computerized tomography (CT) or magnetic resonance imaging (MRI) scanner and facilities capable of managing strokes with fibrinolytic therapy. Modern medicine has seen the development of new advances in pharmacological and surgical interventions that are only available in the hospital setting.

Constantly reevaluate and monitor the patient's airway and neurological system.

6. **Describe common causes of altered mental status.** pp. 196–197

Risk factors differ for the various types of neurological conditions. Strokes are vascular in nature (hemorrhagic or occlusive), and the major risk factors for stroke reflect this: atherosclerosis, heart disease, diabetes, abnormal blood lipid levels, hypertension, sickle cell disease, use of oral contraceptives, and the cardiac dysrhythmia atrial fibrillation. Some chronic conditions such as epilepsy reflect different causes and thus have different risk factors. Epilepsy can develop in patients who have had head trauma, brain tumors, or certain vascular disorders such as stroke. Most cases are considered idiopathic, which means the cause is unknown. Syncope is similar in having very different causes. Syncopal episodes can be due to cardiovascular (such as dysrhythmias or mechanical problems) origin or noncardiovascular (metabolic, neurological, or psychiatric) origin; indeed, many episodes are considered idiopathic even after workup. Headaches tend to be classified as vascular (such as migraine), tension, or organic (the last including headache due to tumor, infection, or other conditions). Some of the risk factors for low back pain are somewhat gender related. Symptoms in women over age 60 years often reflect postmenopausal osteoporosis. Occupations involving exposure to vibrations from vehicles or machinery or jobs requiring repetitive lifting are associated with risk for low back pain. Other causes include compression or trauma to the sciatic nerve or its roots, as can happen with a herniated intervertebral disk. Most cases, though, are also idiopathic.

Common causes of altered mental status are listed in the following four general categories:

- Drugs
  - Depressants (including alcohol)
  - Hallucinogens
  - Narcotics
- Cardiovascular
  - Anaphylaxis
  - Cardiac arrest
  - Stroke
  - Arrhythmias
  - Hypertensive encephalopathy
  - Shock
- Respiratory
  - Chronic obstructive pulmonary disease (COPD)
  - Inhalation of toxic gas
  - Hypoxia
- Infectious
  - AIDS
  - Encephalitis
  - Meningitis
  - Parasites

During history taking and assessment, remember the mnemonic AEIOU-TIPS, and look for signs of these common causes: A (acidosis or alcohol), E (epilepsy), I (infection), O (overdose), U (uremia, or kidney failure), T (trauma, tumor, or toxin), I (insulin, either hypoglycemia or ketoacidosis), P (psychosis or poison), S (stroke, seizure).

7. **Describe the pathophysiology of specific neurologic presentations, including the following:** pp. 190–214

   a. **Altered mental status** pp. 196–197

   Altered mental status is extremely common, as you'll understand when you consider the wide variety of causes. Morbidity and mortality are often correlated to cause. Vigilant assessment and management on your part will optimize your patient's chances, regardless of causes. An alteration in mental status is the hallmark sign of CNS injury or illness; as such, any alteration, be it subtle or as florid as coma, requires evaluation. In coma, the patient cannot be aroused by even powerful external stimuli such as pain. The two mechanisms generally capable of causing altered mental status are structural lesions (such as tumor, trauma, degenerative disease, or another process that destroys or encroaches on the substance of the brain) and toxic-metabolic states (such as the presence of toxins such as ammonia or the absence of vital substances such as oxygen, glucose, or thiamine). Causes of toxic-metabolic disturbances include anoxia, diabetic ketoacidosis, hepatic failure, hypoglycemia, renal failure, thiamine deficiency, and toxic exposure (for instance, cyanide). Some of the most common causes you'll see for altered mental status (meaning they can cause a structural lesion or a toxic-metabolic state) are the following: (1) drugs, including depressants such as alcohol, hallucinogens, and narcotics; (2) cardiovascular, including anaphylaxis, cardiac arrest, stroke, dysrhythmias, hypertensive encephalopathy, and shock; (3) respiratory, including COPD, inhalation of a toxic gas such as carbon monoxide, and hypoxia; and (4) infectious, such as AIDS, encephalitis, and meningitis.

   b. **Chronic alcoholism** p. 197

   Chronic alcoholism interferes with the intake, absorption, and use of thiamine. A significant percentage of alcoholics have thiamine deficiency that can cause Wernicke's syndrome or Korsakoff's psychosis. Wernicke's syndrome is an acute but reversible encephalopathy (brain disease) characterized by ataxia, eye muscle weakness, and mental derangement. Of even greater concern is Korsakoff's psychosis, characterized by memory disorder. Once established, Korsakoff's psychosis may be irreversible.

©2013 Pearson Education, Inc.
Paramedic Care: Principles & Practice, Vol. 4, 4th Ed.

c. Stroke and transient ischemic attack pp. 197–202

Stroke is a general term for injury or death of brain tissue, usually due to interruption of blood flow to that region of the cerebrum. The term "brain attack" is being used more frequently because of some similarities between stroke and heart attack, the latter also being due to oxygen deprivation. You should also realize that there are treatment similarities to heart attacks. Strokes due to thromboembolic causes may be aborted or minimized with use of fibrinolytic agents now used with heart attack (such as tissue plasminogen activator, tPA). The importance to you is that the need for prompt recognition and transport of stroke patients is greater than ever. Stroke patients who may be candidates for fibrinolytic therapy must receive definitive treatment within 3 hours of onset.

Strokes are the third most common cause of death and a frequent cause of considerable disability among middle-aged and elderly persons. Major risk factors include atherosclerosis, heart disease, hypertension, diabetes, abnormal blood lipid levels, use of oral contraceptives, and sickle cell disease. Strokes can be caused either by occlusion of an artery or by hemorrhage. Both interrupt blood flow to distal tissues. An occlusive stroke is any caused by blockage of the artery, resulting in ischemia to brain tissue that may progress to infarction if oxygen deprivation continues long enough. Infarcted brain tissue swells, further damaging nearby tissue that might have only a marginal blood supply itself. If swelling is sufficiently severe, herniation (protrusion of tissue through the foramen magnum, the opening at the base of the skull through which the spinal cord emerges from the cranium) can occur. Occlusive strokes are either thrombotic or embolic in origin.

Thrombotic strokes are due to a thrombus, or blood clot, that forms in and then obstructs a cerebral artery. Thrombosis is often related to atherosclerotic change in the artery. Unsurprisingly, the signs and symptoms of a thrombotic stroke are often gradual in onset. The stroke often occurs at night and is characterized by the patient waking with altered mental status and/or loss of speech, sensation, or motor function. An embolic stroke is caused by a solid, liquid, or gaseous mass that is carried to the site of obstruction from a remote site. The most common brain emboli are blood clots that often arise from diseased blood vessels in the neck (namely, the carotid artery) or from abnormal cardiac contraction. Atrial fibrillation often results in atrial dilation, a precursor to clot formation. Other types of emobli include air, tumor tissue, and fat. Typically, embolic strokes present with sudden onset of severe headaches. Hemorrhagic strokes are due to bleeding within brain tissue, and they can be categorized as intracerebral or subarachnoid.

A transient ischemic attack (TIA) is a temporary manifestation of the signs and/or symptoms of stroke that is due to temporary interference with blood supply to the affected part of the brain. These symptoms may persist for a few minutes or for hours, but they almost always resolve within 24 hours. After the attack (because it reflects ischemia, not infarction), there is no evidence of brain or neurological damage. The most common cause is carotid artery disease (provoking an embolic event). Other causes can be small emboli of different origin, decreased cardiac output, hypotension, overmedication with antihypertensive medications, or cerebrovascular spasm. Part of the importance of recognizing TIAs is that they may be the precursor to a stroke. One-third of TIA patients suffer a stroke soon afterward. A TIA is typically sudden in onset, with specific signs and symptoms depending on the part of the brain involved.

In the prehospital setting, it is virtually impossible to distinguish a TIA from a stroke. While taking the history, try to get the following information: previous neurological symptoms, if any; initial symptoms and their progression; changes in mental status; precipitating factors, if any; dizziness; palpitations; and history of hypertension, cardiac disease, sickle cell disease, or previous TIA or stroke. Because TIAs and strokes are generally indistinguishable in the field, the management is the same.

d. Intracranial hemorrhage p. 197

Hemorrhagic strokes are due to blood within brain tissue, and they can be categorized as intracerebral or subarachnoid. These intracranial hemorrhages often occur with sudden onset of a severe headache. Most intracranial hemorrhages occur in a hypertensive patient when a small vessel deep within brain tissue ruptures. Subarachnoid hemorrhages most commonly result from either congenital blood vessel anomalies or from head trauma. Congenital anomalies include aneurysms and arteriovenous malformations. Aneurysms tend to be on the brain's surface and may hemorrhage into either brain tissue or the subarachnoid space. Hemorrhage within brain tissue may tear and separate normal brain tissue. Release of blood into the ventricles containing CSF may paralyze vital centers. If blood impairs drainage of CSF, the resultant increase in intracranial pressure may cause herniation of brain tissue.

Most intracranial hemorrhages occur in the hypertensive patient when a small vessel deep within the brain tissue ruptures. Subarachnoid hemorrhages most often result from congenital blood vessel abnormalities or from head trauma. Congenital abnormalities include aneurysms (weakened vessels) and arteriovenous malformations (collections of abnormal blood vessels). Aneurysms tend to be on the surface and may hemorrhage into the brain tissue or the subarachnoid space. Arteriovenous malformations may be within the brain, in the subarachnoid space, or both. Hemorrhage inside the brain often tears and separates normal brain tissue. The release of blood into the cavities within the brain that contain cerebrospinal fluid may paralyze vital centers. If blood in the subarachnoid space impairs drainage of cerebrospinal fluid, it may cause a rise in the intracranial pressure. Herniation of brain tissue may then occur.

e. **Seizures and status epilepticus**   pp. 202–205

A seizure is a temporary alteration in behavior due to a massive discharge of one or more groups of neurons in the brain. Seizures can be induced in anyone under certain stressful conditions such as hypoxia or rapidly decreasing blood glucose. Febrile seizures often occur in young children with a sudden increase in body temperature. Structural diseases of the brain such as tumors, head trauma, toxic eclampsia, and vascular disorders can also cause a seizure. Recurrent seizures without such a known cause are termed epilepsy. Epilepsy affects about 2.5 million persons, who may present with a neurological emergency or have another condition complicated by their seizure disorder. Most cases of epilepsy are idiopathic, that is, without known cause, whereas others arise secondary to damage from strokes, head trauma, tumor surgery or radiation, and so on.

Status epilepticus, two or more generalized seizures without intervening return of consciousness, can be a life-threatening emergency. The most common cause in adults with epilepsy is failure to comply with medication regimen. Status epilepticus is a major emergency because it involves a prolonged period of apnea with the possibility of CNS hypoxia.

f. **Syncope**   pp. 205–206

Syncope, or fainting, is characterized by a sudden, temporary loss of consciousness caused by insufficient blood flow to the brain, with recovery almost immediate upon supine positioning. Syncope is very common, accounting for roughly 3 percent of all emergency department visits. It can occur at any age. Symptoms may include prior feelings of dizziness or lightheadedness, or there may be no warning at all. By definition, if return of consciousness does not occur within a few moments, the event is NOT syncope; it is something more serious. There are three pathophysiological mechanisms for syncope: cardiovascular, noncardiovascular, and idiopathic. Cardiovascular causes include dysrhythmias or mechanical problems such as an abnormally functioning heart valve. Noncardiovascular causes include metabolic, neurological, or psychiatric conditions. For instance, hypoglycemia, a TIA, or an anxiety attack may all precipitate syncope. Idiopathic means that there is no known cause even after careful expert evaluation.

g. **Headache**   pp. 206–207

Headaches, either acute or chronic, are a tremendously common complaint. You've probably had problems with a headache at least once. Nearly 45 million Americans suffer from chronic headaches. There three general categories of headache: vascular, tension, and organic. Headaches of vascular origin include migraines and cluster headaches. Migraines occur more commonly in women, whereas cluster headaches occur more commonly in men. Migraines are typically characterized by intense, throbbing pain, sensitivity to light or sound, nausea, vomiting, and sweating. Migraines may last from several minutes to several days. They typically present as one-sided headaches and they may be preceded by an aura. Cluster headaches usually occur as a series of one-sided headaches that are sudden in onset, intense, and continue for roughly 15 minutes to 4 hours. Symptoms may include nasal congestion, drooping eyelid, and an irritated eye. Tension headaches account for a significant percentage of headaches. Most personnel in emergency medicine have had, or will have, a tension headache. Some people experience them on a daily basis. These persons may wake with a headache that worsens over the course of the day. The typical tension headache has a dull, achy pain that feels as if forceful pressure is being applied to the neck or head. The last class of headache, organic headaches, is less common. These headaches occur in association with tumor, infection, or other diseases of the brain, eye, or other body system.

©2013 Pearson Education, Inc.
Paramedic Care: Principles & Practice, Vol. 4, 4th Ed.

h. **Cranial nerve disorders**   pp. 207–208

The 12 pairs of cranial nerves innervate parts of the head, neck, and trunk. The function of these nerves can be sensory (touch, pain, hearing, taste, sight, and smell) or motor. A cranial nerve disorder is one that affects the connection between the cranial nerve centers of the brain and the particular tissues innervated by those nerves. The signs and symptoms of cranial nerve disorders depend on the nerve involved. Although some cranial nerve disorders are common, most are rare. The two most common cranium nerve disorders encountered in emergency medicine are Bell's palsy and trigeminal neuralgia.

- *Bell's palsy.* Bell's palsy is a sudden, unilateral weakness or paralysis of the facial muscles. It is due to a dysfunction of the seventh cranial nerve (facial nerve). The facial nerve controls some of the facial muscles, innervates the salivary and tear glands, and allows the front portion of the tongue to detect taste. In most cases, the cause of Bell's palsy is unknown. It has been associated with a herpes simplex virus infection. Initially, the patient develops pain behind the ear. This may occur over days and then is followed by the rapid development of unilateral facial muscle weakness. This is often alarming for the patient, and many will seek emergency care, fearing the condition is a stroke. The patient may complain of the face feeling numb or heavy. However, sensation remains unaffected. Some patients are unable to close the eye on the affected side. They also blink less often, causing dryness of the eye. In some instances, Bell's palsy may interfere with the normal production of saliva and/or tears, thus causing a dry eye or dry mouth. The diagnosis is made based on the history and physical exam. Treatment sometimes includes the use of antiviral drugs. In most instances, Bell's palsy resolves completely without any residual deficits.

- *Trigeminal neuralgia.* Trigeminal neuralgia, also called *tic douloureux*, is an extremely painful disorder that affects the fifth cranial nerve (trigeminal nerve). The trigeminal nerve is responsible for sensation in the face. Although primarily a sensory nerve, it also has some motor functions (e.g., biting and chewing). The trigeminal nerve has three branches: the ophthalmic nerve, the maxillary nerve, and the mandibular nerve. The pain associated with trigeminal neuralgia arises from the nerve. It is usually a condition of older adults but can be seen at any age. The signs and symptoms of trigeminal neuralgia include painful electrical-shock-type spasms and pain in the distribution of the nerve. The pain is usually localized to one side of the face—often around the eyes, cheek, and lower part of the face. It is sometimes exacerbated by touch or loud sounds. Common activities of daily living, such as brushing one's teeth, chewing, or eating, can trigger trigeminal neuralgia. Trigeminal neuralgia tends to be a chronic condition. Various medications, especially antiseizure drugs, are used in treatment of this condition. In severe cases, surgery may be necessary.

i. **Complaint of "weak and dizzy"**   pp. 208

A frequent problem that paramedics encounter is the patient who is "weak and dizzy" or "weak all over." Generalized weakness and dizziness, although vague, can be symptoms of many diseases. Furthermore, the feeling of being weak or the feeling of being dizzy can be quite disconcerting, especially to the elderly.

j. **Central nervous system neoplasms**   pp. 189–190

Neoplasm is a general term for "new growth," and it is used to describe tumors that arise after birth. Neoplasms of the CNS affect about 40,000 Americans per year. These neoplasms can be divided into benign and malignant tumors based on several characteristics. The cells of a benign tumor generally resemble normal cells, grow relatively slowly, and tend to remain confined to one location. In contrast, malignant tumors of the CNS often have cells that are primitive in appearance and don't resemble normal cells, grow quickly, and may invade adjacent, healthy tissue or spread within the CNS. Both kinds of CNS tumors can be dangerous because any tumor growth can place pressure on other tissues and impair their function and because the pressure cannot be relieved by expansion of the cranial space. In adults, the cranium is rigid and fixed. Pressure exerted by a tumor causes increased intracranial pressure. There are numerous types of brain tumors, and the cause is unknown for most of them.

CNS tumors present with many signs and symptoms dependent on the size, type, and location of the tumor. It isn't your role in the field to diagnose new tumors; rather, you are more likely to have patients with previously diagnosed tumors or patients who present with problems that may reflect a CNS tumor. Common complaints among persons with undiagnosed brain tumors include the following: headache (often severe and recurrent), new-onset seizures, nausea and vomiting, behavioral or cognitive changes, weakness or paralysis of one or more limbs or one side of the face, change in sensation in one or more limbs or one side of the face, new-onset uncoordination, difficulty walking or unsteady gait, dizziness, and double vision.

k. Brain abscess p. 210

A brain abscess is a pocket of pus localized to one area of the brain. They are uncommon, accounting for 2 percent of intracranial masses. Signs and symptoms are similar to those of a neoplasm and include headache, lethargy, hemiparesis (weakness on one side of the body), seizures, rigidity of the neck, and nausea and vomiting. Fever is frequently present, suggesting an infectious cause.

l. Degenerative neurological orders and dementia pp. 210–212

The term *degenerative neurological disease* characterizes diseases that selectively affect one or more functional systems of the CNS. Generally, they produce symmetrical and progressive involvement of the CNS, affect similar areas of the brain, and produce similar clinical signs and symptoms. Examples include Alzheimer's disease, muscular dystrophy, multiple sclerosis, dystonias, Parkinson's disease, central pain syndrome, Bell's palsy, amyotrophic lateral sclerosis, myoclonus, spina bifida, and poliomyelitis. Alzheimer's disease is perhaps the most important of the degenerative disorders because of its frequency and devastating nature. It is the most common cause of dementia in the elderly. Alzheimer's results from neuronal cell death and disappearance in the cerebral cortex, causing marked atrophy of the brain. Initially, patients have problems with short-term memory, and this usually progresses to problems with thought and intellect. Patients also develop a shuffling gait and have stiffness of body muscles. As the disease progresses, the patient develops aphasia and psychiatric problems. In its final stages, the patient may become virtually decorticate, losing all ability to think, speak, and move. Muscular dystrophy (MD) actually refers to a group of genetic diseases characterized by progressive muscle weakness and degeneration of skeletal muscle fibers. The heart and other involuntary muscles are affected in some types of MD. The most common form is Duchenne's MD. Some forms begin in childhood, whereas others do not appear until midlife. Prognosis depends on the type and individual progression of the disorder. Multiple sclerosis (MS) is another common and potentially devastating degenerative disorder. It involves inflammation of certain nerve cells followed by demyelination (loss of the fatty insulation surrounding nerve fibers in the CNS). Prevalence in the United States is approximately 300,000 to 400,000 persons. Most are women who first developed symptoms between ages 20 and 40 years. The pathophysiology of MS involves autoimmune attack against myelin. Signs and symptoms include weakness of one or more limbs, sensory loss, paresthesias, and changes in vision. Symptoms may wax and wane over years, and they may range from mild to severe. Severe cases leave the patient so debilitated she may not be able to care for herself.

The dystonias are characterized by muscle contractions that cause twisting, repetitive movements, abnormal postures, or freezing in the middle of an action. Early symptoms include deterioration in handwriting, foot cramps, or tendency of one foot to drag after walking or running. In some cases, symptoms become more noticeable and widespread over time. In other individuals, there is little or no progression over time. Parkinson's disease is a motor system disorder also called a "shaking palsy." Parkinson's is characterized chemically by a deficiency of dopamine in the CNS, and treatment is generally aimed at increasing levels in the brain. Parkinson's is common, and you will see it in the field. Roughly 500,000 Americans are affected, and more than 50,000 new cases are reported annually. It affects men and women equally and has an average age at onset of 60 years. It usually does not develop in persons under 40. Parkinson's is chronic and progressive, and its signs fall into four categories: tremor (which usually begins in the hand and may progress to involve the arm, a foot, or the jaw), rigidity (resistance to movement among muscles in opposing pairs), bradykinesia (slowing or loss of normal, spontaneous movement), and postural instability (with development of a forward or backward lean, stooped posture, or tendency to fall easily).

Central pain syndrome results from damage or injury to the brain, brain stem, or spinal cord, and it is marked by intense, steady pain that may be described as burning, aching, tingling, or "pins and needles." It occurs in patients who, at some point in the past, have had strokes, multiple sclerosis, limb amputation, or spinal cord injury. Pain medications generally do not provide relief, and patients often rely on sedatives or other means of keeping the CNS free from stress. One example is trigeminal neuralgia, which is caused by abnormal impulse conduction along the trigeminal nerve (cranial nerve V). It often has brief episodes of intense facial pain. The fear of a possible attack may

©2013 Pearson Education, Inc.
Paramedic Care: Principles & Practice, Vol. 4, 4th Ed.

be debilitating. Medications including carbamazepine (Tegretol) may be helpful, and surgery may be indicated for select cases.

Bell's palsy is the most common form of facial paralysis, affecting roughly 40,000 Americans yearly. It results from inflammation of the facial nerve (cranial nerve VII) and is marked by one-sided facial paralysis, inability to close the eye on the affected side, pain, tearing of that eye, drooling, hypersensitivity to sound, and impaired taste. Multiple causes exist, among them head trauma, herpes simplex virus, and Lyme disease. Treatment is usually aimed at protecting the eye. Corticosteroids may be used for inflammation when pain is severe. Most patients recover within three months. Amyotrophic lateral sclerosis (ALS, or Lou Gehrig's disease) affects 20,000 Americans, with roughly 5,000 new cases reported each year. ALS involves progressive degeneration of the nerve cells that control voluntary movement. It is marked by weakness, loss of motor control, difficulty speaking, and cramping. Eventually a weakened diaphragm and intercostal muscles lead to breathing problems. There is currently no effective therapy and no cure, and prognosis continues to be poor, with death within three to five years of diagnosis (often as a result of pulmonary infection). Myoclonus refers to temporary involuntary twitching or spasm of a muscle or muscle group. It is generally considered not a disorder, but a symptom. It occurs with a variety of disorders, including multiple sclerosis, Parkinson's, and Alzheimer's. Pathological myoclonus may limit a person's ability to eat, walk, and talk. Treatment consists of medication that reduces symptoms, often antiepileptic drugs such as clonazepam, phenytoin, and sodium valproate.

Spina bifida (SB) is a congenital neural defect resulting from failure of one or more fetal vertebrae to close properly during development, leaving a portion of the spinal cord unprotected. Long-term effects include impairment in physical mobility, and most individuals have some form of learning disability. The three most common types are myelomeningocele, the most severe form, in which the spinal cord and meninges protrude from the opening in the spine; meningocele, in which the meninges only protrude through the spinal opening; and SB occulta, the mildest form, in which one or more vertebrae are malformed and covered only by a layer of skin. Treatment includes surgery, medication, and physiotherapy appropriate for the extent of deformity. Poliomyelitis (polio) is an infectious disease that sometimes results in permanent paralysis. The acute disease is marked by fatigue, headache, fever, vomiting, stiffness of the neck, and pain in the hands and feet. New cases in the United States are rare because of routine childhood vaccination. However, thousands of prevaccine polio survivors are alive today, and you may see them as patients. Many of these individuals require supportive care.

m. Back pain and nontraumatic spinal disorders   pp. 212–214
Back pain

Low back pain, defined as pain felt between the lower rib cage and the gluteal muscles, often radiating to the thighs, is an extremely common complaint but only occasionally the reason for an EMS call. Men and women are equally affected, but you should keep in mind that back pain in women over 60 years may represent the first sign of osteoporosis, an important medical condition. Vertebral fractures from causes other than osteoporosis are also possible causes. Other causes of low back pain include sciatica, which is reflected as severe pain along the path of the sciatic nerve down the back of the thigh and inner leg. Sciatica may be due to compression or trauma to the sciatic nerve or its roots, perhaps from a herniated intervertebral disk or an osteoarthritic lumbosacral vertebral bone. Sciatica may also be due to inflammation of the nerve secondary to metabolic, toxic, or infectious causes. Pain at the level of L-3, L-4, L-5, and S-1 may be due to inflammation of interspinous bursae. External to the spine are other causes of low back pain: inflammation or sprain of muscles and ligaments that attach to the spine. Most low back pain, though, is found to be idiopathic.

Assessment of back pain is based on chief complaint, history, and physical exam. When the complaint is low back pain, a precise diagnosis is likely to be difficult. Preliminary diagnosis may focus on occupational risk from repetitive lifting or exposure to machinery vibrations. Listen for clues in the history about the nature and timing of the pain and whether the current complaint is acute pain or exacerbation of a chronic condition. Your priorities in the field are to determine whether pain is due to a life-threatening or non-life-threatening condition. Note: The presence of any identifiable neurological deficit may point to a serious underlying cause, as may a gradual onset of pain consistent with degenerative disk disease or tumor growth. The location of the injury may be revealed on exam by a limited range of motion in the lumbar spine; point tenderness on palpation; alterations in sensation, pain, and temperature at a localized point; or pain or paresthesia below a point of injury. Always keep in mind that you are unlikely to be able to determine the cause of the pain in the field. Your primary goal is to look for signs of life-threatening problems and to gather historical and exam information that will be useful to the receiving physician. You will also need to decide, perhaps after consultation with medical direction, whether immobilization (and, if so, to what degree) is necessary during transport.

If there are no clear life-threatening problems requiring intervention, management is primarily aimed at minimizing pain and immobilizing as per local protocol. If there is no historical reason to suspect injury in the past or an underlying condition such as osteoporosis (which makes patients vulnerable to pathological fracture), C-spine immobilization may still be recommended as a comfort measure during transport. Also remember that some patients will require parenteral analgesia and diazepam before they can lie on a stretcher. Consult medical direction if you feel your patient might fit into this category. Last, remember to provide ongoing assessment en route with special attention to the ABCs, vitals, and the possible presence or development of motor or sensory deficits that might indicate a critical condition capable of compromising ventilatory efforts.

Herniated intervertebral disk

Intervertebral disks may rupture due to injury or due to degeneration associated with aging. Degenerative disk disease is most common in patients over 50 years of age. A herniated disk occurs when the gelatinous center of the disk extrudes through a tear in the tough outer capsule, and the resulting pain is due to pressure on the spinal cord or to muscle spasm at the site. The disks themselves are not innervated. Non-injury-related herniation may also be caused by improper lifting. Men aged 30 to 50 years are more prone to herniated disks than are women. Herniation is most common at levels L-4, L-5, and S-1, but it also may occur at C-5, C-6, and C-7.

Spinal cord tumors

A cyst or tumor along the spine or intruding into the spinal canal may cause pain by pressing on the spinal cord, causing degenerative changes in bone, or interrupting blood supply. The specific manifestations depend on location and type of tumor or cyst.

8. **Apply prehospital stroke scoring systems in the assessment of patients with suspected stroke.** pp. 199–202

Standardized scoring systems are now available to aid paramedics in making a field diagnosis of stroke. The two most commonly used are:

- **Los Angeles Prehospital Stroke Screen (LAPSS).** The LAPSS assesses blood glucose levels, facial droop, grip strength, and arm (pronator) drift. Patients meeting the LAPSS criteria should result in activation of the stroke team at the receiving hospital.
- **Cincinnati Prehospital Stroke Scale (CPSS).** The CPSS evaluates facial droop, arm drift, and speech. An abnormal finding on any of these three parameters is associated with a 72 percent probability the patient has suffered a stroke.

9. **Given a variety of scenarios, develop treatment plans for patients with neurologic disorders.** pp. 190–214

The priorities for someone who is unconscious or clearly in urgent distress with neurological difficulties are the same as for a patient who is affected by a potentially life-threatening emergency of another origin. Ensure adequate airway, breathing (ventilation), and circulation. This is particularly important for someone whose emergency may be originating in, or affecting, the CNS. The brain requires a constant supply of oxygen, glucose, and vitamins. After 10 to 20 seconds without blood flow, unconsciousness will occur. Significant deprivation of oxygen (anoxia) or glucose (hypoglycemia) can cause seizures or coma. You should always give high-concentration oxygen to a patient with a neurological emergency and give glucose to any patient found to be hypoglycemic.

Neurological injuries and illnesses usually require treatment as soon as possible to prevent progressive damage. In the case of thromboembolic stroke, this may be particularly true because therapies are coming into use that can minimize the region of brain tissue infarcted in the stroke or even prevent the progression of tissue ischemia to tissue infarction. Patients who show altered mental status and/or any clear neurological impairment (pupillary dilation, especially unilateral; facial drooping; slurred speech; abnormal posturing—if these appear to be new or progressing findings) that may suggest TIA or stroke need immediate intervention and transport. Management of seizures and syncope often mandates prompt intervention and care as well.

You will see many calls for complaints such as low back pain and headache. These conditions may be relatively minor or the signal of a serious underlying disorder. History suggesting new-onset, severe pain, or clearly progressive pain indicates the need for aggressive assessment and management, whereas other patients with chronic pain of either origin also require full assessment but may need only supportive care.

Patients with known CNS neoplasms or degenerative neurological conditions may present with a complaint related to their underlying disease or a problem of completely different origin. Be aware that these persons are always more vulnerable to oxygen or glucose deprivation from another source, such as cardiac disease or diabetes. In addition, remember that some patients will have airways vulnerable to compromise secondary to muscle paralysis or other neurologic causes.

Case Study Review

Reread the case study on page 180 in Paramedic Care: Medicine; *then, read the following discussion.*

This case study demonstrates how paramedics react to a relatively common neurological emergency: a "possible stroke patient." The case study demonstrates how initial impressions, assessment findings, and knowledge of the likely pathophysiology not only reveal diagnosis but directly guide the team in prioritizing transport and in identifying the appropriate receiving center.

Jack and Linda are dispatched to a bank for a man in his 60s with reported (presumably new-onset) neurological signs of right-sided weakness and inability to speak. Because possible stroke is a true emergency, one in which time can make a substantial difference to outcome, it is in the patient's favor that the team can respond within 3 minutes or so of the dispatch.

Their initial impression is of an elderly man sitting upright, with some assistance, in a chair. The neurological deficit of aphasia (inability to speak) appears to be confirmed on attempts to communicate with the patient, and the team realizes that the patient, although unable to speak, appears to be oriented and cooperative. Their attention then turns to airway and breathing as priorities. The man's airway is patent (at the moment), and his respirations are normal.

Blood pressure is measured in the unaffected arm, and it is hypertensive at 160/90. Chronic hypertension is a risk factor for stroke, so it is important for the team to ask about a history of hypertension and any associated medications when they get the opportunity to talk with the patient's family. If none of the bystanders knew the gentleman, and if he seemed lucid, the team might be able to solicit limited information from him via a Medic-Alert tag (if he wears one) and/or via requests for head nodding or for written responses to questions. Changes in his ability to comply with such requests might serve as a signal of decreasing mental status. The rest of his initial physical exam is largely benign except for confirmation of unilateral (right-sided) weakness. You are told that there is marked right-sided weakness, but you aren't told the extent: Does it involve the arm only, or does it also involve the face or the leg, or both? Extent of weakness, as well as any sign of additional extent, is an indicator of stroke progression and also signals that sudden airway compromise may be more likely. The use of the Cincinnati Prehospital Stroke Scale helps identify this patient as having a stroke. All elements of the assessment direct Linda and Jack to the same conclusion, stroke.

Only at this point, after initial assessment, is oxygen started, a heparin lock placed in the unaffected arm, and ECG monitoring begun. The timing of the IV access and ECG monitoring is appropriate, but the team should have considered oxygen supplementation as soon as they knew the patient was unable to talk. Any time advantage in reversal of brain anoxia should be taken. On the other hand, it is a positive sign that pulse oximetry after initiation of oxygen supplementation is 99 percent.

You aren't told what information is elicited regarding personal medical history, but you are told that the ECG shows atrial fibrillation with a ventricular rate of 90. Atrial fibrillation is a risk factor for embolic (occlusive) stroke because small clots form in the heart and break off to enter the systemic circulation. This knowledge increases the importance of timely transport, as well as expedient consideration of appropriate facility, because current guidelines indicate that thrombolytic therapy within the first 3 hours of an embolic occlusion may well be successful in minimizing or preventing infarction of brain tissue.

Indeed, the team packages the patient carefully but expediently and transports him to a facility that can handle a stroke. On arrival, a hemorrhagic stroke of significant magnitude is ruled out via CT scan and the team decides to initiate therapy with tPA. The outcome is positive: The patient's aphasia resolves completely and most of his right-sided weakness reverses. The patient is discharged to a rehabilitation unit for further therapy on his hemiparesis. You don't know how or whether the man's atrial fibrillation (AF) is resolved, but you should assume that in-hospital care would have involved adjustment of medication (if he were taking any for AF) or possible electrical conversion to normal rhythm.

Content Self-Evaluation

MULTIPLE CHOICE

_____ 1. Afferent nerve fibers carry messages to the central nervous system (CNS), whereas efferent fibers carry impulses from the CNS to the rest of the body.
   A. True
   B. False

_____ 2. The two mechanisms that generally cause altered mental status are
   A. occlusive and hemorrhagic strokes.
   B. systemic diseases and drugs or toxic agents.
   C. structural lesions and toxic-metabolic states.
   D. head trauma and CNS disease.
   E. toxic-metabolic states and brain tumors.

_____ 3. Peripheral neuropathy can affect muscle activity, sensation, and reflexes, but not internal organ function.
   A. True
   B. False

_____ 4. The Glasgow Coma Scale assesses eye opening, verbal response, and motor response. Which correlation of score and likely outcome is NOT correct?
   A. Score of 3 or 4, 10 percent favorable outcome
   B. Score of 8 or higher, 94 percent favorable outcome
   C. Score of 5 to 7 that increases to 8 or higher, 80 percent favorable outcome
   D. Score of 5 to 7, 50 percent favorable outcome in adults and 90 percent in children
   E. Score of 5 to 7 that decreases by 1 point, 10 percent favorable outcome

_____ 5. Three interventions that may be indicated in treatment of a patient with altered mental status are
   A. hyperventilation, 50 percent dextrose, and naloxone.
   B. mannitol (Osmotrol), 50 percent dextrose, and naloxone.
   C. 50 percent dextrose, thiamine, and naloxone.
   D. mannitol (Osmotrol), hyperventilation, and 50 percent dextrose.
   E. mannitol (Osmotrol), thiamine, and naloxone.

_____ 6. Management of a patient with a suspected stroke or a suspected TIA is the same because they can rarely be distinguished in the field.
   A. True
   B. False

_____ 7. If a stroke patient is apneic or breathing inadequately, controlled positive pressure at 12 ventilations per minute may be beneficial because it
   A. causes cerebral vasoconstriction, decreasing cerebral swelling.
   B. causes a reflex increase in respiration rate.
   C. eliminates excess CO_2 levels.
   D. increases CO_2 levels toward normal range.
   E. increases the ability of brain cells to take up any available oxygen.

©2013 Pearson Education, Inc.
Paramedic Care: Principles & Practice, Vol. 4, 4th Ed.

8. Which of the following is NOT an element of the Los Angeles Stroke Screen?
   A. Grip strength
   B. Facial droop
   C. Blood glucose level
   D. Arm drift
   E. Speech

9. If a patient meets any of the criteria within the Cincinnati Stroke Screen, that patient's likelihood of suffering a stroke is 100 percent.
   A. True
   B. False

10. Among the many types of epileptic seizures, the most likely to require intervention on your part are
    A. absence seizures.
    B. tonic-clonic seizures.
    C. petit mal seizures.
    D. simple partial seizures.
    E. complex partial seizures.

11. Status epilepticus is considered a serious, but not life-threatening, emergency.
    A. True
    B. False

12. If a patient with suspected syncope does not regain consciousness within a few moments, the event is NOT syncope, but something more serious.
    A. True
    B. False

13. The two most common causes of headache are
    A. vascular and organic.
    B. vascular and neurogenic.
    C. tension and vascular.
    D. tension and organic.
    E. tension and neurogenic.

14. Which one of the following is NOT a degenerative neurological disorder?
    A. Multiple sclerosis (MS)
    B. Parkinson's disease
    C. Bell's palsy
    D. Muscular dystrophy
    E. Vertebral disk disease

FILL IN THE BLANKS

Write the word or words that best complete the following statements in the space(s) provided.

15. Stimulation of the sympathetic nervous system results in increased _____ _____ and dilation of _____ and _____ .

16. The center for speech is located in the _____ lobe of the _____ .

17. The autonomic nervous system regulates _____ physiological processes.

18. Tissues innervated by the sympathetic nervous system include _____ and _____ muscle and some glands.

19. The diencephalon consists of the _____ , the _____ , and the _____ system.

20. The neuronal processes that detect an incoming nerve impulse are the _____ .

21. The peripheral nervous system consists of the _____ _____ _____ and the _____ _____ _____ .

22. The nervous system consists of the _____ _____ _____ and the _____ _____ _____ .

23. In outer-to-inner order, the dura mater, arachnoid membrane, and the pia mater make up the three layers of the _____.

24. The multiple tips of the _____ allow a neuron to send an impulse to more than one other neuron.

25. Actions of the parasympathetic nervous system include decreased _____ _____ and constriction of _____ and _____.

26. The brain stem consists of the _____, the _____, and the _____ _____.

27. Both the brain and spinal cord are bathed in _____ _____.

28. The reticular activating system (RAS), in the lateral portions of the medulla, pons, and midbrain, is responsible for maintaining _____ and the ability to respond to _____.

29. The center form vision is located in the _____ lobe of the _____.

30. The center for motor activity is located in _____ lobes of the _____.

31. The somatic nervous system mediates _____, _____ actions.

32. The junction of two neurons is called a(n) _____, and a(n) _____ enables a nerve impulse to move from one neuron to another.

33. The central nervous system consists of the _____ and _____ _____.

Label the Diagram

The following figure shows the major parts of the brain. Label each part and then match its major function(s) by placing the appropriate letter in the space provided below each label name.

34. _____

Function(s): _____

40. _____

Function(s): _____

Cerebral hemispheres

35. _____

Function(s): _____

36. _____

Function(s): _____

37. _____

Function(s): _____

38. _____

Function(s): _____

41. _____

Function(s): _____

39. _____

Function(s): _____

©2013 Pearson Education, Inc.
Paramedic Care: Principles & Practice, Vol. 4, 4th Ed.

A. adjustment of balance and muscular coordination

B. generates involuntary somatic muscle responses, maintains consciousness

C. contains autonomic centers for cardiovascular, respiratory, and digestive system function

D. contains centers for involuntary somatic and visceral motor activity

E. contains centers for control of emotion, autonomic, and endocrine functions

F. conscious thought, memory storage, and control over voluntary motor activity

G. secretes hormones responsible for regulation of endocrine glands

H. acts as relay and processing center for sensory information

MATCHING

Write the two letters giving the cause and description of the abnormal breathing pattern in the space provided next to the name of the pattern.

A. rapid, deep respirations

B. brain damage due to trauma or cerebral hemorrhage and with chronic hypoxia

C. ineffective thoracic muscular coordination due to CNS damage

D. severe metabolic or CNS conditions

E. rapid, deep, noisy respirations involving hyperventilation

F. prolonged inspiration unrelieved by expiration attempts

G. brief period of apnea followed by increasing depth and frequency of respirations

H. lesion in the CNS

I. poor respirations

J. pattern due to damage in the upper part of the pons

_____ 42. Cheyne-Stokes respiration

_____ 43. Central neurogenic hyperventilation

_____ 44. Kussmaul's respiration

_____ 45. ataxic respirations

_____ 46. apneustic respirations

Write the two letters giving the major cause and characteristic of presentation in the space provided next to the type of stroke to which they apply. A letter may be used more than once.

A. gradual development of signs/symptoms, often first noticed on waking during night

B. congenital blood vessel abnormalities or head trauma

C. sudden onset of severe headache

D. blood clot that forms in an area of a cerebral artery narrowed by atherosclerosis

E. rupture of a small blood vessel within brain tissue

F. lodging of a blood clot, air bubble, tumor tissue, or fat in an artery that is far from its site of origin

_____ 47. Thrombotic stroke

_____ 48. Intracerebral hemorrhage

_____ **49.** Embolic stroke

_____ **50.** Subarachnoid hemorrhage

LISTING

51. The AVPU model for mental status stands for:

A _____

V _____

P _____

U _____

52. Assessment of a patient's cerebral function includes evaluation of emotional state. Fill in a word for each letter of the MTPJ and MA models.

M _____

T _____

P _____

J _____

MA _____

53. Cushing's triad, which is associated with increasing intracranial pressure, consists of what three elements?

1. _____

2. _____

3. _____

54. A mnemonic for the common causes of altered mental status is AEIOU-TIPS. Fill in one or more words for each letter of the mnemonic.

A _____

E _____

I _____

O _____

U _____

T _____

I _____

P _____

S _____

55. Name the two types of occlusive strokes.

_____

_____

56. Name two categories of hemorrhagic strokes.

_____

_____

©2013 Pearson Education, Inc.
Paramedic Care: Principles & Practice, Vol. 4, 4th Ed.

57. List the four main characteristics of Parkinson's disease.

_____

_____

_____

_____

58. List, in increasing order of severity, the three forms of spina bifida.

_____

_____

_____

59. List the two common forms of vascular headache.

_____

_____

Special Project

Distinguishing Different Conditions in the Field

The chapter presented situations in which you might need to distinguish between very different conditions that may have somewhat similar presentations. Complete the following tables to demonstrate your knowledge of these conditions.

Scenario 1: Shock vs. Increased Intracranial Pressure As discussed in Chapter 3, one of the reasons to take vital signs every 5 minutes in patients with suspected CNS injury is that vitals may change quickly, showing signs of instability or of emergence of a diagnostic pattern. Complete the following table to demonstrate the characteristic vital signs in shock and in increased intracranial pressure.

Vital Signs	Shock	Increased Intracranial Pressure
Blood pressure		
Pulse		
Respirations		
Level of consciousness		

Scenario 2: Syncope vs. Tonic-Clonic Seizure As discussed in Chapter 3, you may arrive on the scene after an event has happened or while an event is in progress. In such cases, history from bystanders and, when able, from the patient may be crucial in establishing what underlying condition is present. Complete the following table to demonstrate the different characteristics, or traits, of syncope and of a generalized tonic-clonic seizure.

Trait	Syncope	Tonic-Clonic Seizure
Starting position		
Warning		
Jerking motions		
Return of consciousness		

4 Endocrinology

Review of Chapter Objectives

After reading this chapter, you should be able to:

1. Define key terms introduced in this chapter.

Knowing and being able to apply the key terms in each chapter is critical to understanding chapter concepts. Write the list of key terms. Then write the definition of each one in your own words. Check your understanding by confirming the definitions in the text glossary. Correct any misunderstandings. Create a study aid by writing each key term on the front of an index card and the definition on the back. Use the cards to quiz yourself, or to have someone quiz you.

2. Relate the anatomy and physiology of the endocrine system to the pathophysiology and assessment of patients with endocrine disorders. pp. 220–238

There are eight major structures associated with the endocrine system located throughout the body: the hypothalamus, pituitary gland, thyroid gland, parathyroid glands, thymus, pancreas, adrenal glands, and gonads. The pineal gland is also part of the endocrine system.

The hypothalamus, located deep within the cerebrum of the brain, is the junction between the endocrine system and the central nervous system. About the size of a pea, the pituitary gland is located adjacent to the hypothalamus within the cerebrum. The pineal gland is also located adjacent to the hypothalamus. The double-lobed thyroid gland is located in the neck anterior to and just below the cartilage of the larynx. The parathyroid glands are very small and are found on the posterior lateral surface of the thyroid gland. The thymus is located in the mediastinum just behind the sternum. The pancreas is located in the upper abdomen behind the stomach and between the duodenum and the spleen. The adrenal glands are somewhat triangular in shape and are located on the superior surface of the kidneys. Gonads can be found in the lower pelvis in women, with each ovary resembling an almond in size and shape. In men, the gonads are located in the scrotum.

The endocrine system is closely linked to the nervous system and plays a critical role in our ability to maintain life by regulating many bodily functions through chemical substances called hormones. The endocrine system is made up of ductless glands, which manufacture and secrete hormones that act in adjacent tissues or travel via the bloodstream to target organs or other endocrine glands to produce specific or generalized effects. Hormones regulate metabolic activity, growth, and development, as well as mediate chemical reactions, maintain homeostatic balance, and initiate our adaptive response to stress.

Many people have endocrine disorders that involve excessive or deficient hormone production or function. The incidence of such disorders is widely variable. Some disorders are readily controlled by hormone replacement therapy; others are more complex and thus more difficult to manage. The most common of all of the endocrine disorders is diabetes mellitus, affecting at least 8 million Americans.

Insulin is a glucagon antagonist and lowers the blood glucose level by promoting energy storage. Insulin increases the rate at which various body cells take up glucose by changing the permeability of the cell membranes. These changes also make the cell more permeable to potassium, magnesium, and phosphate ions, as well as many amino acids. Because the liver rapidly breaks down insulin, the hormone must be secreted constantly.

Homeostasis of blood glucose is remarkably effective. In nondiabetics, when blood glucose is high, as after a meal, the beta cells of the pancreas release insulin. Insulin enables cells to use glucose directly as well as to store energy as glycogen, protein, and fat. If you were to draw a venous blood sample to measure fasting blood glucose levels, you'd find the level in healthy individuals is usually between 80 and 90 mg glucose/dL blood. In the first 60 to 90 minutes after a meal the level will increase to approximately 120 to 140 mg/dL before dropping off to near-fasting levels as insulin is released to move the glucose from the bloodstream into the cells. Conversely, when blood glucose levels are low, the alpha cells of the pancreas release glucagon to raise the blood glucose level.

Insulin deficiency contributes to the development of hyperglycemia. Without insulin to facilitate the movement of large glucose molecules across cell membranes, the blood glucose level rises even as the intracellular level of glucose plummets. At the same time, the alpha cells of the pancreas release glucagon to increase blood glucose by stimulating the breakdown of glycogen, as well as stimulating the breakdown of body proteins and fats with subsequent chemical conversion to glucose (gluconeo-genesis). With a rise in blood glucose levels, as is the case in type I diabetes, the body's cells cannot take up circulating glucose. Glucose then spills into urine, leading to a large water loss, via osmotic diuresis, and significant dehydration. This can lead to significant loss of potassium and hypokalemia.

3. **Adapt the scene size-up, primary assessment, patient history, secondary assessment, and use of monitoring technology to meet the needs of patients with complaints and presentations related to endocrine disorders.** pp. 220–238

During the scene size-up, your general impression will be very important, as you will be looking for clues that can indicate the patient's condition. The causes of endocrine disorders are numerous. One of the first questions you will answer will be if there is a history of endocrine disorders such as diabetes or thyroid dysfunction. Evaluate the patient's level of consciousness using the AVPU method, speech, skin appearance, and posture. The patient's emotional status may also provide clues to the patient's cerebral function that may be altered due to hypoxia, hypoglycemia, or hyperglycemia. Complete your primary ABCD assessment and recognize any findings that would indicate an endocrine emergency. Your secondary assessment should include a detailed neurologic exam, accurate history, and physical exam with a full set of vital signs. Initiate all appropriate monitoring devices. For example, alterations in ventilatory function may be observed in a patient experiencing an endocrine emergency. Capnography measures exhaled or end-tidal CO_2 and can assist the paramedic in evaluating the ventilation rate and quality in such a patient. Pulse oximetry is used to monitor a patient's general state of perfusion. Patients with abnormal endocrine function are at risk for vomiting and aspiration, so frequent assessment of the airway, breathing, and circulation is vital. Because hypoglycemia is commonly manifested by neurologic focal deficits, every patient with an abnormal neurologic exam should have his blood glucose measured.

4. **Use a process of clinical reasoning to guide and interpret the patient assessment and management process for patients with endocrine disorders.** pp. 220–238

As a paramedic, it is vital that you develop your clinical reasoning process to quickly recognize and treat acute endocrine conditions to improve patient outcome. This is because diagnosis and treatment with many endocrine emergencies is time sensitive. Develop an organized general impression to rapidly identify signs and symptoms of endocrine emergencies. This will include obtaining an accurate history.

Diabetes mellitus is the most commonly encountered endocrine disorder. Among the predisposing factors that have been identified for this condition are heredity, viral infection, autoimmune antibodies, and obesity. Heredity is also thought to be the key factor in the predisposition for Graves' disease, although autoimmune antibodies are known to trigger the excess production of thyroid hormone. Severe physiological stress has been found to be a common triggering factor for thyrotoxicosis (thyroid storm). On the other hand, hypothyroidism or myxedema may be either congenital or acquired. The risk of adrenal gland disorders is increased by the administration of glucocorticoids, or it may be a consequence of abnormalities of the anterior pituitary gland or the adrenal cortex. Approximately half of all adrenal gland disorders are due to autoimmune disorders or may be aggravated by acute physiological stress.

The primary treatment for endocrine emergencies is to identify and treat reversible causes and to treat serious signs and symptoms. When a reversible cause is not identified, treatment shifts to supportive measures. Management can include oxygenation, ventilatory assistance, fluid resuscitation, IV glucose, suctioning, assisting ventilations, keeping the patient warm, and glucose and ECG monitoring. In addition, based on local protocols, you may be collecting venous blood samples. Make a strong effort to make the patient comfortable, keep NPO, prevent aspiration, and be prepared for seizures. Consider the following:

- *Airway and breathing.* Properly position any patient who, you suspect has an endocrine emergency and protect the airway. Have suction ready. Administer supplemental oxygen if the patient is hypoxic—but only enough to correct hypoxia. Avoid hyperoxia. If the patient is breathing inadequately or is apneic, initiate ventilatory assistance. If an airway problem is detected, first apply basic airway maneuvers such as head positioning or the modified jaw-thrust maneuver. Intubate, if indicated.
- *Circulatory support.* Establish a saline lock. It is important to have an accessible route for medications. Some patients may need volume resuscitation.
- *Pharmacological interventions.* Medications are available to treat signs and symptoms in patients with endocrine emergencies. Medications include dextrose, thiamine, and naloxone (if associated with narcotic overdose).
- *Psychological support.* Patients suffering from an endocrine emergency, acute or chronic, are likely also to suffer depression, anxiety, or anger. The neurological deficits associated with some endocrine emergencies are frightening experiences. Provide the patient with emotional support and explain the treatment regimen. In most cases, it is appropriate to explain to the patient what is occurring and why. Careful explanation and emotional support will help allay anxiety and apprehension. Patients that you treat on the scene for acute hypoglycemia can experience complete resolution of symptoms. Some of these patients may refuse transport. Use therapeutic communication to effectively explain the rationale for transport.
- *Transport considerations.* Assess, provide emergency care, and package the patient as quickly and safely as possible. Rapidly transport any patient with a neurological deficit or altered mental status secondary to endocrine emergencies to an appropriate emergency department, equipped with a computerized tomography (CT) or magnetic resonance imaging (MRI) scanner and facilities capable of managing strokes with fibrinolytic therapy. Constantly reevaluate and monitor the patient's airway, breathing, circulation and neurologic status.

5. **Describe the pathophysiology of specific endocrine problems, including the following:**

a. **Diabetes mellitus types I and II, including hypoglycemic and hyperglycemic diabetic emergencies.** pp. 227–235

Type I diabetes mellitus

Type I diabetes mellitus is characterized by β-cell destruction with very low production of insulin by the pancreas. In many cases, no insulin is produced at all. Type I diabetes is commonly called juvenile-onset diabetes because of the average age at diagnosis. The term insulin-dependent diabetes mellitus (IDDM) is also used because patients require regular insulin injections to maintain glucose homeostasis. This type of diabetes is less common than is type II diabetes, but it is more serious. Diabetes is regularly among the 10 leading causes of death in the United States, and type I diabetes accounts for most diabetes-related deaths.

Heredity is an important factor in determining which persons will be predisposed to development of type I diabetes. The cause of type I diabetes is often unclear. However, viral infection, production of autoantibodies directed against beta cells (immune-related), and genetically determined early deterioration of beta cells are all possible. The immediate cause of the disease is destruction of beta cells.

In untreated type I diabetes, blood glucose levels rise because without adequate insulin, cells cannot take up the circulating sugar. Hyperglycemia in the range of 300 to 500 mg/dL is not uncommon. As glucose spills into urine, large amounts of water are lost, too, through osmotic diuresis. Catabolism of fat becomes significant as the body switches to fatty acids as the primary energy source. Overall, this pathophysiology accounts for the constant thirst (polydipsia), excessive urination (polyuria), ravenous appetite (polyphagia), weakness, and weight loss associated with untreated type I diabetes. Ketosis can occur as the result of fat catabolism and it may proceed to diabetic ketoacidosis.

Type II diabetes mellitus

Type II diabetes mellitus is associated with a moderate decline in insulin production accompanied by a markedly deficient response to the insulin that is present in the body (insulin resistance). Type II diabetes is also called non-insulin-dependent diabetes mellitus (NIDDM), although some type II patients may also require insulin.

Heredity may play a role in predisposition. In addition, obese persons are more likely to develop type II diabetes, and obesity probably plays a role in development of the disease. Increased weight (and increased size of fat cells) causes a relative deficiency in the number of insulin receptors per cell, which makes fat cells less responsive to insulin. In fact, as obesity in children has become more prevalent, so has the occurrence of type II diabetes in children. Previously, type II diabetes was so uncommon in children that it was often called "adult-onset diabetes," a descriptor that is, unfortunately, no longer appropriate.

Type II diabetes is far more common than type I diabetes, accounting for about 80 percent of cases of diabetes mellitus.

Hyperosmolar hyperglycemic coma

This condition is a complication of type II diabetes due to inadequate insulin activity and is marked by high blood glucose, marked dehydration, and decreased mental function. Development of the coma is slower than with ketoacidosis. Early signs include increased urination and thirst. Later signs may include orthostatic hypotension, dry skin, and tachycardia.

This condition is difficult to distinguish from ketoacidosis in the field. Field management focuses on maintaining ABCs and fluid resuscitation.

Diabetic ketoacidosis

Diabetic ketoacidosis is a serious, potentially life-threatening complication of diabetes mellitus. It occurs when profound insulin deficiency is coupled with increased glucagon activity.

The onset is slow, lasting from 12 to 24 hours. In its early stages, the signs and symptoms include increased thirst, excessive hunger, increased urination, and malaise. Increased urination results from the osmotic diuresis accompanying glucose spillage into the urine. Intensified thirst is caused by the body's attempt to replace the fluids lost by increased urination. Nausea, vomiting, marked dehydration, tachycardia, and weakness characterize diabetic ketoacidosis. The skin is usually warm and dry. Coma is not uncommon. The breath may have a sweet or acetone-like character due to the increased ketones in the blood. Very deep, rapid respirations, called Kussmaul's respirations, also occur. Kussmaul's respirations represent the body's attempt to compensate for the metabolic acidosis produced by the ketones and organic acids present in the blood. It may be complicated by several electrolyte imbalances. The most significant is decreased potassium. Decreased potassium (hypokalemia) can lead to serious dysrhythmias or even death.

The approach used with the patient suffering from diabetic ketoacidosis is essentially the same as with any unconscious patient. You should first complete your initial assessment of airway, breathing, and circulation. You will then complete your focused history and physical exam. Pay particular attention to the presence of a Medic-Alert bracelet and/or insulin in the refrigerator. Also, obtain a history from bystanders. The fruity odor of ketones occasionally can be detected on the breath. If possible, complete the rapid test for blood glucose.

It is not uncommon for patients in ketoacidosis to have blood glucose levels well in excess of 300 mg/dL. The field management of such cases is focused on maintenance of ABCs and fluid resuscitation to counteract the patient's dehydration. Treatment should include drawing a red-top tube (or the tube specified by local protocols) of blood. Following this, you should administer 1 to 2 liters of normal saline per protocol. If transport time is lengthy, the medical direction physician may request intravenous or subcutaneous administration of regular insulin. If the blood glucose level cannot be quickly determined, draw a red-top tube of blood for analysis and start an IV of normal saline. Following this, administer 50 mL (25 grams) of 50 percent dextrose solution. This additional glucose load will not adversely affect the ketoacidotic patient because it is negligible compared to the total quantity present in the body. If the patient is alcoholic, consider administering 100 mg of thiamine. Transportation to an appropriate facility should be expedited.

©2013 Pearson Education, Inc.
Paramedic Care: Principles & Practice, Vol. 4, 4th Ed.

Hypoglycemia

Hypoglycemia, or low blood glucose, is a potentially life-threatening medical emergency. Sometimes called insulin shock, it can occur if a patient accidentally or intentionally injects too much insulin, eats an inadequate amount of food after taking insulin, or has overexercised and burned up all available glucose. Untreated, the insulin will cause the blood glucose to drop to a very low level. The longer the period of hypoglycemia persists, the greater the risk that the brain cells will be permanently damaged or even killed.

The signs and symptoms of hypoglycemia are many and varied. An abnormal mental status is the most important and often the earliest sign. In the earliest stages of hypoglycemia, the patient may appear restless or impatient or complain of hunger. As the blood glucose falls lower, he may display inappropriate anger or display a variety of bizarre behaviors. Physical signs may include diaphoresis and tachycardia. If the blood glucose falls to a critically low level, the patient may sustain a hypoglycemic seizure or become comatose. In contrast to diabetic ketoacidosis, hypoglycemia can develop quickly. When encountering a patient behaving bizarrely, you should always consider hypoglycemia.

In suspected cases of hypoglycemia, perform the initial assessment quickly. Inspect the patient for a Medic-Alert bracelet. If possible, determine the blood glucose level. If the blood glucose level is noted to be less than 60 mg/dL, draw a red-top tube of blood and start an IV of normal saline. Next, administer 50 to 100 milliliters (25 to 50 grams) of 50 percent dextrose intravenously. If the patient is conscious and able to swallow, complete glucose administration with orange juice, sodas, or commercially available glucose pastes.

If the blood glucose cannot be obtained and if the patient is unconscious, you should start an IV of normal saline and administer 50 to 100 mL (25 to 50 g) of 50 percent dextrose. Expedite transport to the nearest medical facility. If you suspect alcoholism, administer 100 mg of thiamine before the administration of dextrose.

Hyperglycemia

Diabetes mellitus results from either inadequate amounts of circulating insulin or inadequate utilization of insulin. This means that there is an excess of blood glucose while there is an intracellular deficit. In diabetes, glucose builds up in the bloodstream, especially after meals. The blood glucose level rises higher and returns to normal more slowly in the diabetic than in the nondiabetic. An oral glucose tolerance test uses this phenomenon in the diagnosis of diabetes. The diabetic's inadequate insulin level and impaired glucose tolerance are partly due to the decreased entry of glucose into the cells, thus leaving more glucose in the bloodstream.

The second cause of hyperglycemia in the diabetic results from difficulties with the function of the liver. When blood glucose levels are high, insulin secretion is normally increased and the breakdown of glycogen is decreased. In the diabetic, however, insulin secretion is decreased, and the alpha cells secrete glucagon to stimulate glycogenolysis by the liver, thus raising the blood glucose level.

In type I diabetes the decreased insulin secretion is accompanied by a steady accumulation of glucose in the blood. Hyperglycemia acts like an osmotic diuretic and glucose "spills over" into the urine (glycosuria), pulling large amounts of water with it (polyuria). The body's attempt to dilute the concentration of glucose in the bloodstream results in intracellular dehydration and stimulates thirst (polydipsia). As the cells become glucose-depleted, they begin to use proteins and fats as an energy source, resulting in weight loss and the formation of harmful by-products, such as ketones and organic free fatty acids. The body's response to this state of cellular starvation is to trigger hunger in the patient (polyphagia). If the acids and ketones continue to collect in the blood, severe metabolic acidosis occurs and coma ensues, resulting in serious brain damage or death.

Type II diabetes does not usually result in diabetic ketoacidosis. It can, however, develop into a life-threatening emergency termed hyperglycemic hyperosmolar nonketotic (HHNK) coma. In type II diabetes, when blood glucose levels exceed 600 mg/dL, the high osmolality of the blood causes an osmotic diuresis and marked dehydration of body cells. However, sufficient insulin is produced to prevent the manufacture of ketones and the complications of metabolic acidosis. In this respect, the condition differs from diabetic ketoacidosis.

b. **Thyroid disorders, including hyperthyroidism, thyrotoxicosis, thyrotoxic crisis, hypothyroidism, and myxedema**   **pp. 235–237**

Hyperthyroidism and thyrotoxicosis

Thyrotoxic crisis, more commonly known as "thyroid storm," is a life-threatening medical emergency that can be fatal within as little as 48 hours if not treated. It is usually associated with severe physiological trauma (infection, uncontrolled diabetes mellitus, and so on) or psychological stress. You will also encounter thyroid storm from an accidental or intentional overdose of thyroid hormone. Many patients with thyrotoxicosis have underlying Graves' disease (hyperthyroidism).

The signs and symptoms associated with thyroid storm reflect the patient's profound hypermetabolic state and increased adrenergic response. The patient may be hyperthermic (with temperatures as high as 105°F) and tachycardic (especially common are atrial tachydysrhythmias), with a high pulse pressure and dyspnea. Mental status changes range from agitation and restlessness to delirium and coma. Nausea, vomiting, and diarrhea are also often present. Death often follows heart failure and profound cardiovascular collapse.

Field management is focused on supportive care with oxygenation, ventilatory assistance, fluid resuscitation, and cardiac monitoring, along with expedited transport to definitive care to block the high circulating levels of thyroid hormones.

Hypothyrodism and myxedema

Inadequate levels of the thyroid hormones in adults produce hypothyroidism or myxedema, which results in a generalized decrease in metabolism. Although it may occur in males or females of any age, it is most commonly seen among middle-aged females or as a consequence when surgery or radiation is used to treat hyperthyroidism.

This disorder tends to have a gradual onset, and the initial signs and symptoms tend to be quite subtle and include hoarse voice and slow speech, facial bloating, weakness, cold intolerance, lethargy, and fatigue as well as altered mental states, particularly depression. Additionally, the skin and hair are quite dry and coarse in texture. Patients with hypothyroidism are treated with replacement thyroid hormone, usually synthetic T_4 agents such as levothyroxine (Synthroid). Rarely do these patients require emergency treatment for their hypothyroidism unless it progresses to myxedema coma; however, you will encounter many patients who take thyroid replacement hormones.

Myxedema coma, a life-threatening complication of hypothyroidism, is not uncommon in colder climates but is unusual in warm ones. It is most often seen in older patients who have pulmonary or vascular disease. Other contributing factors include a history of thyroid disease and exposure to cold, infection, trauma, or drugs that suppress the central nervous system, such as sedatives and hypnotics. The mortality rate associated with myxedema coma is high.

Myxedema coma usually has a gradual onset, with lethargy and depression that progress to coma. Other signs and symptoms include extreme hypothermia (temperatures as low as 75°F are not uncommon), low-amplitude bradycardia, carbon dioxide retention, and profound respiratory depression.

Emergency management of myxedema coma is focused on maintenance of the ABCs and, as always, careful monitoring of the patient's cardiac and oxygenation status; most patients will require intubation and ventilatory assistance. Active rewarming is contraindicated because of the risk of cardiac dysrhythmias and the potential to cause vasodilatation, which may contribute to cardiovascular collapse. Although it is appropriate to initiate intravenous access, care must be taken to limit fluids because fluid and electrolyte imbalance is common. Follow local protocols or contact medical direction for specific orders based on your patient's presentation.

Thyrotoxic crisis (thyroid storm)

The mechanisms underlying thyrotoxic crisis are poorly understood. An acute increase in the levels of thyroid hormones does not appear to be the cause. It is more likely that thyroid storm is caused by a shift of thyroid hormone in the blood from the protein-bound (biologically inactive) to the free (biologically active) state.

c. **Adrenal disorders, including Cushing's syndrome and Addison's disease**   **pp. 237–238**

Cushing's syndrome

Chronic high levels of glucocorticoids result in the development of Cushing's syndrome, or hyperadrenalism. Cushing's syndrome may occur as a result of long-term glucocorticoid (steroid) therapy, from abnormalities of the adrenal glands, or from a pituitary tumor triggering excessive

©2013 Pearson Education, Inc.
Paramedic Care: Principles & Practice, Vol. 4, 4th Ed.

secretion of adrenocorticotropic hormone (ACTH), which stimulates the adrenals to produce excessive amounts of glucocorticoids.

Presenting signs and symptoms include weight gain, particularly through the trunk of the body, face, and neck, with a typical "moon-faced" appearance and often a "buffalo hump" due to the fat deposits in these areas; skin changes, such as the thinning of the skin to an almost transparent appearance, a tendency to bruise easily, delayed healing from even minor wounds, and the development of facial hair among women; increased vascular sensitivity; hypertension; mood swings; and memory impairment or decreased ability to concentrate.

Treatment involves removing the cause, such as the surgical removal of a tumor, or adjusting the dosage of glucocorticoids. Although it is unlikely that you would encounter a patient with an acute hyperadrenal crisis, you are very likely to encounter patients who exhibit signs and symptoms of Cushing's syndrome. These patients have a higher incidence of cardiovascular disease, hypertension, and stroke than the general population and are prone to infection. When performing your assessment, be alert for the signs mentioned in the previous section, which are associated with high glucocorticoid levels. Pay particular attention to skin preparation when starting intravenous lines, due to the fragility of these patients' skin and their susceptibility to infection. Your observations noted in your patient care report and relayed to the receiving hospital staff may contribute to the early diagnosis and treatment of this disorder, especially in those patients who do not have a primary care provider whom they see on a regular basis.

Adrenal insufficiency, or Addison's disease

Most commonly, adrenal insufficiency, or Addison's disease, is an idiopathic autoimmune disorder causing atrophy of the adrenal glands and resulting in the inadequate production of the adrenal hormones, such as cortisol, aldosterone, and androgens. Other causes include pituitary or hypothalamic dysfunction; adrenal hemorrhage; infections, such as tuberculosis and acquired immunodeficiency syndrome (AIDS); or sudden cessation of long-term or high-dose therapy with synthetic glucocorticoids.

Chronic adrenal insufficiency is characterized by progressive weakness, fatigue, decreased appetite, and weight loss. Hyperpigmentation of the skin and mucous membranes is one of the earliest signs. The hyperpigmentation tends to be most significant in sun-exposed areas, joints, and pressure points. Patients with Addison's disease are prone to hypotension, hypoglycemia, hyponatremia, and hyperkalemia. About half of the patients will have gastrointestinal problems such as nausea, vomiting, or diarrhea, which will exacerbate the electrolyte imbalances and increase the potential for cardiac dysrhythmias.

Acute adrenal insufficiency, known as Addisonian crisis, is a life-threatening medical emergency characterized by profound hypotension and shock, which can be rapidly fatal. It is most commonly seen in those patients with Addison's disease who have been exposed to stress such as acute infection, trauma, dehydration, or emotional duress. It has been suggested that adrenal insufficiency should be considered in any patient with unexplained cardiovascular collapse. Vomiting and diarrhea tend to increase the volume depletion and subsequent hypotension. It is not uncommon for patients to report abdominal pain, which tends to mimic an acute abdomen. Fever, weakness, and confusion are also common.

Lifelong replacement hormone therapy and careful monitoring of electrolyte levels are used to treat chronic adrenal insufficiency. Most of this is provided by the primary care physician. Patient education is critical to maintenance of well-being. All patients with Addison's disease are advised to wear a Medic-Alert tag in addition to carrying an identification card detailing their current medication regimen and physician's phone number.

Emergency management is focused on maintenance of the ABCs and, as always, careful monitoring of the patient's cardiac and oxygenation status as well as blood glucose level. Hypoglycemia poses its own threat to the patient's well-being, so blood glucose levels should be assessed and 25 to 50 g of 50 percent dextrose should be administered to patients with levels less than 50 mg/dL or those with altered mental status. Obtaining a baseline 12-lead ECG is important due to the potential for dysrhythmias related to electrolyte imbalance. Fluid resuscitation should be aggressive. Follow your local protocol or contact medical direction for specific orders based on your patient's presentation. Immediate transport to an appropriate facility is imperative because definitive treatment includes the administration of glucocorticoids and/or mineralocorticoids in conjunction with correcting other electrolyte or hormonal abnormalities.

6. **Given a variety of scenarios, develop treatment plans for patients with endocrine disorders.** pp. 227–238

The priorities for someone who is clearly in urgent distress due to endocrine difficulties are the same as for a patient who is affected by a potentially life-threatening emergency of another origin. Ensure adequate airway, breathing (ventilation), and circulation. This is particularly important for someone whose emergency may be affecting the CNS. The brain requires a constant supply of oxygen, glucose, and vitamins. Decreased blood glucose is a common cause of altered mental status and unconsciousness from endocrine emergencies. Significant deprivation of oxygen (anoxia) or glucose (hypoglycemia) can cause seizures or coma. Most endocrine disorders in the prehospital setting will require a minimum of supportive measures, such as airway maintenance, oxygenation, ventilatory management, and hemodynamic monitoring. You should always provide oxygen to a patient with neurologic symptoms secondary to endocrine emergencies and give glucose to any patient found to be hypoglycemic.

Hypoglycemic and hyperglycemic emergencies usually require treatment as soon as possible to prevent progressive damage. In the case of diabetic ketoacidosis, this is especially true because the pathologic features of metabolic acidosis, dehydration, and hypokalemia are considered life threatening. Hyperosmolar hyperglycemic state (HHS) is also associated with severe dehydration and requires early fluid volume resuscitation. Hypoglycemia must be recognized early and treated with oral or IV glucose. As the period of hypoglycemia lengthens, the risk of brain cell death increases due to lack of glucose. IM glucagon should also be considered for hypoglycemic patients who cannot take oral medications or for cases in which IV access is delayed.

Cardiac dysfunction is probably the most likely context within which an emergency call may arise from thyrotoxicosis (usually caused by Graves' disease, as noted earlier). Use of Beta-adrenergic blockers such as propranolol may temporarily reduce cardiac stress, but make sure the patient does not have heart failure before considering use. Glucocorticoid therapy (namely, dexamethasone) is sometimes helpful in quickly reducing the level of circulating T_4.

Case Study Review

Reread the case study on pages 219–220 in Paramedic Care: Medicine; *then, read the following discussion.*

This case study draws attention to the assessment and management of a commonly encountered patient presentation, altered mental status, which is subsequently determined to be due to hypoglycemia, a potentially life-threatening endocrine emergency.

Shauna and Steve arrive at the scene of an "unknown medical emergency." Before their entry into the house, they are joined on the scene by two police officers. Many jurisdictions have dispatch protocols in place that specify dual dispatch of EMS and law enforcement personnel for calls of an unknown nature or those where there has been or is a potential for violence.

As is sometimes the case at emergency scenes, the patient may not have placed the call for service. Whenever possible, it is helpful in those situations in which the 911 call has been placed by a third-party caller to be able to interview that individual to obtain information about the situation on your arrival on the scene. In this case, Mrs. Spencer is a concerned neighbor who is able to provide a great deal of information about the usual residents of this home.

The scene size-up and bystander-provided information raise a high index of suspicion about potential dangers, and the police enter the house first to secure the scene. Only after the scene is declared safe do Shauna and Steve enter. It is important to always remember that there is no benefit to be gained by risking your own personal safety. There is truth to the adage that "fools rush in."

Shauna begins her initial assessment of the patient even as she approaches the teenager identified by Mrs. Spencer as Mark McKenzie. Although he is conscious, his responses to Shauna are incoherent. The overturned furniture and disarray on the scene, along with Mark's confusion, lead Shauna and Steve to consider hypoglycemia or drug use as possible causes for the situation. Sudden changes in mental status or bizarre behavior should always make you consider hypoglycemia. Mark's confusion and apparent violent behavior, along with his tachycardia and diaphoresis, are very typical manifestations of hypoglycemia. The decision to gently restrain Mark is based on his lack of appropriate interaction with his environment as well as concern for his own safety and the safety of all of the personnel on the scene.

Routine assessment of oxygen saturation via pulse oximetry and blood glucose level determination via a glucometer reflect the standard of care for any patient presenting with an altered mental status. Most EMS agencies also routinely obtain pretreatment venous blood samples for analysis at the hospital when dealing with patients presenting with altered mental status.

The glucometer reading of "LOW" indicates a blood glucose level that is less than 50 mg/dL, confirming the presumptive diagnosis of hypoglycemia. Prompt and careful administration of 50 percent dextrose intravenously is the treatment of choice. It is imperative that this medication is administered into a patent IV line in a large vein. Localized venous irritation is likely when small veins are used, and if the dextrose should extravasate, tissue necrosis is common.

Mark's prompt improvement in response to the administration of dextrose is fairly typical. It is not uncommon for diabetics to have no recall of the events that transpired while they were hypoglycemic. The arrival of Mark's mother on the scene allows the EMS personnel to get more information about Mark's usual health status. It is not uncommon for diabetics to have some variation in their usual level of control when their insulin dosages have been changed. Although it makes good sense for diabetics to wear some type of medical alert device on their bodies, it is not uncommon for adolescents to be noncompliant with that practice. Follow your agency's protocols regarding "refusal of transport."

Content Self-Evaluation

MULTIPLE CHOICE

_____ 1. Which of the following is an exocrine gland?
A. Pineal
B. Thymus
C. Salivary
D. Parathyroid
E. Adrenal

_____ 2. The term describing the sum of cellular processes that produce energy and molecules needed for growth and repair is
A. anabolism.
B. catabolism.
C. metabolism.
D. homeostasis.
E. physiology.

_____ 3. The gland that is the connection between the endocrine system and the central nervous system is the
A. pituitary.
B. hypothalamus.
C. thymus.
D. pineal.
E. thyroid.

_____ 4. Diabetes insipidus is a disorder associated with carbohydrate metabolism that is similar to diabetes mellitus.
A. True
B. False

_____ 5. Antidiuretic hormone plays a role in maintaining fluid balance by increasing water reabsorption.
A. True
B. False

_____ 6. All of the following are hormones secreted by the anterior pituitary gland, EXCEPT
A. growth hormone.
B. oxytocin.
C. prolactin.
D. adrenocorticotropic hormone.
E. thyroid-stimulating hormone.

7. In children, the thymus secretes a hormone that is critical to the maturation of T-lymphocytes, which play a significant role in
A. maintaining blood calcium levels.
B. cell-mediated immunity.
C. cellular metabolism.
D. carbohydrate metabolism.
E. gluconeogenesis.

8. All of the following are pancreatic hormones, EXCEPT
A. pancreatic polypeptide.
B. glucagon.
C. somatostatin.
D. cortisol.
E. insulin.

9. Homeostasis of blood glucose is controlled by insulin and
A. polypeptide.
B. glucagon.
C. somatostatin.
D. cortisol.
E. thymosin.

10. The substance that the alpha cells of the pancreas secrete when blood glucose levels fall is
A. polypeptide.
B. glucagon.
C. somatostatin.
D. cortisol.
E. insulin.

11. The substance secreted by the beta cells of the pancreas when blood glucose levels rise is
A. polypeptide.
B. glucagon.
C. somatostatin.
D. cortisol.
E. insulin.

12. Insulin's primary function is to
A. metabolize glucose at the cellular level.
B. free glucose from muscle storage sites.
C. promote cell uptake of glucose.
D. store glucose at the cellular level.
E. enhance the function of glucagon.

13. The production of glucose by the processes of glycogenolysis and gluconeogenesis is triggered by
A. polypeptide.
B. glucagon.
C. somatostatin.
D. cortisol.
E. insulin.

14. All of the following are hormones secreted by the adrenal glands, EXCEPT
A. epinephrine.
B. cortisol.
C. somatostatin.
D. norepinephrine.
E. aldosterone.

15. Glucocorticoids play a role in maintaining blood glucose levels by promoting gluconeogenesis and
A. decreasing glucose utilization.
B. increasing glucose utilization.
C. promoting salt and fluid retention.
D. decreasing salt and fluid retention.
E. potentiating the effects of catecholamines.

16. Catecholamines such as epinephrine and norepinephrine are hormones secreted by the adrenal medulla.
A. True
B. False

©2013 Pearson Education, Inc.
Paramedic Care: Principles & Practice, Vol. 4, 4th Ed.

_____ 17. The primary function of aldosterone is to
  A. regulate sodium and potassium excretion.
  B. regulate calcium and magnesium excretion.
  C. promote gluconeogenesis.
  D. inhibit gluconeogenesis.
  E. stimulate glucocorticoid production.

_____ 18. Diabetes mellitus is caused by the inadequate production or activity of
  A. polypeptide.   D. cortisol.
  B. glucagon.   E. insulin.
  C. somatostatin.

_____ 19. Osmotic diuresis, a characteristic of untreated diabetes, contributes to the development of
  A. polydipsia and polyphagia.   D. polyuria.
  B. polydipsia and polyuria.   E. polyphagia.
  C. polyuria and polyphagia.

_____ 20. All of the following are signs and symptoms of diabetic ketoacidosis, EXCEPT
  A. abdominal pain.   D. cold, clammy skin.
  B. deep, rapid respirations.   E. tachycardia.
  C. decreased mental function.

_____ 21. Diabetic ketoacidosis, characterized by high blood glucose and metabolic acidosis, occurs as a
         result of all of the following, EXCEPT
  A. profound insulin deficiency.   D. physiological stress.
  B. decreased glucagon activity.   E. overexertion.
  C. cessation of insulin injections.

_____ 22. Kussmaul's respirations are a primary compensatory mechanism for reducing acidosis in the
         patient with diabetic ketoacidosis.
  A. True
  B. False

_____ 23. The most important sign or symptom associated with hypoglycemia is
  A. tachycardia.   D. polydipsia.
  B. cool, clammy skin.   E. polyphagia.
  C. altered mental status.

_____ 24. Hyperglycemic hyperosmolar nonketotic acidosis differs from diabetic ketoacidosis because
         significant production of ketone bodies is prevented by the action of
  A. polypeptide.   D. cortisol.
  B. glucagon.   E. insulin.
  C. somatostatin.

_____ 25. Even in the absence of a blood glucose level, altered mental status in a known diabetic should
         always be treated with 50 percent dextrose.
  A. True
  B. False

_____ 26. All of the following are signs and symptoms associated with thyrotoxic crisis, EXCEPT
  A. high fever.   D. delirium.
  B. bradycardia.   E. vomiting.
  C. hypotension.

_____ 27. Potential triggers for myxedema coma include all of the following, EXCEPT
  A. excessive thyroid medication.   D. cold environment.
  B. infection.   E. CNS depressants.
  C. trauma.

_____ 28. Signs and symptoms associated with myxedema coma include all of the following, EXCEPT
    A. hypothermia.
    B. decreased mental status.
    C. low-amplitude bradycardia.
    D. CO_2 retention.
    E. seizures.

_____ 29. Long-term exposure to excess glucocorticoids or abnormalities to either the adrenal cortex or pituitary gland may cause hyperadrenalism.
    A. True
    B. False

_____ 30. Addison's disease is characterized by high corticosteroid activity that causes major disturbances in water and electrolyte balance.
    A. True
    B. False

MATCHING

Write the letter of the term in the space provided next to the appropriate definition.

  A. homeostasis

  B. hormone

  C. anabolism

  D. catabolism

  E. antidiuretic hormone

  F. oxytocin

  G. calcitonin

  H. gluconeogenesis

  I. glycogenolysis

  J. Addisonian crisis

_____ 31. Crisis form of shock associated with adrenocortical insufficiency that is characterized by profound hypotension and electrolyte imbalance

_____ 32. Phase of metabolism associated with building molecules of higher complexity

_____ 33. Hormone that increases water reabsorption by the kidneys

_____ 34. Conversion of protein and fat to form glucose

_____ 35. Hormone responsible for lowering blood calcium levels

_____ 36. Phase of metabolism associated with the breakdown of complex molecules

_____ 37. Hormone that causes uterine contraction and lactation

_____ 38. Breakdown of glycogen to form glucose

_____ 39. Chemical substance released to control or affect processes in other organs or body systems

_____ 40. The natural tendency of the body to keep the internal environment and metabolism at a steady, normal level

©2013 Pearson Education, Inc.
Paramedic Care: Principles & Practice, Vol. 4, 4th Ed.

Special Project

Label the Diagram

Write the names of the endocrine glands marked A through I in the figure shown below and then list at least one of the hormones secreted by each gland.

A. _____

B. _____

C. _____

D. _____

E. _____

F. _____

G. _____

H. _____

I. _____

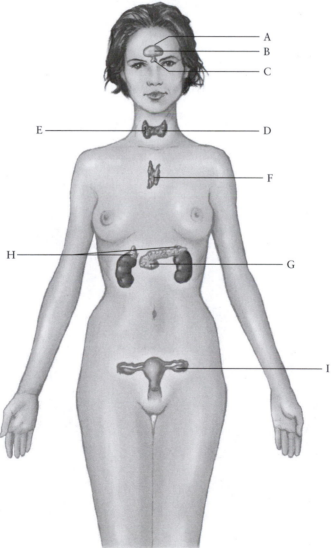

Immunology

Review of Chapter Objectives

After reading this chapter, you should be able to:

1. Define key terms introduced in this chapter.

Knowing and being able to apply the key terms in each chapter is critical to understanding chapter concepts. Write the list of key terms. Then write the definition of each one in your own words. Check your understanding by confirming the definitions in the text glossary. Correct any misunderstandings. Create a study aid by writing each key term on the front of an index card and the definition on the back. Use the cards to quiz yourself, or to have someone quiz you.

2. Relate the anatomy and physiology of the immune system to the pathophysiology and assessment of patients with allergies and anaphylaxis. **pp. 243–251**

The immune system is a complex system responsible for combating infection. Components of the immune system can be found in the blood, the bone marrow, and the lymphatic system. The immune response is a complex cascade of events that occurs following activation by an invading substance.

Following exposure to a particular antigen, large quantities of IgE antibodies are released. These antibodies attach to the membranes of basophils and mast cells, causing them to release histamine, heparin, and other chemicals into the surrounding tissue. The release of these chemical mediators causes a response in the cardiovascular, respiratory, and gastrointestinal systems as well as in the skin.

The signs and symptoms associated with allergy and anaphylaxis are due to the physiological changes triggered by the chemical mediators of the immune response that are released from the basophils and mast cells. Histamine is the primary mediator of all allergic reactions. It is a potent substance that causes bronchoconstriction, vasodilation and increased vascular permeability, and increased intestinal motility. Other chemical substances are also released that have effects similar to or synergistic with histamine, such as slow-reacting substance of anaphylaxis (SRS-A), which results in an asthma-like attack or asphyxia. An allergic reaction is an exaggerated immune response to a foreign protein or other substance; anaphylaxis is an unusual or exaggerated allergic reaction to a foreign protein or other substance.

An antigen (allergen) is any substance that is capable, under appropriate conditions, of inducing a specific immune response. An antibody is a member of a unique class of chemicals that are manufactured by specialized cells of the immune system. The antibody is the principal agent of a chemical attack on an invading substance. Following exposure to an antigen, antibodies are released from cells of the immune system. The antibodies attach themselves to the invading substance so it can be removed from the body by other cells of the immune system.

Allergens can enter the body through various routes, including oral ingestion, inhalation, topically, and through injection or envenomation. The vast majority of anaphylactic reactions result from injection or envenomation.

The signs and symptoms of anaphylaxis begin within 30 to 60 seconds after exposure for the vast majority of patients. The more rapid the onset, the more severe the patient presentation. Respiratory manifestations of anaphylaxis include laryngeal edema and bronchoconstriction. Cardiovascular symptoms include tachycardia plus massive vasodilation resulting in profound hypotension. The combination of respiratory and cardiovascular signs will lead to a rapid deterioration of the patient's mental status. Generalized flushing and urticaria are common, as is angioedema about the head, face, and neck. Nausea, vomiting, and diarrhea may accompany hypermotility of the gastrointestinal tract.

3. **Adapt the scene size-up, primary assessment, patient history, secondary assessment, and use of monitoring technology to meet the needs of patients with complaints and presentations related to allergies and anaphylaxis.** pp. 247–248

During the scene size-up, your general impression will be very important, as you will be looking for clues that can rapidly indicate the patient's condition. As a paramedic, you will adapt your assessment process to rapidly identify signs and symptoms of anaphylaxis and severe allergic reactions. These conditions are time sensitive and must be treated quickly for patient survival. The causes of anaphylaxis and severe allergic reactions are numerous. One of the first questions you will answer will be whether there is a history of allergies or anaphylaxis. Common allergens include drugs, foods, animals, insects, fungi and molds, and radiology contrast materials. Evaluate the patient's level of consciousness using the AVPU method, as well as speech, skin appearance, and posture. The patient's appearance and work of breathing will also provide clues to the patient's level of hypersensitivity reaction. Complete your primary ABCD assessment and recognize any findings that would indicate anaphylaxis or a severe allergic reaction. Your secondary assessment should include a detailed exam of the skin, respiratory system, and cardiovascular system; accurate history; and physical exam with a full set of vital signs. Initiate all appropriate monitoring devices. For example, alterations in ventilatory function may be observed in a patient experiencing an allergic reaction or anaphylaxis. Capnography measures exhaled or end-tidal carbon dioxide (CO_2) and can assist the paramedic in evaluating the ventilation rate and quality in such a patient. Pulse oximetry is used to monitor a patient's general state of perfusion. Patients in anaphylaxis are at risk for respiratory distress, respiratory arrest, and anaphylactic shock, so frequent assessment of the airway, breathing, and circulation is vital. Because the treatment for anaphylaxis and severe allergic reaction includes epinephrine, every patient who receives epinephrine must have continuous cardiac monitoring and transport.

4. **Use a process of clinical reasoning to guide and interpret the patient assessment and management process for patients with allergies and anaphylaxis.** pp. 247–251

As a paramedic, it is vital that you develop your clinical reasoning process to quickly recognize and treat severe allergic reactions and anaphylaxis to improve patient outcome. This is because diagnosis and treatment with many hypersensitivity reactions is time sensitive. Develop an organized general impression to rapidly identify signs and symptoms of allergies and anaphylaxis. This will include obtaining an accurate history and a detailed physical exam.

The central physiological action in severe allergic reaction and anaphylaxis is the massive release of histamine and other chemical mediators of the immune system. The resultant bronchospasm, airway edema, peripheral vasodilation, and increased capillary permeability can take a patient from his usual state of health to the brink of death in mere seconds. This chemically caused transformation is readily evident in the patient's clinical presentation: air hunger, dyspnea, angioedema, tachycardia, and hypotension. Your timely intervention is imperative to your patient's survival.

The first priority in the management of allergic reactions and anaphylaxis is to establish and maintain the patient's airway. Administer oxygen immediately along with ventilatory support as needed. You should be prepared to intubate, recognizing that laryngeal edema may change the size and appearance of the airway. Establish vascular access as soon as possible and be prepared to run crystalloid solutions wide open if the patient is hypotensive.

Epinephrine is the drug of choice for severe allergic reaction and anaphylaxis. In mild to moderate cases, administer 0.3 to 0.5 mg of 1:1,000 epinephrine subcutaneously or IM; in severe reactions and anaphylaxis, administer 0.3 to 0.5 mg of intravenous 1:10,000 epinephrine. Remember that the effects of epinephrine wear off quickly, so be prepared to repeat boluses in 3 to 5 minutes. It may be necessary to establish a continuous epinephrine infusion.

Antihistamines, such as diphenhydramine, are widely used for the management of allergic reactions due to their ability to block histamine receptors. The usual dosage is 25 to 50 mg given either intravenously or intramuscularly. It may also be helpful to administer beta agonist agents via hand-held nebulizer to help reverse bronchospasm. Adult patients should receive 0.5 mL of albuterol in 3 mL of normal saline.

Selective histamine blockers have been available for the last 15–20 years. These are primarily H_2 blockers and are used to treat ulcer disease. Blockage of the H_2 receptors decreases gastric acid secretion. However, H_2 receptors are also present in the peripheral blood vessels. Administration of H_2 blockers conceivably will reverse some of the vasodilation associated with anaphylaxis. The two most frequently used H_2 blockers are cimetadine (Tagamet) and ranitidine (Zantac). Typically, 300 mg of cimetadine or 50 mg of ranitidine are administered by slow intravenous push (over 3–5 minutes).

Corticosteroids are important in the treatment and prevention of anaphylaxis. Although they are of little benefit in the initial stages of treatment, they help suppress the inflammatory response associated with these emergencies. Commonly used corticosteroids include methylprednisolone (Solu-Medrol), hydrocortisone (Solu-Cortef), and dexamethasone (Decadron).

Severe and prolonged anaphylactic reactions may require the use of potent vasopressors to support blood pressure. Use these medications in conjunction with first-line therapy and adequate fluid resuscitation. Commonly used agents include dopamine, norepinephrine, and epinephrine. These medications are prepared as infusions and are continuously administered to support blood pressure and cardiac output.

As is always the case, your management approach should be dictated by local protocols. Other medications that may be used to manage severe anaphylaxis include corticosteroids, such as SoluMedrol, to suppress the inflammatory response, or vasopressors, such as dopamine, to enhance cardiac output. Remember that volume resuscitation with isotonic fluids before initiating vasopressor therapy is important.

5. **Given a variety of scenarios, develop treatment plans for patients with allergies and anaphylaxis.** pp. 247–251

The priorities for someone who is clearly in urgent distress due to an allergic reaction or anaphylaxis are the same as for a patient who is affected by a potentially life-threatening emergency of another origin. Ensure adequate airway, breathing (ventilation), and circulation. This is particularly important for someone whose emergency may be affecting the respiratory and cardiovascular systems. Most hypersensitivity reactions in the prehospital setting will require a minimum of supportive measures, such as airway maintenance, oxygenation, ventilatory management, and hemodynamic monitoring. You should always provide oxygen to a patient with signs and symptoms of a hypersensitivity reaction and give epinephrine to patients in anaphylaxis. Common manifestations of mild (nonanaphylactic) allergic reactions include itching, rash, and urticaria. Patients with simple itching and nonurticarial rashes may be treated with antihistamines alone. In addition to antihistamines, epinephrine is often necessary for the treatment of urticaria.

Any patient suffering an allergic reaction who exhibits dyspnea or wheezing should receive supplemental oxygen. This should be followed by intramuscular epinephrine 1:1,000. Lesser allergic reactions that are not accompanied by hypotension or airway problems can be adequately treated with epinephrine 1:1,000 administered intramuscularly. Epinephrine 1:1,000 contains 1 mg of epinephrine in 1 mL of solvent. When administered into the muscle tissue, the drug is absorbed more slowly and the effect prolonged. The intramuscular dose is the same as the subcutaneous dose formerly used (0.3–0.5 mg). The intramuscular route should not be used in severe anaphylaxis for which, as noted earlier, IV epinephrine should be administered.

Case Study Review

Reread the case study on page 242 in Paramedic Care: Medicine; *then, read the following discussion.*

This case study draws attention to the typical presentation and management for a patient experiencing severe anaphylaxis.

The majority of fatal anaphylaxis cases in the United States are attributed to injections, usually of penicillin. It is for this reason that patients receiving injections in an outpatient setting are asked to remain on site for at least 20 to 30 minutes afterward to ensure the availability of emergency care should the need arise. In this case, the injection was an immunization received just 15 minutes earlier. The patient's immediate response was a red rash and generalized itching that quickly progressed to marked respiratory compromise and cardiovascular collapse. The clinic staff had administered oxygen via a nasal cannula and was setting up an IV.

With the arrival of Steve and Beth on the scene, appropriate emergency care was quickly initiated; the nasal cannula was replaced with high-concentration oxygen via nonrebreather mask, keeping an ET kit readily accessible. Beth established vascular access and initiated fluid resuscitation to correct massive vasodilation, while Steve administered epinephrine intramuscularly to counteract the immune system response. Although the patient showed improvement within 2 minutes of the epinephrine administration, Steve knew that the medication wears off quickly and was prepared to administer IV 1:10,000 epinephrine in case the improvement did not continue. Diphenhydramine was also administered to block the histamine receptors. All of these efforts were effective in reversing the anaphylaxis, and the patient was treated in the emergency department (ED) with corticosteroids to suppress the immune response and additional IV fluids, and was released within 2 hours.

Subsequent questioning at the hospital revealed that this patient had received a tetanus injection at the clinic and that he had a similar reaction with a prior tetanus immunization. This situation highlights the importance of patient education about the potential for repeat and possibly more severe allergic reactions. It also underscores the importance for every health care professional to carefully question patients about allergies or untoward responses to medication prior to administering any drug.

Content Self-Evaluation

MULTIPLE CHOICE

_____ 1. The type of immunity resulting from a direct attack on a foreign substance by specialized cells of the immune system is known as
   A. humoral.
   B. cellular.
   C. natural.
   D. acquired.
   E. genetic.

_____ 2. The unique class of chemicals that are manufactured by specialized cells of the immune system to attack invading foreign proteins is
   A. allergens.
   B. antigens.
   C. toxins.
   D. antibodies.
   E. pathogens.

_____ 3. Any substance that is capable, under appropriate conditions, of inducing a specific immune response is a(n)
   A. immunoglobulin.
   B. antigen.
   C. toxin.
   D. antibody.
   E. pathogen.

©2013 Pearson Education, Inc.
Paramedic Care: Principles & Practice, Vol. 4, 4th Ed.

4. The type of immunity that is present at birth and has no relation to a previous exposure to a particular antigen is
- **A.** humoral.
- **B.** cellular.
- **C.** natural.
- **D.** acquired.
- **E.** genetic.

5. The type of immunity that develops over time as a result of exposure to an antigen is
- **A.** humoral.
- **B.** cellular.
- **C.** natural.
- **D.** acquired.
- **E.** genetic.

6. An allergic reaction is best defined as an exaggerated, sometimes potentially life-threatening response by the immune system to a foreign substance.
- **A.** True
- **B.** False

7. All of the following are common allergens, EXCEPT
- **A.** insect stings.
- **B.** drugs.
- **C.** antibodies.
- **D.** seafood.
- **E.** radiology contrast materials.

8. Most anaphylactic reactions occur as a result of
- **A.** inhalation.
- **B.** ingestion.
- **C.** injection.
- **D.** topical exposure.
- **E.** genetics.

9. The antibody most commonly associated with hypersensitivity reactions is
- **A.** IgA.
- **B.** IgD.
- **C.** IgE.
- **D.** IgG.
- **E.** IgM.

10. The primary chemical mediator of an allergic reaction is
- **A.** heparin.
- **B.** histamine.
- **C.** SRS-A.
- **D.** basophil.
- **E.** the mast cell.

11. All of the following are physiological effects associated with the release of the chemical mediators of anaphylaxis, EXCEPT
- **A.** bronchodilation.
- **B.** vasodilation.
- **C.** increased intestinal motility.
- **D.** increased vascular permeability.
- **E.** secretion of gastric acids.

12. Urticaria, a wheal and flare reaction characterized by red raised bumps that appear on the skin, is due to
- **A.** bronchodilation.
- **B.** vasoconstriction.
- **C.** increased intestinal motility.
- **D.** increased vascular permeability.
- **E.** secretion of gastric acids.

13. The first-line parenteral drug for the management of anaphylaxis is
- **A.** oxygen.
- **B.** diphenhydramine.
- **C.** epinephrine.
- **D.** methylprednisolone.
- **E.** albuterol.

14. The first priority when responding to a patient with an anaphylactic reaction is to
- **A.** protect the airway.
- **B.** administer diphenhydramine.
- **C.** stabilize the cervical spine.
- **D.** assure scene safety.
- **E.** establish vascular access.

_____ **15.** Hypotension that is seen in severe anaphylaxis is due to

    A. internal hemorrhage.   **D.** vasodilation.

    B. inadequate oxygenation.   **E.** gastrointestinal hypermotility.

    C. bradycardia.

MATCHING

Write the letter of the drug in the space provided next to the phrase that best describes its action.

A. dopamine

B. epinephrine

C. diphenhydramine

D. methylprednisolone

E. albuterol

_____ **16.** Beta agonist that reverses bronchospasm

_____ **17.** Blocks histamine receptors

_____ **18.** Suppresses inflammatory response

_____ **19.** Sympathetic agonist that improves cardiac output

_____ **20.** Potent vasopressor to support blood pressure

Special Project

Completing Tables

A. _Complete the following table by listing the common systemic signs and symptoms associated with allergies and anaphylaxis._

System	Signs and Symptoms
Skin	
Respiratory system	
Cardiovascular system	
Gastrointestinal system	
Nervous system	

B. _Complete the following table by listing the actions associated with each drug._

Drug	Action
Albuterol	
Diphenhydramine	
Dopamine	
Epinephrine	
Methylprednisolone	

©2013 Pearson Education, Inc.
Paramedic Care: Principles & Practice, Vol. 4, 4th Ed.

6

Gastroenterology

Review of Chapter Objectives

After reading this chapter, you should be able to:

1. **Define key terms introduced in this chapter.**

   Knowing and being able to apply the key terms in each chapter is critical to understanding chapter concepts. Write the list of key terms. Then write the definition of each one in your own words. Check your understanding by confirming the definitions in the text glossary. Correct any misunderstandings. Create a study aid by writing each key term on the front of an index card and the definition on the back. Use the cards to quiz yourself, or to have someone quiz you.

2. **Identify patients with risk factors for gastrointestinal emergencies.** **p. 271**

   Many of the most common risk factors are self-induced by patients, and they include excessive alcohol consumption and tobacco use, stress, ingestion of caustic substances, and poor bowel habits. Because of the various risk factors and possible causes of gastrointestinal (GI) emergencies, it is particularly important that you know how to complete a thorough focused history and examination before making a field diagnosis, how to assess the seriousness of the emergency, and possible prevention strategies to minimize organ damage.

   Although patients should never be stereotyped based on race or sex, both appear to be risk factors for several gastroenterological problems. Because of this, you should consider racial and gender differences as they may affect various disease states. For example, acute pancreatis affects males more commonly than females. The hospitalization rate for acute pancreatitis per 100,000 patients is three times higher in black patients when compared to their white counterparts.

   Cholecystitis also seems to have racial and gender predilections. Pima Indians and Scandinavians have the highest risk for gallstones and, subsequently, cholecystitis. In the United States, whites have a higher incidence of cholecystitis than blacks. Asians and sub-Saharan Africans have an extremely low risk of cholecystitis. Cholecystitis is two to three times more frequent in females than in males.

3. **Relate the anatomy and physiology of the gastrointestinal system to the pathophysiology and assessment of patients with gastrointestinal disorders.** **pp. 256–259**

   The GI tract is a long system that extends from the mouth to the anus and is divided structurally and functionally into different parts. In general, the GI system is divided into the upper and lower GI tracts. The upper GI tract includes the mouth, esophagus, stomach, and duodenum, whereas the lower GI tract includes the remainder of the small intestine and the large intestine, rectum, and anus. In the upper GI tract, food is ingested and preliminary physical and chemical digestion is begun. In the lower GI tract, digestion of food is completed, nutrients are absorbed into the body, and remaining fiber, intestinal bacteria, and other materials are eliminated through the anus as feces. In addition, three additional organs, the liver, gallbladder, and pancreas, are intimately associated with the GI system both structurally (through connections with the duodenum) and functionally. The vermiform appendix, a blind sac found at the junction of the small and large intestines, does not have any apparent physiological role in GI function but is important to you because of the inflammatory condition appendicitis, which you will see in patients in the field.

Sudden-onset, or acute, pain can be caused by a variety of mechanisms, one of which is inflammation. Inflammation of hollow organs such as the appendix or gallbladder produces pain that is characteristically poorly localized and crampy in nature (visceral pain). When inflammation is widespread within the abdomen, as happens after an inflamed appendix ruptures, inflammation of the peritoneal membrane (peritonitis) results in pain that is usually localized and sharp in nature (somatic pain). It is important for you to become familiar with the different types of pain because they often represent progressive stages in an inflammatory condition—for example, pain from appendicitis that changes from visceral to somatic pain over time.

4. **Adapt the scene size-up, primary assessment, patient history, secondary assessment, and use of monitoring technology to meet the needs of patients with complaints and presentations related to gastrointestinal disorders.**   pp. 257–259

During the scene size-up, your general impression will be very important, as you will be looking for clues that can indicate the patient's condition. The causes of GI disorders are numerous. One of the first questions you will answer will be if there is a history of GI disease such as gastroesophageal reflux disease (GERD), diverticulosis, pancreatitis, or cholecystitis. Evaluate the patient's level of consciousness using the AVPU method, as well as speech, skin appearance, and posture. The patient's emotional status may also provide clues to the patient's developing condition that may be altered due to pain, volume loss, or hemorrhage.

Complete your primary ABCD assessment and recognize any findings that would indicate a GI emergency. Always start with the least invasive step, visual inspection. This includes checking patient appearance and positioning as well as visually inspecting the abdomen for signs of distention or discoloration. Your secondary assessment should include an abdominal assessment, accurate history, and physical exam with a full set of vital signs. Initiate all appropriate monitoring devices. For example, alterations in ventilatory function may be observed in a patient experiencing a GI emergency associated with sever hemorrhage or volume loss. Capnography measures exhaled or end-tidal carbon dioxide (CO_2) and can assist the paramedic in evaluating the ventilation rate and quality in such a patient. Pulse oximetry is used to monitor a patient's general state of perfusion. Be sure to get a complete set of baseline vital signs early in the process. Changes in vitals along with alterations in mental status may indicate early shock due to hemorrhage or other processes. Auscultation and percussion often do NOT provide useful information in the field; however, if you do auscultate, be sure to do so before palpating in order to avoid perturbation in abdominal sounds. Palpation with gentle pressure should start in the *least* affected area and move toward the point of greatest pain. Remember to immediately stop palpation if you feel any pulsation. Further palpation may cause rupture of the affected blood vessel or organ.

Patients with abdominal pain are at risk for vomiting, aspiration, and hypovolemic shock, so frequent assessment of the airway, breathing, and circulation is vital. Abdominal pain and nausea/vomiting are also commonly associated with acute coronary syndromes (ACS) in special populations such as women, the elderly, and diabetics. Therefore, it is important to perform appropriate electrocardiogram (ECG) monitoring, including a 12-lead/15-lead or 18-lead ECG, as part of your assessment.

5. **Use a process of clinical reasoning to guide and interpret the patient assessment and management process for patients with gastrointestinal disorders.**   pp. 257–259

As a paramedic, it is vital that you develop your clinical reasoning process to quickly recognize and treat acute GI emergencies to improve patient outcome. This is because diagnosis and treatment with many acute GI emergencies is time-sensitive. Develop an organized general impression to rapidly identify signs and symptoms of GI emergencies. This will include obtaining an accurate history.

Local inflammation within the GI tract often produces visceral pain associated with sympathetic nervous system stimulation (which typically results in nausea, vomiting, diaphoresis, and tachycardia). General inflammation within the abdomen often includes bacterial or chemical irritation of the peritoneum (the origins of peritonitis) and is thus associated with increasingly widespread somatic pain. Peritonitis (inflammation of the peritoneum) often represents the end stage of a generalized inflammatory or hemorrhagic process; as such, it is often associated with the most significant physical signs, including altered vitals or overt shock. Because pain associated with peritonitis is often very severe, it is typical to find the patient lying with knees to chest because this position minimizes stretch on the already inflamed peritoneum.

Assessment includes initial size-up, SAMPLE focused history with attention to current complaint, personal medical and family history, and physical examination. History of present illness will reveal whether the condition is acute, chronic, or an acute flare-up of a chronic problem. The relation of pain (if any) with last oral intake may suggest ulcers (in which eating typically relieves pain) or, in contrast, cholecystitis (where pain may worsen after eating, particularly a fatty meal). The presence of chest pain rather than abdominal pain (or in addition to abdominal pain) may mean a condition has generated referred pain; examples include GERD, gastric or duodenal ulcers, and cholecystitis. A change in nature of pain from visceral to somatic may infer a progression of abdominal pathology. Always remember before starting the physical exam that the majority of GI emergencies entail bleeding from the upper or lower GI tract. Watch for changes in vital signs that may indicate hemorrhage and shock. Evaluate your visual inspection of the abdomen, as well as an examination of any vomitus or stool.

The primary treatment for GI emergencies is to rapidly identify signs and symptoms of GI emergencies that can lead to shock. In cases not associated with alarm symptoms and shock, pain management and supportive measures are appropriate. Management of patients presenting with signs and symptoms of shock can include oxygenation, ventilatory assistance, fluid resuscitation, suctioning, assisting ventilations, keeping the patient warm, and ECG monitoring. In addition, based on local protocols, you may be initiating an additional IV. Make a strong effort to make the patient comfortable, keep NPO, prevent aspiration, and be prepared for developing shock. Consider the following:

- *Airway and breathing.* Position any patient that you suspect has a GI emergency in the position most comfortable for the patient. Protect the airway. Because nausea and vomiting are common in patients with abdominal pain, you should have an emesis container close and have suction ready. Keep the patient NPO.
- *Circulatory support.* Establish at least one IV access based on your local protocols. It is important to have an accessible route for fluid volume resuscitation and medications. Some patients may need an additional IV if rapid blood loss is possible, such as in patients with esophageal varices or upper GI bleeding.
- *Pharmacological interventions.* Medications are available to treat signs and symptoms in patients with GI emergencies. When calling for orders, consider that the initial dose may not sufficiently alleviate the patient's nausea or pain. Request an initial dose and a prn dose with your initial contact with medical direction. This will keep you from being unprepared or having to call again later. Medications vary, but can include antiemetics, non-narcotic analgesics, narcotic analgesics, H2 blockers, and proton-pump inhibitors, to name a few.
- *Psychological support.* Patients suffering from a GI emergency, acute or chronic, are likely also to suffer anxiety, depression, or anger. The experiences associated with GI emergencies are often frightening for patients because the pain is often intense and many patients believe the abdominal pain is associated with internal hemorrhage. Some GI symptoms may be perceived as embarrassing to patients, such as lower GI bleeds or diarrhea resulting in fecal incontinence. Provide the patient with effective therapeutic communication and emotional support and explain the treatment regimen. In most cases, it is appropriate to explain to the patient what may be occurring and why. Careful explanation and emotional support will help allay anxiety and apprehension.
- *Transport considerations.* Assess, provide emergency care, and transport the patient as quickly and safely as possible. Rapidly transport any patient who is at risk for shock or is demonstrating signs of shock secondary to a GI emergency. Constantly reevaluate and monitor the patient's airway, breathing, circulation, and neurologic status. In addition, reevaluate the patient's nausea and pain scale. Provide additional antiemetics and analgesics as appropriate.

6. **Describe the pathophysiology of specific gastrointestinal problems, including problems in the following classifications:**

   a. **Upper gastrointestinal tract disorders** pp. 259–264

   The six most common causes of hemorrhage in the upper GI tract are (in descending order) peptic ulcer disease, gastritis, variceal rupture, Mallory-Weiss syndrome (esophageal laceration, generally secondary to vomiting), esophagitis, and duodenitis. Note that ulcers and gastritis account for 75 percent of cases (with 50 percent due to ulcers). Irritation and erosion of the GI lining is the most common pathophysiological basis for bleeding, and involvement of the stomach lining underlies 75 percent of upper GI bleeds. Because most such cases involve chronic, low-level hemorrhage, many patients can be cared for on an outpatient basis. However, brisk upper GI bleeds may be life threatening. Assessment findings that can help to distinguish the severity of the bleed include presence and severity of hematemesis (vomiting of blood) and/or melena (passage of partially digested blood represented as dark, tarry stools). Look for subtle signs of shock and manage accordingly. Besides shock, another potentially grave complication of some bleeds is airway compromise due to aspiration of vomitus (when vomiting is present). Be sure to support the airway, and beware of vomiting in patients who are lying in a supine position. A patient with pain characteristic of peritonitis, especially with discoloration or bulging of the abdomen, may have life-threatening blood loss. General management centers on airway, oxygenation, and circulatory status. Position the patient to minimize risk of aspiration, provide high-concentration oxygen, and start a large-bore IV line. Base your fluid resuscitation on patient condition and response to treatment.

   b. **Lower gastrointestinal tract disorders** pp. 264–270

   Hemorrhage from the lower GI tract is most common in association with chronic medical conditions and the anatomical changes of advancing age. The most common causes include diverticulosis, colorectal lesions, and inflammatory bowel disease. Remember that lower GI bleeds rarely result in the massive hemorrhage that can be associated with esophageal or stomach pathology. Assessment should establish whether the problem is new in onset or chronic (be sure to look for scars from previous surgical procedures). Questions about stool or inspection of stool may show melena, which usually indicates a slow lower GI bleed, or bright red blood, which indicates severe hemorrhage with rapid passage through the intestines or a source in the distal colon. Distal GI causes include hemorrhoids and rectal fissures. Be sure to assess for abdominal signs such as discoloration or bulging and maintain ongoing checks for signs of early shock. General management centers on the patient's physiological status. Watch airway and oxygenation closely, and use oxygen if necessary. Establish IV access and fluid resuscitation based on patient's findings or shift in findings over time. If there are any signs of significant blood loss, be sure one IV line is available for blood transfusion.

   c. **Accessory organ diseases** pp. 270–273

   The GI tract has three closely associated organs, the liver, gallbladder, and pancreas, as well as the small structure called the vermiform appendix. Accessory organ emergencies can arise in all four locations.

   A review of specific illnesses follows.

Acute gastroenteritis p. 262

Acute gastroenteritis involves inflammation of the stomach and intestines associated with sudden-onset vomiting, diarrhea, or both. It is very common; the underlying inflammation causes erosion of the mucosal and submucosal layers of the GI tract with blood loss and damage to the intestinal villi. Triggers can include alcohol or tobacco use, use of nonsteroidal anti-inflammatory agents, stress, and GI or systemic infection. The most common and striking finding is copious volumes of watery diarrhea secondary to damage to the intestinal lining. Diarrhea may contain blood.

   In general, patients are often febrile and suffering from general malaise as well as nausea and vomiting. Watch for any signs of early shock such as altered mental status, development of pale, clammy skin, or changes in vitals. Abdominal tenderness is common; distention is uncommon unless significant amounts of gas are in the intestines. In cases of severe dehydration, watch for problems such as cardiac dysrhythmia secondary to electrolyte disturbance. Management is supportive and palliative, with any needed support for airway (position to minimize odds of aspiration), oxygenation, or circulation. Fluid resuscitation via oral or IV route may be indicated. Be sure you take appropriate precautions during patient care to prevent spread of any possible infectious disease.

©2013 Pearson Education, Inc.
Paramedic Care: Principles & Practice, Vol. 4, 4th Ed.

Acute hepatitis
p. 273

Acute hepatitis, inflammation of the liver, can result from any injury to liver cells associated with an infectious or inflammatory process. Viral hepatitis is the most common form, and alcoholic hepatitis secondary to cirrhosis is also common. Symptoms range from mild manifestations to overt liver failure and death, and mortality is high due to the wide range of potential causes. You will find that presentation often parallels the severity of hepatitis. Common complaints include right upper quadrant tenderness not relieved by eating or antacids and development of clay-colored stools (this secondary to decreased bile production). If bilirubin retention exists, scleral icterus and jaundice may be present. Palpation may reveal liver enlargement, and fever may be due to infection or tissue necrosis. Presence of cool, clammy, diaphoretic skin suggests hemorrhage of a hepatic lesion. Secure ABCs and establish IV access. Be particularly careful in consideration of use of any pharmacological agent because liver failure may impair drug metabolism. Never forget to use personal protective equipment (PPE) and to use body substance isolation (BSI) precautions.

Appendicitis
p. 270

Appendicitis is inflammation of the vermiform appendix. You will encounter acute appendicitis in the field, most commonly in older children and young adults. Untreated appendicitis can result in rupture with subsequent peritonitis. The pathophysiology has parallels to that of diverticulitis. The appendix becomes obstructed with fecal material, and the resultant inflammation and infection cause the characteristic discomfort, which may present initially as periumbilical, visceral pain, but later becomes the well-known somatic, right lower quadrant pain. Somatic pain or signs of peritonitis suggest significant inflammation with ischemia or infarction of the appendix or appendiceal rupture, respectively. Other findings such as fever, anorexia, and nausea or vomiting relate to the stage of appendiceal inflammation. Exam findings range from vague abdominal discomfort on palpation (in early cases) to clear peritonitis. Management during transport centers on positioning for comfort, managing airway to avoid aspiration, and establishing IV access. Monitor as you would for bowel obstruction and be aware of any early signs of shock.

Bowel obstruction
p. 268

Bowel obstruction involves partial or complete blockage of a portion of the small or large intestine. Rapid diagnosis and treatment are essential to avoid complications such as bowel infarction. The four most common causes are hernias, intussusception, volvulus, and adhesions. The most common site is the small intestine due to smaller diameter and greater length and motility of intestinal loops. Chronic obstruction is often due to a progressive process such as tumor growth or adhesions. Acute obstruction may be due to ingestion of a foreign body or incarceration and strangulation of a hernia or loop of intussuscepted bowel. Findings suggestive of obstruction include pain (which is often diffuse and visceral in nature) and vomiting. The character of the vomitus (for example, feces-like material) may suggest the approximate site of the obstruction. Significant ischemia or infarction is suggested by findings of early or overt shock. Visual inspection may reveal distention, peritonitis, or free air within the abdomen. Ask about scars that indicate prior surgery and look for discoloration that may indicate the presence of free blood in the abdominal cavity. Palpation may be useful in localizing discomfort, but only use light pressure because heavier pressure may cause rupture of the obstructed segment. Treatment depends on the patient's physiological status, with attention and support of the ABCs. Remember to place one IV line capable of blood transfusion if there are any indications of significant hemorrhage.

Cholecystitis
p. 271

Roughly 90 percent of cases of cholecystitis, inflammation of the gallbladder, are due to gallstones. Cholecystitis caused by stones can be acute or chronic. In both cases, the basic pathophysiology involves obstruction of the flow of bile by gallstones, with resultant inflammation of the gallbladder. Bacterial infection can also cause chronic cholecystitis. An acute attack is characterized by right upper quadrant pain, often with referred pain in the right shoulder. The right subcostal region may be tender due to muscle spasm. Sympathetic nervous stimulation may cause pale, cool, clammy skin. Prehospital care centers on palliation of distress and monitoring of ABCs with use of oxygen if needed and with establishment of IV access.

Chronic gastroenteritis   p. 263

Gastroenteritis, inflammation of the stomach and intestines, is characterized by longer-term changes in the mucosa, thus distinguishing it from acute gastroenteritis. Gastroenteritis is usually due to microbial infection, with viral infection most common. However, patients with bacterial infection are usually the sickest. Common findings are fever, nausea, vomiting, diarrhea, lethargy, and, in the most severe cases, shock. Infection with *Helicobacter pylori* (the most common infectious cause in the United States) commonly presents with heartburn, abdominal pain, and the presence of gastric ulcers. Management includes appropriate infection precautions and patient care centered on monitoring of ABCs and transport. When outbreaks are associated with natural disaster or other possible contamination of water supply, be sure to protect yourself by use of proper sanitation and protection of water and food supplies.

Colitis   p. 265

Colitis is a general term for inflammation of the large intestine. Ulcerative colitis, which you may see in the field, is an inflammatory bowel disease that frequently affects relatively young people (with average age of 20 to 40 years at onset). Mild disease may only affect the distal colon, and it may present in the field with bloody diarrhea and discomfort. More severe disease may affect the entire colon, and this may present with severe, bloody diarrhea, electrolyte disturbances, or even hypovolemic shock. Management is tied to the patient's condition and includes appropriate support of oxygenation and circulation. If the patient has bouts of nausea and vomiting, beware of possible aspiration and airway compromise. Any patient who presents with a lower GI bleed or colicky, visceral-type pain should be transported for diagnostic evaluation.

Crohn's disease   p. 266

Crohn's disease, like ulcerative colitis, is an inflammatory bowel disease. However, the pathological inflammation can occur anywhere in the GI tract, from the mouth to the rectum. After inflammation damages the mucosa and submucosa, granulomas form that further damage the wall of the GI tract. Patients with Crohn's frequently have narrowing of damaged segments, occasionally to the point of complete obstruction. Other findings include diarrhea and intestinal or perianal abscesses or fistulas. Because of the variety of sites involved in different patients, as well as the variety of complications due to progressive damage, prehospital diagnosis is nearly impossible. You should remember that an acute flare-up of symptoms accompanied by absence of bowel sounds suggests intestinal obstruction, which is a surgical emergency. Because significant hemorrhage is unusual, however, hypovolemic shock is infrequent among these patients. Prehospital management is largely palliative, with specific monitoring and support of the ABCs. Evidence of obstruction or shock includes oxygen and circulatory support, including IV access and fluid resuscitation.

Diverticulitis   p. 267

Diverticulitis represents inflammation secondary to infection of diverticula, the outpouchings of intestinal mucosa and submucosa common in older Americans. Diverticulitis frequently starts with occlusion of a diverticulum by fecal material followed by bacterial infection. Complications include colonic hemorrhage or perforation. Common presenting signs of diverticulitis include low-grade fever, nausea and vomiting, and point tenderness on palpation. Because roughly 95 percent of cases involve the sigmoid colon, another name for this condition is "left-sided appendicitis." Management is supportive, with attention to the ABCs. Signs of shock suggest significant hemorrhage.

Esophageal varices   p. 261

A varix is a swollen vein, and esophageal varices (plural) are usually due to hypertension in the portal system. Varices are subject to rupture and hemorrhage, and mortality in these cases exceeds 35 percent. The most common cause is liver damage secondary to alcohol consumption (via cirrhosis of the liver and portal hypertension). The other common cause is ingestion of caustic substances, which damage the esophagus directly and eventually cause rupture of an esophageal vein. Initial presentation of rupture features painless bleeding with evolution of signs of hemodynamic instability. Hematemesis can be both forceful and large in volume. Clotting time increases as high portal pressure backs up blood into the spleen, destroying platelets. Because tamponade isn't possible in the prehospital setting, management centers on rapid transport, with care focusing on aggressive airway management (including orotracheal intubation if needed), use of high-concentration oxygen, and IV fluid resuscitation.

©2013 Pearson Education, Inc.
Paramedic Care: Principles & Practice, Vol. 4, 4th Ed.

Hemorrhoids
p. 268

Hemorrhoids are small masses of swollen veins in the rectum or anus (internal and external hemorrhoids, respectively). Most are of unknown origin and occur in midlife, although some result from recognizable causes such as pregnancy or portal hypertension. In addition, external hemorrhoids can be caused by heavy lifting with straining. Although hemorrhoids frequently bleed during defecation, particularly in the setting of constipation, significant hemorrhage is rare. The typical cause for your call will be distress over the presence of bright red blood with defecation. The physical findings are usually benign, with hemodynamic stability and absence of signs of shock (skin is warm and dry, tachycardia is consistent with anxiety). Emotional assurance and monitoring for continued physiological stability (due to possibility that bleeding is first sign of a lower GI bleed) is usually sufficient during transport. Signs of significant bleeding associated with hemorrhoids in an alcoholic patient warrant closer monitoring and transport for immediate care.

Pancreatitis
p. 272

Pancreatitis is inflammation of the pancreas. The four main pathological types are metabolic, mechanical, vascular, and infectious. Metabolic causes (specifically, alcoholism) account for over 80 percent of cases. Alcohol causes deposition of platelet plugs in the acini. As flow of digestive secretions from the pancreas is impaired, digestive enzymes become activated while within the pancreas, damaging pancreatic tissue. Progression of this chronic damage can lead to hemorrhage, which presents as sudden-onset nausea, vomiting, and severe pain that is in the left upper quadrant and may radiate to the back or the epigastric region. Mechanical pancreatitis is due to gallstones or elevated serum lipids. As digestive secretions accumulate behind the obstruction, pancreatic tissue damage occurs, edema develops, and blood flow is secondarily impaired, causing further damage due to ischemia. Mechanical pancreatitis is often acute in onset. Vascular causes of pancreatitis include thromboembolism and ischemia secondary to shock. Findings of mild pancreatitis include visceral pain, often epigastric in location, abdominal distention, nausea and vomiting, and elevated blood amylase and lipase. Findings in severe pancreatitis include refractory hypotensive shock, blood loss, and respiratory failure. As with other conditions involving hemorrhage, management of severe pancreatitis centers on support of ABCs, including use of high-concentration oxygen and appropriate IV access.

Peptic ulcers

Peptic ulcers, created secondary to mucosal erosion by gastric acid, can occur anywhere in the GI tract and are particularly common in the duodenum and stomach. You will see ulcer cases and GI problems complicated by the presence of peptic ulcers. Pathophysiology includes genetic predisposition (seen as positive family history), as well as risk factors such as stress, use of nonsteroidal anti-inflammatory drugs, acid-stimulating products such as alcohol and nicotine, and chronic infection with *H. pylori*. The common mechanism is a breach of the mucous layer that protects the mucosa from the acid secreted in the stomach. Findings can vary widely. Chronic pain is typically worst when the stomach is empty and is relieved by eating or drinking coating liquids such as milk. Acute pain, particularly when somatic in character, may suggest rupture of the ulcer with hemorrhage into the abdomen. Bleeds manifest similarly to other upper GI hemorrhages and are handled similarly. In severely ill patients, appearance suggests severity of distress (such as lying still with knees drawn to chest), and there are often signs of shock. Management depends on physiological status and involves monitoring of ABCs with appropriate intervention for possible or overt shock.

7. **Given a variety of scenarios, develop treatment plans for patients with gastrointestinal disorders.** pp. 257–272

The priorities for someone who is clearly in urgent distress due to GI disorders are the same as for a patient who is affected by a potentially life-threatening emergency of another origin. Ensure adequate airway, breathing (ventilation), and circulation. This is particularly important for someone whose emergency may be affecting the respiratory and cardiovascular system. Intractable nausea and vomiting can cause respiratory distress. This is especially true for the patient with an underlying pulmonary disease. Also, persistent vomiting can cause alterations in heart rate and blood pressure, produce dramatic volume losses, and place the patient to be at risk for aspiration. Most GI disorders in the prehospital setting will require a minimum of supportive measures, such as airway maintenance, oxygenation, ventilatory management, and hemodynamic and cardiac monitoring. You should always provide oxygen, allow a position of comfort, initiate an IV, and treat nausea, vomiting, and pain.

Although there are some conditions, such as Crohn's disease, in which bleeding rarely leads to hypovolemic shock, you should always be prepared to treat shock. Cases that seem to represent progressive, nonhemorrhagic conditions such as appendicitis, cholecystitis, or diverticulitis should also be monitored for stability and signs of acute events such as rupture or hemorrhage. Also, be aware that GI emergencies often present in older patients with coexisting conditions, and monitor cardiopulmonary status and other organ function carefully. Take close note of conditions such as alcoholism, consider GI problems associated with them (such as hepatitis, pancreatitis, or esophageal varices), and adjust assessment and treatment accordingly.

Case Study Review

Reread the case study on pages 255–256 in Paramedic Care: Medicine; *then, read the following discussion.*

This case study demonstrates how paramedics react to a life-threatening emergency of unknown origin, treat each critical problem as it appears with focus on the ABCs, and transport the patient to an appropriate emergency facility. In addition to noting how the teams react to the patient's presentation and assessment, note how clues to the GI origin of his condition emerge from the assessment and history known to the emergency department (ED) staff.

George and Stephanie's dispatch is one you will encounter often, the "unknown medical emergency." Although the study doesn't say which equipment they are transferring for use in the house, you know they should be prepared to support the basic ABCs (airway, breathing, circulation) in a patient who may be gravely ill and have cardiopulmonary compromise either as part of the primary complaint or secondary to shock of some type.

The only information they get on the scene is from a hysterical spouse, and it is nonspecific except for the mention of blood. George and Stephanie consider the possibility of self-inflicted injury or violence, as well as accidental trauma, and call for police backup, which arrives with little delay. By the time the deputy sheriff arrives, the team is ready to enter the house, having donned appropriate protective gear (because of the blood) and gathered equipment useful in trauma and medical settings.

Their readiness means there is no further delay in initiating critical care and assessment. The patient has his spine immobilized and is then moved to a position that is protective of his airway and allows assessment. The first findings, about respirations and pulse, indicate the man is physiologically unstable; the same is inferred from an apparently large volume of blood found on the floor. Note that the team instinctively looks for sites of external hemorrhage and finds none.

The paramedics' next actions go to the central focus of any severe emergency: the ABCs. As they attempt to stabilize the airway through intubation, the patient vomits. Ready suction prevents aspiration of the vomitus and provides a clue to the GI origin of the hemorrhage. The vomited material turns out to be bright red blood. Intubation in the face of the intact gag reflex and active vomiting is achieved with rapid-sequence intubation, and oxygen supplementation is begun with a bag-valve unit. IV access is secured, and an initial fluid bolus is given. The scenario doesn't give the bore of the needle, but you should assume one or two IV lines will be established as soon as possible, with at least one line of caliber sufficient to support blood transfusion.

Vital signs confirm that the patient is physiologically unstable (tachycardia, but no sign of dysrhythmia yet) and in hypovolemic shock (tachycardia, depressed blood pressure), and the physical finding of diminished breath sounds with crackles (rales) at the bases suggests that the patient may have already aspirated blood. Even if aspiration hasn't occurred, the pulmonary findings indicate compromised function.

You don't know whether the wife gave any historical information or not, and you don't know whether she came to the hospital in a separate vehicle. If she were capable of giving any historical information, one of the team members should have questioned her at the home or while en route about the patient's medical history, particularly whether he had any GI conditions or comorbid conditions (such as alcoholism) that may have led to GI hemorrhage. (Note that the patient was middle-aged, not elderly, which may increase the importance of asking about comorbid conditions because you cannot assume any age-related organ dysfunction.)

©2013 Pearson Education, Inc.
Paramedic Care: Principles & Practice, Vol. 4, 4th Ed.

The history is revealed at the nearby emergency facility, when staff members recognize the patient as a man with alcohol-induced problems that they have previously treated. The comorbid conditions of portal hypertension and liver failure are identified. Initial assessment by the surgical resident reveals the cause of the life-threatening upper GI hemorrhage, a ruptured esophageal varix. The ED staff further supports treatment of shock and rushes the patient for definitive therapy of the bleed in the surgical suite.

George and Stephanie close the call by learning more about the pathophysiology of the underlying conditions and the probable trigger for the variceal rupture (forceful vomiting in the setting of portal hypertension). The attending physician also lets them know that the rapidity and correctness of their care may have saved the patient's life.

Content Self-Evaluation

MULTIPLE CHOICE

_____ 1. Which of the following statements about gastrointestinal (GI) emergencies is NOT true?
   A. GI emergencies account for about 5 percent of all annual visits to the emergency department.
   B. The majority of GI emergencies entail GI hemorrhage.
   C. The number of GI emergencies is expected to rise, in part due to aging of the population.
   D. The risk factors for GI emergencies are well known, and most (such as familial predisposition to GI conditions) are out of control of the patient.
   E. The number of GI emergencies is expected to rise, in part due to delays in seeking treatment by patients who treat themselves as long as symptoms allow.

_____ 2. Risk factors for GI disease include excessive use of alcohol and tobacco, stress, ingestion of caustic substances, and poor bowel habits.
   A. True
   B. False

_____ 3. Which of the following statements about physical examination of the abdomen is NOT true?
   A. Visual inspection should always be done first.
   B. Palpation should always precede auscultation.
   C. Of auscultation, percussion, palpation, and visual inspection, palpation may be most likely to produce a lot of useful information.
   D. Discoloration of the skin (specifically, ecchymosis) may indicate where hemorrhage has occurred into the abdominal cavity.
   E. Abdominal distention may be an ominous sign, suggesting either free air in the abdomen or loss of a large amount of circulating volume.

_____ 4. Three organs intimately associated with the GI tract are the
   A. teeth, tongue, and epiglottis.
   B. appendix, gallbladder, and parotid gland.
   C. cystic duct, bile duct, and common bile duct.
   D. appendix, rectum, and anus.
   E. liver, pancreas, and gallbladder.

_____ 5. The chief function of the upper GI tract is digestion, whereas the chief functions of the lower GI tract are absorption of nutrients and excretion of wastes.
   A. True
   B. False

_____ 6. Major causes of upper GI hemorrhage include all of the following, EXCEPT
   A. gastritis.   D. peptic ulcers.
   B. rupture of an esophageal varix.   E. Mallory-Weiss syndrome.
   C. gastroenteritis.

_____ 7. Severe, potentially life-threatening upper GI hemorrhage is common with
   A. variceal and hemorrhoidal rupture and bleeding.
   B. peptic ulcer disease and Crohn's disease.
   C. esophageal varices and hepatic cirrhosis.
   D. esophageal varix rupture and esophageal Mallory-Weiss tears.
   E. eroded gastric ulcers and eroded ulcerative colitis lesions.

_____ 8. Blood is indicated by melena, stool containing small or large amounts of bright red blood, and hematochezia, dark, tarry, foul-smelling stool.
   A. True
   B. False

_____ 9. Of acute gastroenteritis and gastroenteritis, gastroenteritis is the more likely to be caused by microbial infection.
   A. True
   B. False

_____ 10. Conditions that routinely call for the paramedic to take infectious precautions include
   A. hepatitis and cirrhosis.
   B. peptic ulcer disease and gastroenteritis.
   C. cholecystitis and pancreatitis.
   D. gastroenteritis and appendicitis.
   E. hepatitis and gastroenteritis.

_____ 11. Patients with peptic ulcer disease typically have worsening of pain after eating, whereas patients with cholecystitis typically have relief of pain after eating.
   A. True
   B. False

_____ 12. Any patient who presents with lower GI bleeding or colicky abdominal pain should be transported to the emergency department for evaluation.
   A. True
   B. False

_____ 13. Conditions that typically have lesions in the rectum and anus include
   A. diverticulosis and hemorrhoids.
   B. ulcerative colitis and Crohn's disease.
   C. ulcerative colitis and hemorrhoids.
   D. volvulus and intussusception.
   E. hernias and hemorrhoids.

_____ 14. Among the most common causes of bowel obstruction are
   A. intestinal tumors, volvulus, and hernias.
   B. intussusception, volvulus, and hemorrhoids.
   C. adhesions, hernias, and intestinal tumors.
   D. hernias, volvulus, and adhesions.
   E. appendicitis, volvulus, and diverticulitis.

_____ 15. Acute pancreatitis is most commonly caused by
   A. excessive use of alcohol and tobacco.
   B. gallstones and excessive use of alcohol.
   C. infectious GI disease and gallstones.
   D. drug toxicity and excessive use of alcohol.
   E. vascular disease causing ischemia and gallstones causing obstruction of the pancreatic duct.

©2013 Pearson Education, Inc.
Paramedic Care: Principles & Practice, Vol. 4, 4th Ed.

MATCHING

Write the letter of the type of pain in the space provided next to the appropriate description of the pain.

A. somatic

B. peritonitis

C. visceral

D. radiated

E. referred

_____ **16.** Pain originating in the walls of hollow organs that is typically produced by the processes of inflammation, distension, or ischemia

_____ **17.** Pain perceived in a location other than the one from which it originates

_____ **18.** Pain frequently characterized by the patient as sharp and well localized

_____ **19.** Condition caused by presence of free blood or GI contents within the abdominal cavity, which is typically perceived by the patient as somatic pain that is eased in a knee-chest position

_____ **20.** Pain frequently originating in the capsules of solid organs and typically perceived by the patient as sharp or tearing in character

_____ **21.** Pain between the shoulder blades that may be produced by a dissecting abdominal aorta

_____ **22.** Pain that an appendicitis patient may perceive when the inflamed appendix ruptures

_____ **23.** Pain that seems to the patient to move from one location to another

Write the letter of the signs or symptoms in the space provided next to the condition to which they apply.

A. epigastric pain, abdominal distension, and nausea and vomiting

B. colicky, lower left quadrant pain, low-grade fever, nausea and vomiting

C. blood loss, refractory shock, and respiratory failure

D. upper right quadrant tenderness, fever, nausea and vomiting

_____ **24.** Hepatitis

_____ **25.** Mild pancreatitis

_____ **26.** Diverticulitis

_____ **27.** Severe pancreatitis

FILL IN THE BLANKS

28. Define the SAMPLE history format by filling in the missing terms:

S _____

A _____

M _____

P _____

L _____

E _____

29. Any case of abdominal pain lasting over _____ in duration is considered a surgical emergency and the patient should be transported to an appropriate facility.

30. Upper GI hemorrhage is defined as bleeding in the GI tract proximal to the _____ _____ _____, whereas lower GI hemorrhage is defined as bleeding in the GI tract distal to it.

Special Project

History Taking

Examine the responses noted in a patient's history of her present illness and fill in the type of question beside the response. Question types are drawn from the OPQRST-ASPN history format discussed in the text.

For the previous half hour to hour, pain has been constant and close to a 9 (out of 10) in intensity.
_____

Nausea without vomiting has been present, along with no appetite, since the discomfort began.
_____

Patient remembers it was about 10:00 P.M. when she first realized her abdominal pain was significant (7 hours ago). _____

Pain is now constant and sharp, like a knife. _____

Pain was poorly localized last evening, but became localized to the right lower quadrant overnight; however, it has become generalized over the abdomen within the last half hour or so.
_____

Patient first noticed some vague, generalized discomfort yesterday afternoon at some point before dinnertime. _____

Currently, there is almost nothing that relieves the pain. Patient does best when lying very still with knees drawn toward chest. _____

There is no pain associated with urination, and no pain has been perceived outside of the abdomen.
_____

Consider the patient's history of present illness given above with the information placed in the order below. Then give a probable field diagnosis.

Patient first noticed some vague, generalized discomfort yesterday afternoon at some point before dinner. Nausea without vomiting has been present, along with no appetite, since the discomfort began.

Patient remembers it was about 10:00 P.M. when she first realized her abdominal pain was significant (roughly 7 hours ago). Pain was poorly localized last evening, but became localized to the right lower quadrant overnight; however, it has become generalized over the abdomen within the last half hour or so. There is no pain associated with urination, and no pain has been perceived outside of the abdomen.

For the previous half hour to hour, pain has been constant and close to a 9 (out of 10) in intensity. Pain is now constant and sharp like a knife. Currently, there is almost nothing that relieves the pain. Patient does best when lying very still with knees drawn toward chest.

Probable field diagnosis: _____

©2013 Pearson Education, Inc.
Paramedic Care: Principles & Practice, Vol. 4, 4th Ed.

7

Urology and Nephrology

Review of Chapter Objectives

After reading this chapter, you should be able to:

1. **Define key terms introduced in this chapter.**

   Knowing and being able to apply the key terms in each chapter is critical to understanding chapter concepts. Write the list of key terms. Then write the definition of each one in your own words. Check your understanding by confirming the definitions in the text glossary. Correct any misunderstandings. Create a study aid by writing each key term on the front of an index card and the definition on the back. Use the cards to quiz yourself, or to have someone quiz you.

2. **Describe the roles of diabetes and gender in the risk for urinary system disorders.** **pp. 294–295**

   A urinary tract infection (UTI) affects the urethra, bladder, or kidney, as well as the prostate gland in men. UTIs are extremely common, accounting for over 6 million office visits yearly. Almost all UTIs start with pathogenic colonization of the bladder by bacteria that enter through the urethra. Thus, females in general are at higher risk because of their relatively short urethras. Other groups at risk for UTI are paraplegic patients or patients with nerve disruption to the bladder, including some diabetic persons. Any condition that promotes urinary stasis (incomplete urination with urine remaining in the bladder that may serve as nutrition for pathogens) places a person at higher risk. Pregnant women often have urinary stasis due to pressure from the gravid uterus. People with neurological impairment (some patients with spina bifida or with diabetic neuropathy, for example) also tend to have urinary stasis, which predisposes them to infection. The use of instrumentation in patients who require bladder catheterization places them at even higher risk of UTIs. In females, infection may begin when gram-negative bacteria normally found in the bowel (that is, the enteric flora) colonize the urethra and bladder. Symptomatic urethritis, inflammation secondary to urethral infection, is very uncommon. More often you will see joint symptomatic infection of the urethra and bladder (urethritis and cystitis, respectively). Sexually active females are at higher risk, which may be attributed to use of contraceptive devices or agents, to the introduction of enteric flora during intercourse, or both.

   Renal (kidney) and urological (urinary tract) disorders are very common, affecting about 20 million Americans, so you will definitely see emergencies related to these disorders in the field. The seriousness of these disorders is demonstrated by two statistics: Roughly 250,000 Americans have the most severe form of long-term kidney failure (end-stage failure) and require either dialysis or transplantation to live. More than 50,000 Americans die annually from some form of kidney disease. Some emergencies are not necessarily life threatening but are very painful to experience and common in the population. Over 500,000 persons are treated annually for kidney stones. Persons most at risk for severe kidney problems include older patients, persons with diabetes mellitus, persons with chronic hypertension, and individuals with more than one risk factor. The two risk factors most significant for end-stage renal failure are hypertension and diabetes, which account for more than half of all cases. The risk factors for kidney stones are very different. Some kinds of stones follow a familial pattern, suggesting genetic predisposition. Other risk factors include physical immobilization, use of certain medications (anesthetics, opiates, and psychotropic drugs), and metabolic disorders such as gout. Finally, urinary tract infection, which accounts for over 6 million office visits yearly, has identified risk factors: female gender, paraplegic persons and others (notably some persons with diabetes) with nerve disruption to the bladder, pregnancy, and regular use of instrumentation such as catheters.

3. **Relate the anatomy and physiology of the urinary system to the pathophysiology and assessment of patients with urologic and renal disorders.**   pp. 279–296

The two major organs of the urinary system are the kidneys and the urinary bladder. Two major structures are the ureters and the urethra. The kidney is the critical organ of the urinary system. The kidneys perform the vital functions of the urinary system, which include:

- Maintenance of blood volume with proper balance of water, electrolytes, and pH
- Retention of key substances such as glucose and removal of toxic wastes such as urea
- Major role in regulation of arterial blood pressure
- Control of the development of red blood cells

The first two roles are achieved through the production of urine in the kidneys. The kidneys' role in regulation of blood pressure is achieved in part through control of the body's fluid volume. In addition, they produce an enzyme called renin, which acts to activate a hormone (chemical messenger) called angiotensin, which is part of a hormonal pathway that acts to retain water in the body (increase blood pressure).

The structural and functional unit within the kidney is the nephron, and each kidney contains about 1 million nephrons, establishing the functional reserve that most people take for granted. Blood is filtered into the first part of the nephron, the glomerulus, and then moves through a length of specialized tubule. As the fluid moves through the parts of the tubule, movement of water and some materials out of the tubule and into the blood occurs (reabsorption), as does movement of some materials out of blood and into the tubule (secretion). The kidneys can maintain an exquisitely fine control over the relative activity of reabsorption and secretion for virtually every substance that is filtered into the glomerulus. The ability of the kidney to retain glucose, excrete wastes such as urea, and thus perform all of its vital roles is extraordinary, and life depends upon it. When kidney function is too low or nonexistent, an individual will die unless the function is replaced through artificial dialysis or through kidney transplantation. The final role of the kidney, control over development of red blood cells, is achieved through production and release of a hormone called erythropoietin, which stimulates red blood cell synthesis in the bone marrow.

Each ureter runs from a kidney to the bladder, and urine moves out of the kidney through them to reach the bladder. Because ureters are very small in internal diameter, they can become blocked by internal objects such as kidney stones. The bladder is a muscular sac that expands to hold urine. During urination, stored urine is eliminated from the bladder (and the body) through the tube called the urethra.

In women, the structures of the urinary system and the reproductive system are completely separate. In men, however, reproductive fluid (semen) is also eliminated from the body through the urethra. Thus, consideration of symptoms of urinary tract trouble in men is sometimes more complex than consideration of the same problem in women. For instance, infection in a man's urethra can come directly through sexual activity.

The genitourinary systems of men include some specifically reproductive organs and structures: the testes (the primary male reproductive organs, which produce testosterone and sperm cells) and tubing called the epididymis and vas deferens, through which sperm cells leave the testes and move toward the urethra. Sperm leaves the vas deferens to enter the urethra as it passes through the substance of the other male reproductive organ, the prostate gland, which produces fluid that mixes with sperm to produce semen, the male reproductive fluid. The prostate will be important to you in field work because it surrounds the first part of the male urethra. Prostate enlargement, which occurs routinely with age, can compress the urethra to the point of closure. This can result in retention of urine and a medical emergency call.

©2013 Pearson Education, Inc.
Paramedic Care: Principles & Practice, Vol. 4, 4th Ed.

The focused history will often provide clues to the severity and duration of acute renal failure (ARF). For instance, if the patient complains of inability to void for a number of hours associated with a feeling of painful bladder fullness, the cause may simply be acute obstruction at the bladder neck or urethra. In contrast, a patient with poor mentation may be unable to give a coherent history, and a family member will tell you that the patient has felt increasingly ill for several days and has not urinated at all within the past 12 hours or so. Questions likely to provide useful information include the following:

- *When was the decrease or absence of urine first noticed, and has there been any observed change in output since the problem was first noted? What was the patient's previous output?* The last question may be useful because patients with chronic renal failure due to inadequate renal function can develop ARF as a complication.
- *Has the patient noted development of edema (swelling) in the face, hands, feet, or torso? How about feelings of heart palpitations or irregular rhythm? Has a family member or friend noticed decreased mental function, lethargy, or overt coma?* If the patient continued to consume fluids after ARF developed, retention of water and Na^+ can lead to visible edema in a relatively short time. Retention of K^+ can lead to hyperkalemia, a condition that can be lethal, especially in a person with previously compromised heart function. Increasingly poor mentation can be a sign of metabolic acidosis.

The focused physical examination may be helpful in assessing the degree of ARF present, the antecedent condition, and any immediate threats to life. Impaired mentation or clear decreases in consciousness in a person with previously good mental function suggest severe ARF and a potential threat to life. In a patient without evidence of shock, cardiovascular findings may include hypertension due to fluid retention, tachycardia, and electrocardiogram (ECG) evidence of hyperkalemia. If the ARF is due to shock, profound hypotension may be present, accompanied by tachycardia and hyperkalemia.

General visual inspection will usually show pale, cool, moist skin; if shock is not present, these findings may still represent homeostatic shunting of blood to the internal organs, including the kidneys. Look for edema in the face, hands, and feet. Examination of the abdomen will reveal very different findings dependent on the cause of ARF. As with any abdominal complaint, look for scars, ecchymosis, and distention. If the abdomen is distended, note whether the swelling is symmetric. Palpate for pulsing masses, which may indicate an abdominal aortic aneurysm. Auscultation is rarely helpful in renal and urological emergencies, and bowel sounds may be muffled if ascites (fluid within the abdomen) are present.

4. **Adapt the scene size-up, primary assessment, patient history, secondary assessment, and use of monitoring technology to meet the needs of patients with complaints and presentations related to urologic and renal disorders.** pp. 274–296

During the scene size-up, your general impression will be very important, as you will be looking for clues that can indicate the patient's condition. The causes of urology and nephrology emergencies are numerous. One of the first questions you will answer will be whether there is a history of chronic renal or urological disease such as chronic renal failure (CRF), kidney stones, frequent UTIs, or prostate enlargement. Also ask about major risk factors such as diabetes and hypertension. Evaluate the patient's level of consciousness using the AVPU method, as well as speech, skin appearance, and posture. The patient's emotional status may also provide clues to the patient's developing condition that may be altered due to metabolic acidosis, pain, fluid retention, or electrolyte imbalances.

Recall Chapter 6, Gastroenterology, in which you learned about the focused history relating to abdominal pain that might be gastrointestinal (GI) in origin. The technique is similar when the GI system is not the focus of attention. For example, initial questioning still follows the OPQRST format (shown below with some specific questions in parentheses):

– Onset of pain (Sudden or slow? Activity at the time?)
– Provocation or palliation of pain (Pain on urination, inability to void or void normally, and palliation with walking all may suggest urinary tract origin.)
– Quality of the pain (Visceral pain is common with urinary emergencies; a change to somatic pain, particularly flank pain, may suggest ureteral obstruction by a stone.)

- Region where pain is felt, along with any radiation of pain (Listen for suggestions of referred/radiated pain; in postpubertal women, be sure to get menstrual history and follow-up comments suggesting OB/GYN problems)
- Severity of pain currently and over time (Most urinary conditions don't cause the abrupt switch to somatic pain—with increase in severity—seen with a ruptured appendix, for instance.)
- Time over which pain has been felt (Note that any patient with pain lasting over 6 hours is considered a surgical emergency and requires transport to an appropriate facility for evaluation. When in doubt, consider the case a potential surgical emergency and treat/transport as such.)

Additional questions center on:

- Previous history of similar event (Note that kidney stones and infections may be recurrent problems; family history may also be helpful.)
- Nausea/vomiting (Because nausea and vomiting can be caused purely by autonomic nervous system discharge, this is not necessarily a sign localizing to the GI system; nausea and vomiting are common with severe pain associated with kidney stones.)
- Changes in bowel habits (Diarrhea may suggest a GI condition; constipation may be less helpful as a clue to the origin of a problem.)
- Weight loss (Loss over hours to days suggests dehydration, whereas longer-term loss suggests chronic illness or GI dysfunction.)
- Last oral intake, include beverages (Learning this is necessary for possible surgical cases; timing of a meal may also suggest acute-onset problem or aggravation of an existing one.)
- Chest pain (Consider myocardial infarction [MI] but also consider referred pain; note that diabetic persons may not have typical pain pattern during MI due to neuropathy.)

5. **Use a process of clinical reasoning to guide and interpret the patient assessment and management process for patients with urologic and renal disorders.** pp. 283–296

As a paramedic, it is vital that you develop your clinical reasoning process to quickly recognize and treat acute urological and renal emergencies to improve patient outcome. This is because diagnosis and treatment with many acute renal emergencies is time-sensitive. The longer nephron dysfunction occurs, the more likely that irreversible kidney damage will result. Develop an organized general impression to rapidly identify signs and symptoms of urologic and renal emergencies. This will include obtaining an accurate history.

Timing of voiding difficulty can provide vital information. A normal history with sudden-onset inability to void may suggest distal obstruction, whereas feeling ill over a number of days with some decrease in voiding may suggest chronic renal problems with an acute aggravation. Ask for renal history. Some triggers of acute renal failure may be obvious: dehydration secondary to diarrhea, hemorrhage, shock, sepsis. Visual inspection may reveal cool, pale, moist skin (which suggests shunting of blood to core, including kidneys, if shock is absent) and edema in the hands, feet, or face. Physical findings may reveal the trigger for the failure: A distended, discolored abdomen may suggest severe intra-abdominal hemorrhage with hypoperfusion to the kidneys.

The physical exam includes overall impressions as well as examination of the abdomen. Elements include both patient appearance and posture/activity. Walking often suggests urinary origin: Walking that relieves pain may suggest a kidney stone, and walking hunched up in a febrile person complaining of back pain may suggest kidney infection. Additionally, altered level of consciousness in the absence of fever may suggest hemorrhage and evolution of hypovolemic shock. Hemorrhage should lead you to consider GI or reproductive (OB) emergencies. Patients undergoing dialysis may have chronic changes in mental status during dialysis; try to discern whether the level you see is the norm for that person or represents an acute or subacute change. Also consider the apparent state of the patient's health and personal appearance, which can often give leads to a chronic condition or one of acute onset. Skin color and appearance can suggest chronic anemia (pale, cool, dry skin), shock (pale, clammy skin), or fever (dry, flushed).

Examination of the abdomen was covered in Chapter 6. Percussion may be very useful in the setting of urology. Pain on percussion of the flanks may suggest kidney inflammation and infection, and pain on percussion of the pelvic rim may suggest problems in the bladder. Remember that pregnancy may

©2013 Pearson Education, Inc.
Paramedic Care: Principles & Practice, Vol. 4, 4th Ed.

also be found during physical examination as you palpate above the pelvic rim. A ruptured ectopic pregnancy may be suggested by lower quadrant pain that increases with palpation and evidence of hemorrhage. In older men, palpation above the pelvic rim may reveal the enlarged, fluctuant mass of an obstructed bladder due to prostatic hypertrophy. In all men, exam includes examination of the scrotum and penis. Urethral discharge may suggest infection. Scrotal masses may be painful (such as infectious epididymitis) or nonpainful (testicular cancer, which is most common in young men, or a varicocele). Ask questions about acute or longer-term presence of any mass. For men with an apparently obstructed bladder, find out when they last urinated and whether there had been any change in pattern.

Generally, nephrological and urological emergencies don't produce acute abnormalities on exam, unlike GI emergencies. However, pain from an inflamed or infected kidney may be felt in the flank, and pelvic pain may suggest bladder origin or a reproductive problem in either a man or woman. Always consider possible miscarriage from either an ectopic pregnancy or an intrauterine one in girls and women of childbearing age.

As noted in Chapter 6, many GI emergencies feature hemorrhage, and discernment through vital signs and physical exam of likely hemorrhage is an important first step in looking for system of origin. Examination of vomitus or diarrhea is also helpful. Gross examination of urine may not be helpful; however, gross blood is consistent with kidney stones in an otherwise appropriate presentation, and cloudiness of urine may represent the large numbers of white cells that may be present in pyelonephritis. Remember the typical pain patterns: GI emergencies often start with visceral pain (frequently located higher than in urinary tract conditions) and progress to somatic pain if an inflamed or damaged structure ruptures; postrupture peritonitis is not unusual. In contrast, most urological/nephrological emergencies feature visceral pain felt in the pelvis or male scrotum. Somatic-like pain felt in the flank, shoulder, or neck may suggest a kidney stone. Tenderness in the lower back at the costovertebral angle may suggest pyelonephritis, particularly if systemic signs of infection are present. If the urinary system appears likely, be sure to address the issue of renal function. Prevention strategies to prevent further loss of nephrons are vital to implement expediently.

Acute renal failure is defined as a sudden (over a period of a day or days) drop in urine output to less than 400 to 500 mL per day. Low urine output is oliguria, whereas no urine output is anuria. Chronic renal failure is inadequate kidney function due to the permanent loss of nephrons (usually representing a loss of at least 70 to 80 percent of total nephrons). When metabolic instability sets in (around 80 percent loss), the condition is termed end-stage renal failure, and either dialysis or kidney transplantation is required to survive. If onset is acute and without evidence of distal obstruction, prerenal ARF may be suggested. Be sure to treat any identifiable potential trigger condition and aggressively protect fluid volume and oxygenation. Always remember that prerenal ARF may be reversible if you act quickly and correctly; this is still true in patients with chronic renal failure. Quick action may also preserve remaining function if renal causes are suspected. Renal causes may require the hospital setting for definitive treatment, but the treatment staples are the same as for prerenal. If history or exam suggests postrenal obstruction, be sure to get as much information as possible for use by hospital staff. For instance, known cancer in the abdomen or pelvis may suggest bilateral ureteral obstruction. Advanced age in men may suggest acute renal retention secondary to prostate enlargement, and history in boys or men of recent sexual activity, recreational drugs, or parties may suggest the possible presence of a foreign body in the urethra.

Management for renal calculi, as always, begins with the ABCs. Position for comfort, but be ready for vomiting, particularly if pain is severe or last oral intake is recent. IV access may be needed for analgesic administration (if needed and appropriate per local protocol) or fluid to promote urine formation and movement of the stone through the urinary tract.

The common pathophysiology for all types of stones rests on an imbalance of water and relatively insoluble substances in the kidney filtrate. The type and size of stone, as well as current site in the urinary tract, may be discerned from personal and family history, as well as physical examination. Assessment for treatment (before and during transport) focuses on nature, site, and severity of pain. A urine sample may reveal blood in the presence of any type of stone. A urine sample may be particularly valuable from a female patient because of inclusion of infection in the differential diagnosis, especially when bladder symptoms are present. Because passage of the stone is the ultimate goal, IV fluid may be beneficial as soon as it can be started, as it promotes urine formation. Analgesia may be necessary, dependent on the individual patient and local protocol. Management centers on monitoring and support of the ABCs. Positioning may help the patient with severe pain; be prepared in case the patient vomits.

Analgesics are usually unnecessary; severely painful cases of pyelonephritis may be the exception. As with renal stones, hydration to increase and dilute urine flow is generally helpful. Use of IV fluid eliminates the risk of vomiting and satisfies treatment guidelines for possible surgical cases.

Lower UTIs typically arise from infection that has entered via the urethra and has damaged tissue in the lower urinary tract. Hydration increases urine formation and promotes a more dilute urine (in a patient with normal renal function), and so it may help ease the symptoms of urgency, frequency, and pain in the patient with a lower UTI. Lack of systemic signs indicates that normal monitoring of ABCs is probably sufficient before and during transport. Patients with pyelonephritis (upper UTI) are more likely to show fever and other signs of systemic infection. IV hydration is also indicated for the same reasons and because IV access may be needed if physiological instability develops or the patient is deemed later to be a surgical case. Transport for diagnosis and definitive treatment (appropriate antibiotic therapy) provides the link to long-term care.

6. **Describe the pathophysiology of specific urologic and renal problems, including the following:**

   a. **Acute renal failure**   pp. 286–289
   There are three types of acute renal failure (ARF) based on pathophysiology: prerenal, renal, and postrenal. You may see all three types in the field. Remember that acute renal failure may be reversible if recognized and treated early enough.

   Prerenal ARF is due to insufficient blood flow to the kidneys. This type accounts for 40 to 80 percent of cases, and it is the most likely to be reversible if perfusion is restored. Common causes in the field include cardiac failure (often an MI), hemorrhage, dehydration, shock, and sepsis, as well as anomalies of a renal artery or vein.
   Renal ARF is due to a pathological process within the kidney tissue itself. The three general causes are damage to small vessels and/or glomeruli, tubular cell damage, and interstitial damage. In each type, nephron function is lost.
   Postrenal ARF is due to obstruction at some point distal to the kidneys: both ureters, the bladder outlet, or the urethra. Postrenal ARF may be reversible if the obstruction is identified and removed before permanent kidney damage occurs.

   b. **Chronic renal failure**   pp. 289–293
   The three processes that can underlie chronic renal failure are the same as those producing acute renal failure: damage to small blood vessels or glomeruli, tubular cell injury, and damage to interstitial tissue. In each case, surviving nephrons adapt by structural changes that increase function, but these changes damage the nephrons themselves over time, leading to greater loss of nephron numbers. Common causes of damage to blood vessels and glomeruli include systemic hypertension, atherosclerosis, diabetes, and systemic lupus erythematosus, an autoimmune disease. Causes of tubular cell injury include nephrotoxic drugs and heavy metals and distal obstruction with backup of urine into the kidney. Finally, interstitial damage can be caused by infections, including pyelonephritis and tuberculosis.

   c. **Complications related to hemodialysis and peritoneal dialysis**   pp. 291–293
   Renal dialysis is artificial replacement of some of the kidneys' vital functions. Two different technologies, hemodialysis and chronic ambulatory peritoneal dialysis, are widely used. Both rely on the physiological principles of osmosis and equalization of osmolarity across a semipermeable membrane. As blood flows over such a membrane, many critical substances such as urea and sodium, potassium, and hydrogen ions move from the blood into the hypoosmolar solution, the dialysate, thus reducing the concentrations in the blood. The overall effect is to lessen or eliminate temporarily volume overload and toxically high blood concentrations of electrolytes, urea, and other substances.

   In hemodialysis, the patient's blood is passed through a machine containing a semipermeable membrane. Vascular access is established through a permanent anastamosis of an artery and vein in the forearm. If such a fistula is not possible, an indwelling catheter may be placed in the internal jugular vein. In chronic ambulatory peritoneal dialysis, the peritoneal membrane is used as the semipermeable membrane and dialysate solution is introduced into, and then removed from, the abdominal cavity via an indwelling catheter.

©2013 Pearson Education, Inc.
Paramedic Care: Principles & Practice, Vol. 4, 4th Ed.

Complications common to both forms of dialysis include physiologically destabilizing shifts in blood volume and composition and blood pressure during and shortly after dialysis. Other complications common to both forms include shortness of breath or dizziness and neurological abnormalities ranging from headache to seizure or coma. Hypotension may represent dehydration, hemorrhage, or infection. Shortness of breath or chest pain may reflect cardiac dysrhythmias, ischemia, or even MI. In many cases the neurological abnormalities represent shifts in the chemical milieu of the brain. Seizures are usually responsive to benzodiazepines.

Complications specific to hemodialysis include bleeding at the needle puncture site, local infection, and stenosis or obstruction of the internal fistula. Under normal flow conditions, you will hear or feel a bruit or thrill. Leading complications requiring hospitalization include thrombosis, infection, and development of an aneurysm. The latter are particularly common in patients in whom artificial graft material was used to construct the fistula. The most common complications in patients undergoing chronic ambulatory peritoneal dialysis include infection in the catheter or tunnel containing the catheter, or in the peritoneum itself. Because the incidence of peritonitis is roughly one episode per year, you may find the signs of peritonitis in this patient group.

d. Renal calculi pp. 293–294

Renal calculi (calculus, singular) are crystal aggregations in the kidney's urine-collecting system. The same condition is referred to as nephrolithiasis. Although overall morbidity and mortality are low, brief hospitalizations are common for patients because of the severity of the pain as stones move through the renal pelvis, ureter, bladder, and urethra.

Some kinds of stones form as part of a systemic metabolic disorder such as gout (excess uric acid) or primary hyperparathyroidism (excess calcium). Most stones, however, form due to a more general imbalance between the amount of water flowing through the kidney tubing and the mineral ions, uric acid, and other relatively insoluble substances that are dissolved in that water. Trigger events for stone formation include change in diet, activity, or climate, all of which can alter water conservation or the amount of one or more such substances in the blood, and thus the filtrate. Calcium stones are the most common and are most frequently seen in men aged 20 to 30 years. This type of stone is likely to recur and is likely to be found in a family history. Struvite stones are also common; their formation is often related to chronic urinary tract infection or frequent bladder catheterization. Perhaps because of the tie to infection, these stones are more common in women. Struvite stones can grow to fill the renal pelvis; in such cases, they present a "staghorn" appearance on x-rays. The less common stones are made of uric acid or cystine. Uric acid stones can occur in the presence of gout (about 50 percent of cases); they are also more common in men and tend to occur in families. Cystine stones are the least common, and they are associated with excess cystine in filtrate. There is probably at least a partial genetic predisposition, and they are known to occur in families.

e. Priapism p. 294

Priapism is a painful and prolonged erection of the penis. Priapism affects only the *corpora cavernosa*. The *corpora spongiosum* remains flaccid. Although in many instances the cause is unclear, priapism has been associated with certain disease processes. The most common cause of nontraumatic priapism is sickle cell disease, in which sickling of erythrocytes prevents normal venous drainage of the penis. Other causes of priapism include leukemia, multiple myeloma, tumors, spinal cord injury, spinal anesthesia, carbon monoxide poisoning, malaria, and black widow spider bites. Priapism has also been associated with use of the following drugs: psychotropic omeprazole, hydroxyzine, prazosin, calcium channel blockers, anticoagulants, cocaine, marijuana, ethanol, and MDMA (ecstasy). Some of the erectile dysfunction drugs, especially vardenafil (Levitra), have been associated with priapism.

f. Testicular torsion p. 294

Testicular torsion is the twisting of the spermatic cord, which cuts off the blood supply to the testicle and surrounding structures within the scrotum. This results in severe testicular pain and associated abdominal pain. Certain men are predisposed to testicular torsion as a result of inadequate connective tissue within the scrotum (bell-clapper deformity). However, it can also result from trauma to the scrotum—particularly if significant swelling occurs. It can also occur after strenuous exercise or may not have an obvious cause. Testicular torsion is more common during infancy and at the beginning of adolescence, although it can occur at any age.

The signs and symptoms of testicular torsion include the sudden onset of severe testicular pain (usually limited to one testicle). The testicle is exquisitely tender and swollen. The testicle is often high in the scrotum (when compared to the other testicle) because of shortening of the spermatic cord that is due to twisting. Nausea, vomiting, and dizziness are common. The patient may also report blood in the semen.

g. Urinary tract infection pp. 294–296

Infection of the urinary tract implies infection in the urethra, bladder, or kidney, or the prostate gland in men. Urinary tract infections (UTI) are extremely common, accounting for about 6 million office visits per year, and you will see them in the field.

Because bacteria usually enter via the urethra, infections are more common in women (who have a much shorter urethra), paraplegic patients or others who require catheterization, and diabetic persons who have neuropathy involving the bladder. UTIs are generally divided into those affecting the lower urinary tract (namely, urethritis, cystitis, and prostatitis) and those of the upper urinary tract (pyelonephritis). Lower UTIs are much more common because of bacterial entrance via the urethra and NOT commonly via the bloodstream. Sexually active females may be at higher risk due to indirect factors (use of contraceptives vaginally and unintentional introduction of enteric flora into the urethra), and direct sexual transmission of infection can occur in males. Pyelonephritis usually occurs due to an infection that ascends through the urinary tract. The infectious inflammation can affect the interstitium, nephrons, or both. Incidence is highest during pregnancy and among the sexually active, paralleling the epidemiology of lower UTIs. Intrarenal abscesses can result, and rupture with spillage of contents into adjacent perirenal fat can cause formation of a perinephric abscess. Note that the likely pathogens are distinctly different in community-acquired and nosocomial infections.

7. Given a variety of scenarios, develop treatment plans for patients with urologic and renal disorders. pp. 283–296

The priorities for someone who is clearly in urgent distress due to urologic or renal disorders are the same as for a patient who is affected by a potentially life-threatening emergency of another origin. You must know how to respond properly and quickly to each major type of urinary or genitourinary emergency. Implementing effective prevention strategies, procedures that minimize further loss of any existing kidney function, is vital for patient outcome. Ensure adequate airway, breathing (ventilation), and circulation. This is particularly important for someone whose emergency may be affecting the respiratory and cardiovascular system. Nausea and vomiting that is commonly associated with urologic disorders can cause respiratory distress. This is especially true for the patient with an underlying pulmonary disease. Fluid retention and anemia often associated with acute renal failure can cause respiratory distress and cardiovascular compromise. Prolonged fluid volume overload and anemia can cause acute heart failure. Most urologic and renal disorders in the prehospital setting will require a minimum of supportive measures such as airway maintenance, oxygenation, ventilatory management, and hemodynamic and cardiac monitoring. You should always provide oxygen, allow a position of comfort, initiate an IV, and treat nausea, vomiting, and pain. Be cautious with IV fluids, as even small boluses can be excessive for patients with acute renal failure or a history of chronic renal failure. Saline locks often offer the best alternative.

Because acute renal failure can cause life-threatening metabolic complications (consider the key role of the kidneys in regulation of fluid volume, electrolytes, and pH), provide close monitoring and support of the ABCs. High-concentration oxygen should be used, and patient positioning and IV fluid resuscitation are important. In general, you want to protect fluid volume and cardiovascular function to minimize damage due to renal hypoperfusion and eliminate or reduce exposure to any potentially nephrotoxic drug. Drug information may be available from medical direction; likewise, specific advice for care of dialysis patients may also be obtained before or during transit. Long-term management will focus on dialysis (either hemodialysis or chronic ambulatory peritoneal dialysis, dependent on individual circumstances) or transplantation.

Immediate management is similar to that for acute renal failure. Focus on close monitoring and support of the ABCs with high-concentration oxygen, positioning to support blood flow to internal organs and the brain, and administration of IV fluid if hypovolemia is suggested. Chief prevention strategies are protection of fluid volume and cardiovascular function with correction of major electrolyte

©2013 Pearson Education, Inc.
Paramedic Care: Principles & Practice, Vol. 4, 4th Ed.

disturbances as merited by individual findings and the philosophy of erring on the side of conservative treatment. Close monitoring of the ECG may give you time to adjust and respond to cardiac problems caused by fluid overload or electrolyte disturbances. Life-threatening conditions should always be treated and lesser conditions or complications noted for consideration by the receiving staff. Where possible, be sure your impressions clearly note which conditions have been chronic (or the norm) for the patient and which findings represent acute changes. As indicated and allowed by medical direction, fluid lavage may be considered for patients who use peritoneal dialysis.

Case Study Review

Reread the case study on pages 277–278 in Paramedic Care: Medicine; *then, read the following discussion.*

This case study demonstrates how paramedics react to a stressful medical emergency involving severe pain of unknown origin. In addition to noting how the team reacts to the patient's presentation and assessment, note how clues to the nephrological origin of his condition emerge from the assessment and history.

Rachel and Jack receive a call that is nonspecific but concerning: A man has fallen and cannot get up. Jack and Rachel have almost no information before arriving at the scene. They do not know the age of the patient, whether traumatic injury is involved, or the nature of the underlying cause of the fall. In their first moments at the house they realize that they are dealing with a relatively young, apparently healthy man who is having an acute episode of severe pain and apparently is not getting up because of the pain.

Their initial actions center on historical questions about the pain and on an initial physical assessment. The patient tells them that the pain was of sudden onset and is very severe. His concerns about the possible cause of his problem give them an immediate clue. He tells them there is a family history of kidney stones and that his brother had one recently, and he is concerned that he could be suffering from one. At the time this information is received, a urine specimen is obtained that appears to have blood in it.

You aren't told whether there are any significant findings on physical exam, so the assumption is that the exam was largely benign. You do know that the patient's vital signs are consistent with pain and stress: a relatively high blood pressure (at least if the patient isn't chronically hypertensive), tachycardia, and brisk respirations with good SaO_2.

The team secures IV access, administers Zofran, starts oxygen supplementation, and transports to the emergency department, where a diagnostic IVP shows complete ureteral obstruction due to an apparent radiopaque renal stone. Treatment centers on rest, gentle analgesia, and IV fluid to promote urine formation and flow. Finally, a visible stone is passed, David's pain subsides, and he can go home.

Although you aren't told about predischarge counseling, you do know that calcium-containing stones, the most common kind, tend to appear in men of approximately his age group, tend to run in families, and tend to recur in an affected individual. The patient should learn about the pathophysiology of stones and any dietary, physical, or other lifestyle modifications that might help reduce the likelihood of recurrence.

Content Self-Evaluation

MULTIPLE CHOICE

_____ 1. The major functions of the urinary system include all of the following, EXCEPT
  A. maintenance of blood volume.
  B. control of development of white blood cells.
  C. regulation of arterial blood pressure.
  D. maintenance of the balance of electrolytes and blood pH.
  E. removal of many toxic wastes from the blood.

_____ 2. BUN, or blood urea nitrogen, and creatinine are both measured in the blood as part of the assessment of kidney function.
  A. True
  B. False

3. The enzyme that is produced by the kidney and is part of the physiological response to low blood pressure is called
   A. aldosterone.
   B. angiotensin.
   C. erythropoietin.
   D. renin.
   E. progesterone.

4. The urethra in men is much shorter than it is in women, and this is one reason why there is a gender difference in the incidence of lower urinary tract infections.
   A. True
   B. False

5. Sperm cells are eliminated from a man's body after they move out of the testicles and pass through the following structures in first-to-last sequence.
   A. Vas deferens, epididymis, urethra
   B. Ureter, epididymis, vas deferens, urethra
   C. Epididymis, vas deferens, urethra
   D. Epididymis, vas deferens, prostate gland, urethra
   E. Vas deferens, epididymis, prostate gland, urethra

6. Typical questions to ask when obtaining a focused history related to abdominal pain include all of the following, EXCEPT
   A. previous history of similar event?
   B. sudden or gradual unintended weight loss?
   C. presence of chest pain?
   D. last oral intake?
   E. last date of sexual activity, if sexually active?

7. Indications that a woman's abdominal pain might be of obstetric (pregnancy-related) origin include all of the following, EXCEPT
   A. known pregnancy or last menstrual period not in immediate past.
   B. frequency and urgency of urination.
   C. indications of intra-abdominal hemorrhage.
   D. presence of blood in the vagina and on the vulva.
   E. palpation of the uterus above the pelvic rim.

8. Patients most at risk for kidney disorders are the elderly; persons with diabetes mellitus, hypertension, or both; and patients with more than one risk factor.
   A. True
   B. False

9. Oliguria is defined as low urine output (roughly 400 to 500 mL daily or less), whereas anuria is complete absence of urine output.
   A. True
   B. False

10. The two factors responsible for more than half of all cases of end-stage renal failure are
    A. damage due to nephrotoxic drugs and other substances and hypertension.
    B. pyelonephritis and diabetes mellitus.
    C. diabetes mellitus and hypertension.
    D. infections and glomerulonephritis.
    E. atherosclerosis and hypertension.

11. Common elements of uremia include all of the following, EXCEPT
    A. peptic ulcer.
    B. hyperkalemia and metabolic acidosis.
    C. easy bleeding and bruising.
    D. hypoglycemia.
    E. chronic anemia.

©2013 Pearson Education, Inc.
Paramedic Care: Principles & Practice, Vol. 4, 4th Ed.

_____ 12. Always be alert for development of physiological instability in patients with chronic renal failure, regardless of initial presentation.
   A. True
   B. False

_____ 13. Which of the following statements about kidney stones is NOT true?
   A. Renal calculi and nephrolithiasis are synonymous terms for kidney stones.
   B. Brief hospitalization for kidney stones is common because of the severity of pain while a stone is being passed.
   C. Immobilization and use of opiates and psychotropic drugs are risk factors for stones.
   D. Calcium and uric acid stones tend to run in families, suggesting a genetic link.
   E. Calcium stones are associated with chronic urinary tract infection or frequent bladder catheterization.

_____ 14. Male patients with kidney stones rarely have referred pain in the testicle on the affected side.
   A. True
   B. False

_____ 15. Risk factors for urinary tract infection include all of the following, EXCEPT
   A. female gender.
   B. pregnancy.
   C. advanced age.
   D. persons requiring routine bladder catheterization.
   E. persons with conditions causing urinary stasis.

MATCHING

Write the letter of the medical specialty in the space provided next to its definition.

A. nephrology

B. urology

_____ 16. Medical specialty pertaining to the kidneys

_____ 17. Surgical specialty pertaining to the urinary system

Write the letter of the description of the cause of acute renal failure (ARF) in the space provided next to the appropriate type of ARF.

A. injury to the nephrons, interstitial tissue, or both

B. hypoperfusion due to hypovolemia or compromised cardiovascular function

C. obstruction of both ureters or at the level of the bladder neck or urethra

_____ 18. Prerenal ARF

_____ 19. Postrenal ARF

_____ 20. Renal ARF

Write the letter of the organ or structure in the space provided next to the infection/inflammation that can affect that organ or structure.

A. urethra

B. prostate gland

C. urinary bladder

D. kidney

_____ **21.** Cystitis

_____ **22.** Pyelonephritis

_____ **23.** Urethritis

_____ **24.** Prostatitis

FILL IN THE BLANKS

Use the following list of terms relating to the structure and physiology of the kidney to fill in the blanks in the following statements. Note that not all terms will be used. One or more may be used multiple times.

secretion	nephron	filtrate
Bowman's capsule	distal tubule	descending loop of Henle
reabsorption	ascending loop of Henle	proximal tubule
urine	glomerulus	
water	sodium and chloride ions	

25. The successive parts of the nephron tubule are the _____, the _____, the _____, and the _____.

26. Filtration, the first process in formation of urine, occurs when blood is filtered through the capillaries of the glomerulus and into _____. This fluid, called _____, then passes into the proximal tubule.

27. The hormone aldosterone increases reabsorption of _____ and _____ in the distal tubule and collecting duct.

28. In the process of _____, substances such as potassium and hydrogen ions are transported from the blood into the tubule.

29. Fill in the blanks below to show the components of the OPQRST focused history about pain.

O. _____

P. _____

Q. _____

R. _____

S. _____

T. _____

Use the following list of terms relating to dialysis to fill in the blanks in the statements below. Note that not all terms will be used. One or more may be used multiple times.

infection	semipermeable membrane
artificial graft	arteriovenous fistula
filtrate	peritonitis
dialysate	

30. Two components necessary for either form of dialysis are a(n) _____ and a(n) _____.

31. In chronic ambulatory peritoneal dialysis, the peritoneum is used as the _____.

©2013 Pearson Education, Inc.
Paramedic Care: Principles & Practice, Vol. 4, 4th Ed.

32. In hemodialysis, vascular access is achieved through a(n) _____ connecting an artery and vein or a(n) _____.

33. _____ is a complication common to both kinds of dialysis.

LABEL THE DIAGRAMS

Supply the missing labels for the figure showing the major organs and structures of the urinary system by writing the appropriate letters in the spaces provided.

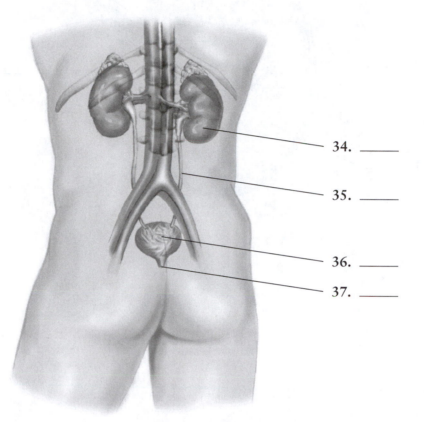

34. _____

35. _____

36. _____

37. _____

A. urethra

B. urinary bladder

C. ureter

D. kidney

Supply the missing labels for the figure showing the internal structure of the kidney by writing the appropriate letters in the spaces provided.

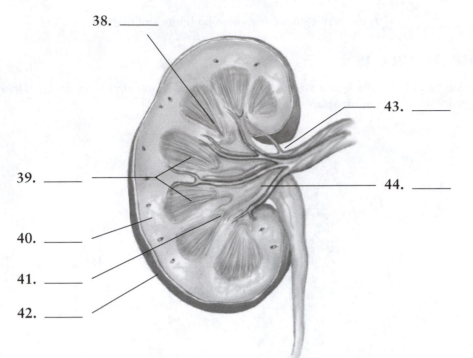

38. _____

43. _____

39. _____

44. _____

40. _____

41. _____

42. _____

A. medulla

B. pyramid

C. cortex

D. papilla

E. hilum

F. renal pelvis

G. renal capsule

©2013 Pearson Education, Inc.
Paramedic Care: Principles & Practice, Vol. 4, 4th Ed.

Special Project

Making the Call

You are called to the home of a patient who is familiar to you as an individual with end-stage renal failure. The call is for "passing out" during home peritoneal dialysis (chronic ambulatory peritoneal dialysis [CAPD]). When you reach the residence, the middle-aged man is awake and alert and has finished his dialysis session. When asked about the recent event, he says he does not usually faint during dialysis, although he commonly feels dizzy.

He says he has felt more tired over the past few days and that he is experiencing more abdominal discomfort during his dialysis sessions. He denies recent illness or injury to his abdomen, although he says he thinks he may have had a low-grade fever on the preceding evening. He admits to more soreness around the catheter entrance site than normal but says he isn't in constant pain and is fairly comfortable as he moves around in the house.

His vital signs are normal.

During your visual inspection of the man's abdomen, you note the end of a catheter protruding with obvious reddening, swelling, and discharge around the entrance site.

1. Based on what you know about chronic ambulatory peritoneal dialysis, what equipment is visible and invisible beneath the skin of the patient's abdomen?

2. Based on the history and physical findings, what is the probable nature of the underlying problem?

3. What equipment or bodily structures may be affected by the problem?

4. What precautions, if any, should you take during transport of this patient to an appropriate medical facility?

Toxicology and Substance Abuse

Review of Chapter Objectives

After reading this chapter, you should be able to:

1. Define key terms introduced in this chapter.

Knowing and being able to apply the key terms in each chapter is critical to understanding chapter concepts. Write the list of key terms. Then write the definition of each one in your own words. Check your understanding by confirming the definitions in the text glossary. Correct any misunderstandings. Create a study aid by writing each key term on the front of an index card and the definition on the back. Use the cards to quiz yourself, or to have someone quiz you.

2. Describe the epidemiology of toxicologic disorders and substance abuse.   **p. 300**

Toxicological emergencies are defined as those relating to exposure to a toxin, which is a chemical substance that causes adverse effects within the exposed individual. The term *toxin* includes drugs and poisons. Over the years, both the number and severity of toxicological emergencies have increased, so this is an area with which you must become familiar and must take steps to remain current in your knowledge. The estimated number of poisonings is over 4 million per year (and the term *poisonings* excludes drug overdoses). Roughly 10 percent of all EMS calls involve toxic exposures. About 70 percent of all accidental poisonings involve children under the age of 6 years; however, these poisonings tend to be relatively mild, accounting for only 5 percent of fatalities. Adult poisonings and drug overdoses are less frequent, but they account for over 90 percent of hospital admissions for toxic exposures and 95 percent of the fatalities in this category.

3. Describe the role of poison control centers in surveillance and management of toxicologic emergencies.   **p. 301**

Poison control centers (PCCs) assist in the treatment of poison victims and provide information on new products and new treatment recommendations. They are usually based in major medical centers serving large populations, and many have computer systems that allow staff to rapidly and accurately access information. Centers are available to you 24 hours a day, 7 days a week. Take the time to memorize the telephone number of the PCC center serving your area. Your PCC center can help you determine the potential toxicity for your patient when you give the PCC the following information: type of agent, amount and time of exposure, and physical condition of the patient. With this information, you may be able to start the current, definitive treatment in the field. The PCC can notify the receiving facility before you get the patient there.

4. **Describe the routes by which toxins can enter the body.** pp. 301–302

There are four routes of entry into the body: ingestion, inhalation, surface absorption, and injection. Ingestion via the mouth is the most common route of entry for toxic exposure. Inhalation of a poison into the lungs results in rapid absorption from the alveolar air into the blood. Causative agents are in the form of gases, vapors, fumes, or aerosols. Surface absorption applies to cases in which entry is through the skin or mucous membranes. Injection applies when the toxic agent is injected under the skin, into muscle, or directly into the bloodstream.

5. **Explain the general principles of assessment and management of toxicologic emergencies.** pp. 302–337

With each route of entry, there is a general pattern of possible toxic effects depending on the type and amount of agent involved. Immediate effects involve the tissues exposed to the toxic agent during entry. Delayed, systemic effects are related to absorption into the bloodstream and circulation throughout the body. In ingestion, corrosive agents can cause immediate injury through burns of the lips, oral mucous membranes, tongue, throat, and esophagus. Delayed effects can arise from absorption via the small intestine into the blood with effects on distant organs and tissues. In inhalation, immediate injury can occur from irritation of the airways, resulting in extensive edema and damaged tissue. Delayed, systemic effects occur when the agent travels through the bloodstream and interacts with distant organs and tissues. In surface absorption, immediate injury can occur in the involved skin or mucous membranes. Delayed effects again relate to absorption into the bloodstream. With injection, immediate injury is seen as irritation at the injection site, usually visible as red, irritated, edematous skin. Delayed, systemic effects are again due to distribution throughout the body via the bloodstream.

Certain basic principles of assessment apply to most toxicological emergencies. For instance, maintain a high index of suspicion that a poisoning or drug overdose may have occurred. During scene size-up, look for potential dangers to yourself and other rescuers, such as a threat of violence from suicidal patients and the threat of accidental injection from used needles that may be hidden on the patient or at the scene. In cases with chemicals and hazardous materials, it is crucial that you use the proper clothing and equipment. Be sure that such articles are distributed to team members who have been trained in their use.

Assessment of the patient begins with a history if the patient appears to be able to give one. Critical questions include what kind of toxin the patient was exposed to and when exposure occurred (so you have clues for likelihood of immediate or delayed effects or both). Physical involves a rapid head-to-toe exam with full vital signs.

In accordance with your local protocols, relay information to the PCC. Generally speaking, you never want to delay initiation of supportive or definitive care or transport because of delays in sending information to, or receiving information from, the PCC. Time is of the essence, literally. Ongoing assessment is particularly important for this group of patients, because they can deteriorate rapidly. Repeat initial assessment and vitals every 5 minutes for critical or unstable patients and every 15 minutes for stable patients. Specific assessment findings are given for each type of agent.

The preliminary steps of management include securing rescuer safety and removing the patient from any toxic environment. Support ABCs as you would with any other patient, keeping in mind that damage may have occurred to the mouth, pharynx, and/or airway in inhalation injury, and to the mouth and pharynx in ingestion incidents. The direct access to the cardiovascular system that occurs with injection cases may also complicate support of the ABCs.

The first management step specific to toxicological emergencies is decontamination, that is, minimization of toxicity by reducing the amount of toxin absorbed into the body. Decontamination involves three steps. The first is reduction of intake of toxin (steps will be route specific, such as removal from fume-filled atmosphere in inhalation, removal of clothes and cleansing of skin in surface absorption, removal of stinger in injection, and so on).

©2013 Pearson Education, Inc.
Paramedic Care: Principles & Practice, Vol. 4, 4th Ed.

The second step is reduction of absorption after the toxin is in the body, and this usually applies to ingestion incidents. The most common method entails use of activated charcoal to bind molecules of the toxin to it and prevent absorption into the bloodstream. Gastric lavage (stomach pumping) is of limited use as a step to reduce absorption. Lavage must be done within about 1 hour of exposure to be effective, and its possible complications (aspiration and perforation) are significant. Lavage is uncommon except in specific circumstances, for example, when the toxin doesn't bind to activated charcoal or when the toxin has no antidote. The third step in decontamination is enhanced elimination of toxin from the body. Cathartics enhance gastric mobility and thus may shorten the time the toxin is in the GI tract. Know the limitations in use of cathartics in your area, especially among pediatric patients, in whom they can induce severe electrolyte disturbances. Whole bowel irrigation with use of a gastric tube seems to be effective and carries few potential complications; however, its use is limited to only a few centers.

The third management step specific to toxicological emergencies is use of an antidote, a substance that neutralizes the specific toxin and counteracts its effects in the body. There are not many antidotes, and few are 100 percent effective. Your best guide is to be thoroughly knowledgeable with your local protocols, the directions given by the PCC, and counsel given by medical direction.

6. **Explain principles of management of poisoning by each of the following routes:**

   a. **Ingested toxins** pp. 301, 303–305

   Ingestion is the most common route of poisoning that you will see. Frequently ingested poisons include household products, petroleum-based agents such as gasoline and paint, cleaning agents such as alkalis and soaps, cosmetics, drugs (prescription, nonprescription, and illicit), plants, and foods. Some poisons can remain in the stomach for several hours, which may permit removal of the poison from the stomach and the body before systemic absorption can occur via passage through the small intestine. In at least one case, ingestion of aspirin, removal from the stomach is difficult because the ingested tablets bind together to form one large bolus. Useful questions for historical assessment include: (1) What did you ingest? (Obtain samples or containers whenever possible.) (2) When did you ingest the substance? (3) How much did you ingest? (4) Did you drink any alcohol? (5) Have you attempted to treat yourself (including induction of vomiting)? (6) Have you been under mental health care, and, if so, why (answer may indicate potential for suicide)? (7) What is your weight?

   Physical exam is especially important because history may be unavailable or unreliable. Your exam should provide physical evidence of intoxication and discover comorbid conditions that may affect treatment or response. Pay particular attention to skin, eyes, mouth, chest, circulation status, and abdomen. Be aware that a patient may have ingested multiple substances. Management centers on prevention of aspiration, intubation where necessary (rapid-sequence intubation may be required to avoid patient's clamping down on tube), use of high-concentration oxygen, and IV access for volume replacement and possible IV drug administration. Remember that it is always important to have ongoing cardiac monitoring and reassessment of vital signs.

   b. **Inhaled toxins** pp. 301, 305

   Toxic inhalations can be self-induced or due to accidental exposure. Commonly inhaled poisons include toxic gases, carbon monoxide, ammonia, chlorine, freon, toxic vapors, fumes, or aerosols (from products such as paint and other hydrocarbons, glue, and so on), carbon tetrachloride, methyl chloride, tear gas, mustard gas, amyl nitrite, butyl nitrite, and nitrous oxide. Inhaled toxins primarily cause direct injury in the respiratory system, and these problems may be most severe in patients who inhaled a chemical or propellant concentrated in either a paper or plastic bag.

   Given the pathophysiology of inhaled toxins, you should look for signs/symptoms related to three major systems: the central nervous system (dizziness, headache, confusion, hallucinations, seizures, or coma), the respiratory system (tachypnea, cough, hoarseness, stridor, dyspnea, retractions, wheezing, chest pain or tightness, crackles, or rhonchi), and the heart (dysrhythmias). Management starts with protecting yourself from any toxins in the atmosphere and removal of the patient from the injurious environment. Follow these guidelines: Wear protective clothing, use appropriate respiratory protection, and remove the patient's contaminated clothing. Then you can perform the initial assessment, history, and physical examination, focusing on the central nervous system, respiratory system, and cardiac system. Support ABCs as you would with any other patient, keeping in mind that damage may have occurred to the mouth, pharynx, and/or airway as a direct, immediate injury. Contact medical direction and your PCC according to your particular protocols.

c. **Surface-absorbed toxins**   pp. 301, 306

For surface absorption, the most common contacts are with poisonous plants such as poison ivy, poison sumac, and poison oak. Many toxic chemicals can be absorbed through the skin. Organophosphates, which are used as pesticides, are easily absorbed through the skin and mucous membranes, as is cyanide. The signs and symptoms vary widely depending on the toxin involved. Whenever you suspect surface absorption, take the following general steps: (1) wear protective clothing; (2) use appropriate respiratory protection; (3) remove the patient's contaminated clothing; (4) perform initial assessment, history, and physical exam; (5) initiate supportive measures; and (6) contact the PCC and medical direction.

d. **Injected toxins**   pp. 302, 325–326

Females in the insect class *Hymenoptera*—honeybees, hornets, yellow jackets, wasps, and fire ants—are common causes of injection injury. In addition, spiders, ticks, snakes, and certain marine animals are known causes of toxic exposure by injection. In addition to intentional injections, most poisonings by injection involve bites and stings from insects and animals. Be alert for the possibility of allergic reactions or anaphylaxis. Over time, beware of delayed systemic reactions. General principles of field management include the following: (1) protection of all rescue personnel because the culprit organism may still be in the area; (2) removal of the patient from danger of repeated injection (particularly in the case of yellow jackets, wasps, or hornets); (3) whenever possible and safe, obtain the injury-causing organism and bring it to the emergency department; (4) perform initial assessment and rapid physical exam; (5) prevent or delay further absorption of the poison; (6) initiate supportive measures as needed; (7) watch for anaphylaxis; (8) transport as rapidly as possible; and (9) contact the PCC and medical direction per protocols.

7. **Explain the specific considerations in the pathophysiology, assessment, and management of exposure to the following specific toxins and toxidromes:**

a. **Carbon monoxide**   pp. 306–315

Carbon monoxide (CO) is a tasteless, odorless gas that is often created by incomplete combustion. Because of its chemical structure, it has an affinity for hemoglobin over 200 times greater than that of oxygen. Once carbon monoxide has bound to hemoglobin, it is very difficult to displace and it causes an effective hypoxia. Because of the variability of signs and symptoms (depending on dose and duration of exposure), many people ignore poisoning until toxic levels are in the blood. Early symptoms resemble those of the flu. Combining likely causes of carbon monoxide generation with early symptoms raises this red flag. Beware of carbon monoxide poisoning in multiple patients living together in a poorly heated and ventilated space who have "flu-like" symptoms. Specific signs and symptoms include headache, nausea and vomiting, confusion or other manifestation of altered mental status, and tachypnea. Ensure safety of rescuing personnel. Remember, carbon monoxide is an odorless, tasteless gas that you can neither observe nor sense. Carry a high index of suspicion for this danger to protect you and fellow rescuers. Remove the patient(s) from contaminated area and have the fire service begin immediate ventilation of affected area. Provide supportive care of the patients, including high-concentration oxygen via nonrebreather device and consider continuous positive airway pressure (CPAP). Be prepared to treat seizures and cardiac dysrhythmias.

b. **Cyanide**   pp. 315–316

Cyanide can enter the body by different routes depending on the product in which it is found. It is present in household items such as rodenticides and silver polish, as well as in foods such as fruit pits and seeds. It can be liberated into inhalable form through burning of nitrogen-containing products such as plastics, silks, or synthetic carpets. (Cyanide poisoning should be suspected in all inhalation injuries associated with fire.) Cyanide also forms in patients on long-term therapy with nitroprusside. Regardless of entry, cyanide acts extremely quickly as a cellular asphyxiant, inhibiting the vital process of cellular respiration. Signs and symptoms include a burning sensation in mouth and throat, headache, confusion, combative behavior, hypertension, and tachycardia, followed by hypotension and further dysrhythmias, seizures and coma, and pulmonary edema. Management relies on removal from the source, immediate supportive measures, and treatment with a cyanide antidote. The most effective antidote for cyanide poisoning is hydroxocohalamin (Cyanokit™). It converts cyanide to vitamin B_{12}, a harmless substance. Note: Cyanide is rapidly toxic, so it is crucial you be familiar with a cyanide antidote kit if your unit carries one.

c. Cardiac medications
pp. 316–317

The number of available cardiac medications grows continually, and many classes exist, including antidysrhythmics, beta blockers, calcium channel blockers, glycosides, angiotensin-converting enzyme (ACE) inhibitors, and so on. General pharmacology includes regulation of heart function by reducing heart rate, suppressing automaticity, reducing vascular tone, or some combination of these. Although overdose can be intentional, it often is due to an error in dosage. At the level of overdose, signs and symptoms include (1) nausea and vomiting; (2) headache, dizziness, and confusion; (3) profound hypotension; (4) cardiac dysrhythmias (usually bradycardic); (5) cardiac conduction blocks; and (6) bronchospasm and pulmonary edema (especially with beta blockers). Management centers on initiating standard toxicological emergency assessment and treatment immediately. Severe bradycardia may not respond well to atropine, so you should have an external pacing device at hand. Some cardiac medications have antidotes; these include calcium for calcium channel blockers, glucagon for beta blockers, and digoxin-specific Fab (Digibind) for digoxin. Contact medical direction before giving any of these antidotes.

d. Caustic substances
pp. 317–318

Caustic substances can either be acids or alkalis, and such substances are common at home and in the industrial workplace. Strong caustics can cause severe burns at the site of contact; if ingested, they can cause tissue destruction at the lips, mouth, esophagus, and more distal regions of the gastrointestinal (GI) tract. Strong acids by definition have a pH less than 2; they are found in plumbing solutions and bathroom cleaners. Contact usually produces immediate, severe pain due to tissue coagulation and necrosis. Often this type of burn produces an eschar over the site, which may act as a shield to protect deeper tissues from damage. Because the substance is in the stomach much longer than the esophagus, the stomach is the more likely to sustain damage. Immediate or delayed hemorrhage is possible, as is perforation. Absorption of acids into the bloodstream produces acidosis, which needs to be managed along with the local, direct effects. Strong alkaline agents by definition have a pH greater than 12.5; they are present in solid or liquid form in household products such as drain cleaners. These agents cause local injury through liquefaction necrosis. Because of a delay in pain sensation, these agents are often present longer at the site of contact, allowing for greater tissue damage and deeper tissue injury. Solid products can stick to the oropharynx or esophagus, causing bleeding, perforation, and inflammation of central chest structures. Liquid alkalis are more likely to injure the stomach because, like the liquid strong acids, they pass quickly through the esophagus. Within one to two days of exposure to a strong alkali, complete loss of mucosal tissue can occur, followed either by gradual healing or further bleeding, necrosis, and stricture formation.

Assessment findings include facial burns; pain in the lips, tongue, throat and/or gums; drooling and trouble swallowing; hoarseness, stridor, or shortness of breath; and shock from bleeding and vomiting. Both assessment and initiation of management must be rapid and aggressive to avoid significant morbidity and mortality. As with other toxicological situations, protect yourself and initiate standard toxicological assessment and treatment. Pay particular attention to the airway. Injury to the oropharynx and/or larynx may make airway control and ventilation very difficult and may go so far as to require cricothyrotomy. Because caustic substances do not adhere to activated charcoal, there is no indication for it. It is controversial whether ingestion of milk or water acts effectively to coat the stomach lining or dilute the caustic. It is clear that rapid transport is essential. Hydrofluoric acid, which is used to clean glass in laboratory settings and in etching glass in artwork, is a specific example of a strong acid that can be lethal in even small exposure doses. Management specific to this agent is immersion of the exposed limb in iced water with magnesium sulfate, calcium salts, or benzethonium chloride.

e. Hydrofluoric acid
p. 318

Hydrofluoric (HF) acid deserves special attention because it is extremely toxic and can be lethal despite the appearance of only moderate burns on skin contact. HF acid penetrates deeply into tissues and is inactivated only when it comes in contact with *cations* such as calcium. Calcium fluoride is formed by this inactivation and settles in the tissue as a salt. The removal of calcium from cells causes a total disruption of cell functioning and can even cause bone destruction as calcium is leeched out of the bones. Death has been reported from exposure of < 2.5 percent body surface area to a highly concentrated solution.

Signs and symptoms of HF acid exposure include burns at the site of contact, dyspnea, confusion, palpitations, and muscle cramps. Management begins by protecting you, your patient, and your team from exposure. Initiate supportive measures to maintain adequate oxygenation, ventilation, and cardiovascular status. Remove any exposed clothing to limit exposure. Thoroughly irrigate the affected area with water. In addition, immerse the affected limb in iced water with magnesium sulfate, calcium salts, or benzethonium chloride. Transport the patient immediately for definitive care.

f. **Alcohol, chronic alcoholism, and withdrawal syndromes**   **pp. 335–337**

Ethyl alcohol is the form of alcohol in beverages, and it is the single most common substance of abuse among Americans. Alcoholism, dependence on alcohol, progresses in much the same way as drug dependence, discussed earlier in the chapter. The early symptoms of alcohol use, especially at low doses, include loss of inhibitions and emotionally excitatory effects, which can cause some of the aberrant behaviors associated with alcohol intoxication. Once ingested, alcohol is completely absorbed from the stomach and intestinal tract within approximately 30 to 120 minutes. After absorption, it is widely distributed in blood to all body tissues, and concentrations of alcohol in the brain rapidly approach the level in the blood. Alcohol's major physiological effects are as a central nervous system (CNS) depressant: toxicity can include stupor, coma, and death. Because the liver is the major site of detoxification within the body, compromise of liver function increases the course and severity of alcohol intoxication.

Another significant health effect is peripheral vasodilation, which results in flushing of the skin and a feeling of warmth. In cold conditions, this can increase loss of body heat and help to produce hypothermia. Alcohol-related diuresis is due to inhibition of vasopressin, a hormone responsible for homeostasis of water balance. The dry mouth associated with hangovers may in part be due to the alcohol-induced dehydration. Methanol, wood alcohol, is so toxic it is not safe for human consumption. However, methanol toxicity can occur either as an accident or because an alcoholic individual could not obtain ethyl alcohol. Methanol causes visual disturbances, abdominal pain, and nausea and vomiting even at low doses. Occasionally, methanol-toxic patients complain of headache or dizziness or present with seizures and obtundation. Ethylene glycol, a related compound, can also be involved in toxic emergencies. It produces similar symptoms, but its CNS effects, including hallucinations, coma, and seizures, present at even earlier stages.

Assessment findings in an individual with chronic alcoholism include poor nutrition, alcoholic hepatitis, liver cirrhosis with subsequent esophageal varices, loss of sensation in the hands and feet, loss of cerebellar function shown as poor balance and coordination, pancreatitis, upper GI hemorrhage (which is often fatal), hypoglycemia, subdural hematoma secondary to falls, and rib and extremity fractures, also secondary to falls. When you are in the field, keep in mind that conditions such as a subdural hematoma, sepsis, and diabetic ketoacidosis can, along with other conditions, mimic alcohol intoxication. For instance, the breath odor of ketoacidosis can resemble that of alcohol.

Abrupt discontinuance of alcohol by a dependent individual may provoke a withdrawal syndrome that can prove to be potentially lethal. Withdrawal symptoms can occur several hours after sudden abstinence and last up to five to seven days. Common signs and symptoms include a coarse tremor of hands, tongue, and eyelids; nausea and vomiting; general weakness; increased sympathetic tone; tachycardia; sweating; hypertension; orthostatic hypotension; anxiety; irritability or depressed mood; and poor sleep. Seizures may occur, as can delirium tremens (DTs). DTs usually develop on the second or third day of withdrawal and are characterized by a decreased level of consciousness associated with hallucinations and misinterpretation of nearby events. Both seizures and delirium tremens are ominous signs.

Alcohol intoxication, whether acute or chronic, should not be underestimated as a toxic emergency. In cases of suspected alcohol abuse, manage as follows: (1) Establish and maintain the airway, (2) determine if other drugs or substances are involved, (3) start an IV with lactated Ringer's solution or normal saline, (4) use a Chemstrip and give 25 g $D_{50}W$ if the patient is hypoglycemic, (5) administer 100 mg thiamine IV or IM, (6) maintain a sympathetic and supportive attitude with the patient, and (7) transport to emergency department for further care. Note: Medical direction may suggest diazepam in severe cases of seizure or hallucination.

©2013 Pearson Education, Inc.
Paramedic Care: Principles & Practice, Vol. 4, 4th Ed.

g. **Hydrocarbons** p. 319

Numerous household substances contain hydrocarbons, organic compounds composed primarily of carbon and hydrogen. Hydrocarbons include kerosene, naphtha, turpentine, mineral oil, chloroform, toluene, and benzene, and they are found in lighter fluid, paint, glue, lubricants, solvents, and aerosol propellants. Exposure can be via ingestion, inhalation, or surface absorption. Signs and symptoms of hydrocarbon exposure vary according to agent, dose, and route of exposure, but common problems include burns due to local contact, respiratory signs (wheezing, dyspnea, hypoxia, or pneumonitis from aspiration or inhalation), CNS signs (headache, dizziness, slurred speech, ataxia, and obtundation), foot and wrist drop with numbness and tingling, and cardiac dysrhythmias. Research has shown that less than 1 percent of hydrocarbon poisonings require physician care. In cases in which you know the agent in question and in which the patient is asymptomatic, medical direction may permit the patient to stay at home. On the other hand, hydrocarbon poisonings can be very serious. If the patient is symptomatic, does not know the causative agent, or has taken a specific agent (such as halogenated or aromatic hydrocarbon compounds) that requires GI decontamination, standard toxicological emergency procedures and prompt transport are indicated.

h. **Tricyclic antidepressants** p. 319

The tricyclic antidepressants were standard therapy for depression for years, despite concerns that their generally narrow therapeutic window made accidental toxic-level exposure, as well as intentional overdose, potentially common. Despite the introduction of newer, safer antidepressants, several tricyclics are still in use for depression, as well as chronic pain syndromes and migraine prophylaxis. Agents still in use include amitriptyline (Elavil), amoxapine, clomipramine, doxepin, imipramine, and nortriptyline. Signs and symptoms on assessment include dry mouth, blurred vision, urinary retention, and constipation. Late into overdose, you may find confusion and hallucinations, hyperthermia, respiratory depression, seizures, tachycardia and hypotension, and cardiac dysrhythmias (such as heart block, wide QRS complex, and torsade de pointes). In addition to standard toxicological procedures, cardiac monitoring is critical because dysrhythmias are the most common cause of death. If you suspect a mixed overdose with a benzodiazepine, DO NOT use flumazenil because it might precipitate a seizure. If significant cardiac toxicity is evident, sodium bicarbonate may be used as an additional therapy; contact medical direction as needed.

i. **Monoamine oxidase inhibitors** pp. 319–320

Monoamine oxidase inhibitors (MAO inhibitors) have been used historically as psychiatric agents, primarily as antidepressants. Recently they have found limited use as treatment for obsessive-compulsive disorder. These drugs have always had relatively limited usage for several reasons. They have a narrow therapeutic index, multiple drug interactions, potentially serious interactions with foods rich in tyramine (for instance, red wine and cheese), and high morbidity and mortality in overdose incidents. The pharmacology of MAO inhibitors directly affects CNS neurotransmitters. The drugs inhibit the breakdown of norepinephrine and dopamine while increasing the molecular components necessary to produce more. Remember that overdose with this group of drugs is very serious, even though symptoms may not appear for up to 6 hours. Assessment findings include headache, agitation, restlessness, tremor, nausea, palpitations, tachycardia, severe hypertension, hyperthermia, and eventually bradycardia, hypotension, coma, and death. Newer MAO inhibitors have been introduced into the marketplace; they appear to be less toxic and avoid the food interactions that involved the older generation of MAO inhibitors. They are reversible in effect; however, overdose outcome data are not yet available for these drugs. Management includes reversal if the drug is in the newer class of reversible MAO inhibitors, prompt institution of standard toxicological procedures, and, if needed, symptomatic support for seizures and hyperthermia with use of benzodiazepines. If a vasopressor is needed, use norepinephrine.

j. **Newer antidepressants and serotonin syndrome** pp. 320–321

In the recent past, numerous new antidepressants that are not related to the tricyclics have been introduced. Because of their high safety profile in both therapeutic and overdose amounts, these drugs have virtually replaced the tricyclics in clinical practice. This group includes trazodone (Desyrel), bupropion (Wellbutrin), and the large group of drugs known as selective serotonin reuptake inhibitors (SSRIs). Drugs in this group include Prozac, Luvox, Paxil, and Zoloft. Their pharmacology, as indicated by group name, centers on prevention of reuptake of serotonin from neural synapses in the brain, theoretically raising the amount of serotonin available to modulate brain function. The usual signs and symptoms in overdose cases are generally mild, including drowsiness, tremor, nausea and vomiting, and sinus tachycardia. Occasionally trazodone and bupropion cause CNS depression and seizures, but deaths are rare, and they have been reported in situations with mixed overdoses and multiple ingestions. You should know that the SSRIs have been associated with serotonin syndrome, a constellation of signs/symptoms correlated with increased serotonin level and triggered by increasing the dose of SSRI or adding a second drug such as a narcotic or another antidepressant. Serotonin syndrome is marked by the following: (1) agitation, anxiety, confusion, and insomnia; (2) headache, drowsiness, and coma; (3) nausea, salivation, diarrhea, and abdominal cramps; (4) cutaneous piloerection and flushed skin; (5) hyperthermia and tachycardia; and (6) rigidity, shivering, incoordination, and myoclonic jerks. Because of the lower morbidity and mortality in these drugs compared with overdoses with the older antidepressants, standard toxicological emergency procedures suffice. The patient should discontinue all serotonergic drugs, and you should institute supportive measures. Benzodiazepines or beta blockers are occasionally used to improve patient comfort, but they are rarely given in the field.

k. Lithium p. 322

Lithium is the most effective drug used in the treatment of bipolar disorder (a psychiatric disorder also known as manic depression). Pharmacology is unclear. However, it is known that lithium has a narrow therapeutic index, making toxicity relatively common during normal use and in overdose situations. Assessment findings of toxicity include thirst and dry mouth, tremor, muscle twitching, increased reflexes, confusion, stupor, seizures, coma, nausea, vomiting, diarrhea, and bradycardia and dysrhythmias. Lithium overdose should be treated primarily with supportive measures. Use standard toxicological procedures but remember that activated charcoal does not bind lithium and should not be used. Alkalinization of the urine with sodium bicarbonate and diuresis with mannitol may increase elimination of lithium, but severe toxicity requires hemodialysis.

l. Salicylates p. 322

Salicylates are some of the most common over-the-counter drugs taken and among the most common taken in overdose. They include aspirin, oil of wintergreen, and some prescription combination medications. About 300 mg/kg aspirin can cause toxicity. In these amounts, the salicylate inhibits normal energy production and acid buffering in the body, resulting in metabolic acidosis that further injures other organ systems. Assessment findings include tachypnea, hyperthermia, confusion, lethargy and coma, cardiac failure and dysrhythmias, abdominal pain and vomiting, and noncardiogenic (inflammatory) pulmonary edema and adult respiratory distress syndrome. The findings of chronic overdose are somewhat less severe and tend not to include abdominal complaints. It is thus difficult to distinguish chronic overdose from early acute overdose or acute overdose that has progressed past the initial abdominal irritation stage. In all cases, management of salicylate poisoning should be treated with use of standard toxicological emergency procedures. Activated charcoal definitely reduces drug absorption and should be used. If possible, learn the time of ingestion because blood levels measured at the right interval can be indicative of the expected degree of injury. Most symptomatic patients require generous IV fluids and may need urine alkalinization with sodium bicarbonate. Severe cases may require dialysis.

m. Acetaminophen pp. 322–323

Acetaminophen (paracetamol, Tylenol) has few side effects in normal dosage, and it is one of the most commonly used drugs in America for fever and pain. It is also a common ingredient in combination medications and is found in some prescription combination medications. In large doses, acetaminophen can be very dangerous. A dose of 150 mg/kg is considered toxic and may result in death secondary to liver damage. A highly reactive metabolite is responsible for most adverse effects, but this is avoided in most cases by detoxification. When large amounts enter the body in overdose, this detoxification system is overloaded and gradually depleted, leaving the metabolite in the circulation to cause liver necrosis. It is important for you to learn and remember that the signs and symptoms of toxicity appear in four stages: stage 1—0.5 to 24 hours after ingestion, marked by nausea, vomiting, weakness, and fatigue; stage 2—24 to 48 hours, marked by abdominal pain, decreased urine, and elevated liver enzymes; stage 3—72 to 96 hours, marked by liver function disruption; and Stage 4—4 to 14 days, marked by gradual recovery or progressive liver failure. Field management relies on standard toxicological procedures. Again, it is important to find time of ingestion because this may allow blood levels to be drawn at a time appropriate to predict potential injury. An antidote (*N*-acetylcysteine, or NAC, Mucomyst) is available and highly effective. However, NAC is usually given based on clinical and lab studies and in the hospital setting.

Nonsteroidal anti-inflammatory agents (called NSAIDs) are a large, commonly used group of drugs such as naproxen sodium, indomethacin, ibuprofen, and ketorolac (Toradol). Overdose is common, and assessment findings include headache, ringing in the ears (tinnitus), nausea, vomiting, abdominal pain, swelling of the extremities, mild drowsiness, dyspnea, wheezing, pulmonary edema, and rash and itching. There is no specific antidote for NSAID toxicity, so use general overdose procedures, including supportive care and transport to the emergency department for evaluation and any necessary symptomatic treatment.

o. **Theophylline** pp. 323–324

Theophylline is a member of the group of drugs called xanthines. It is generally used by patients with asthma or chronic obstructive pulmonary disease (COPD) because it has moderate bronchodilation and mild anti-inflammatory effects. It has a narrow therapeutic index and high toxicity, so it has been used less frequently recently. Thus, it is not a factor as often as it once was in overdose injuries. Assessment findings include agitation, tremors, seizures, cardiac dysrhythmias, and nausea and vomiting. Theophylline can cause significant morbidity and mortality. In an overdose setting, you must start toxicological emergency procedures immediately. Theophylline is on a short list of drugs that have significant enterohepatic circulation. Thus, activated charcoal in multiple doses over time will continuously remove more and more theophylline from the body. Dysrhythmias should be treated according to ACLS procedures.

p. **Metals (iron, lead, mercury)** p. 324

With the exception of iron, heavy metal overdose is rare. Metals that can cause toxicity include lead, arsenic, and mercury, all of which affect numerous enzyme systems in the body and thus cause a variety of symptoms. Some also have direct local effects when ingested and they accumulate in various organs.

Iron. The body needs only small daily amounts of iron; excess amounts are easily obtained through nonprescription supplements and multivitamins. Children have the tendency to overdose on iron by taking too many candy-flavored chewable vitamins containing iron. Symptoms occur when more than 20 mg/kg of elemental iron are ingested. Excess iron causes GI injury and possible hemorrhagic shock, especially if it forms concretions (lumps formed when tablets fuse together). Patients with significant iron ingestions may have visible tablets or concretions in the stomach or small intestine on x-ray. Other signs and symptoms include vomiting (often hematemesis) and diarrhea, abdominal pain, shock, liver failure, metabolic acidosis with tachypnea, and eventual bowel scarring and possible obstruction. It is essential to start standard toxicological procedures promptly. Because iron inhibits GI motility, tablets remain in the stomach for a long time and may possibly be easier to remove via gastric lavage (especially if concretions are not present). Because activated charcoal does not bind metals, it should not be used for iron overdose or for any other metal overdose. Deferoxamine, a chelating agent, may be used in iron overdose as an antidote because it binds iron such that less enters the cells to cause damage.

Lead and Mercury. Both metals are found in varying amounts in the environment. Lead was often used in glazes and paints before its toxic potential was realized. Mercury is a contaminant from industrial processing and is also found in some thermometers and temperature-control switches in homes. Both acute and chronic overdose are possible with both metals. Signs and symptoms of heavy metal toxicity include headache, irritability, confusion, coma, memory disturbance, tremor, weakness, agitation, and abdominal pain. Chronic poisoning can result in permanent neurological injury, which makes it crucial that heavy metal levels be monitored in the environment of a patient with toxicity. You need to remember the signs and symptoms of heavy metal poisoning and promptly institute standard procedures. Although activated charcoal is not helpful, various chelating agents (such as DMSA, BAL, and CDE) are available and may be used in definitive management in the hospital.

q. **Contaminated food** pp. 324–325

Food poisoning can be due to a variety of causes, including bacteria, viruses, and bacterial-associated chemical toxins. All notoriously produce varying degrees of gastrointestinal distress. Bacterial food poisonings range in severity. Bacterial exotoxins (secreted by bacteria) and enterotoxins (exotoxins associated with GI diseases) cause nausea, vomiting, diarrhea, and abdominal pain. Food contaminated with the bacteria *Shigella*, *Salmonella*, or *E. coli* can produce more severe reactions, often leading to electrolyte imbalance and hypovolemia. The world's most toxic poison is produced by *Clostridium botulinum,* and exposure presents as severe respiratory distress or even arrest. Fortunately, botulism rarely occurs except in cases of improper food storage procedures such as canning. A variety of seafood poisonings result from toxins produced by dinoflagellate-contaminated shellfish such as clams, mussels, oysters, and scallops. This exposure syndrome is called paralytic shellfish poisoning and can lead to respiratory arrest in addition to the GI symptoms. Toxicological emergencies can also arise from toxins found within commonly eaten fish. Bony fish poisoning (Ciguatera poisoning) is most frequent in fish caught in the Pacific Ocean or along the tropical reefs of Florida and the West Indies. Ciguatera may have an incubation period of 2 to 6 hours before producing myalgia and paresthesia. Scombroid (histamine) poisoning results from bacterial contamination of mackerel, tuna, bonitos, and albacore. Both Ciguatera and scombroid poisoning cause the standard GI symptoms; scombroid poisoning also produces immediate facial flushing due to histamine-induced vasodilation.

Except for botulism, food poisoning is rarely life threatening and treatment is largely supportive. In cases of suspected food poisoning, contact PCC and medical direction, and take the following steps: (1) perform necessary assessment, (2) collect samples of suspected food source, and (3) support ABCs with airway maintenance, high-concentration oxygen, intubation or assisted ventilation as needed, and establish IV access. In addition, consider administration of antihistamines (especially in seafood poisonings) and antiemetics.

r. **Poisonous plants and mushrooms**   p. 325

Plants, trees, and mushrooms are common contributors to accidental toxic ingestions. You should know that many decorative home plants can present a toxic danger to children. Most PCCs distribute pamphlets that list relevant household plants. In nature, it is impossible to identify all toxic plants and mushrooms. A general approach for you to take is to obtain a sample of the offending plant if possible, trying to find a complete leaf, stem, or flower. Mushrooms are very difficult to identify from small pieces. Because many ornamental plants contain irritating material, be sure to examine the patient's mouth and throat for redness, blistering, or edema. Identify other findings during the focused physical exam. Mushroom poisonings generally involve a mistake in identification of edible mushrooms or accidental ingestion by children. Mushrooms in the class *Amanita* account for over 90 percent of deaths; they produce a poison that is extremely toxic to the liver and carry a mortality rate of about 50 percent. Signs and symptoms of poisonous plant ingestion include excessive salivation, lacrimation, diaphoresis, abdominal cramps, nausea, vomiting, and diarrhea, as well as decreasing levels of consciousness, eventually progressing to coma. Contact the PCC if at all possible for guidance on management. If contact isn't possible, follow the procedures outlined under food poisoning (text pages 00–00).

s. **Animal and insect bites and stings**   pp. 326–331

Spider and snake bites can be common and significant toxicological emergencies in certain parts of the country. The brown recluse spider lives in southern and midwestern states. It is found in large numbers in Tennessee, Arkansas, Oklahoma, and Texas. It has also been reported in Hawaii and California. The brown recluse is about 15 mm in length, generally lives in dark and dry locations, and can often be found in or around a house. The bites themselves are usually painless, and bites often occur at night while the victim is asleep. The initial, local reaction occurs within minutes and consists of a small erythematous macule surrounded by a white ring. Over the next 8 hours or so, localized pain, redness, and swelling develop. Tissue necrosis develops over days to weeks. Other symptoms include fever, chills, nausea, vomiting, joint pain, and, in severe cases, bleeding disorders (namely, disseminated intravascular coagulation [DIC]). Treatment is largely supportive, and there is no antivenin. Antihistamines may reduce systemic reactions and surgical excision may be required for necrotic tissue. Black widow spiders live in all parts of the continental United States and are often found in woodpiles or brush. The female spider bites, and the venom is very potent, causing excessive neurotransmitter release at the synaptic junctions. Immediate, local reactions include pain, redness, and swelling. Progressive muscle spasms of all large muscles can develop and are usually associated with severe pain. Other systemic symptoms are nausea, vomiting, sweating, seizures, paralysis, and decreased level of consciousness. Field treatment is largely supportive, with reassurance an important factor. IV muscle relaxants may be needed for severe spasms. If medical direction orders it, you may use diazepam or calcium gluconate. Calcium chloride is ineffective and should not be used. Because hypertensive crisis is possible, monitor blood pressure (BP) carefully. Transport as rapidly as possible so antivenin can be given in the hospital.

There are several thousand snake bites annually in the United States, but few deaths. The assessment findings depend on snake, location of the bite, and the type and amount of venom injected. Two families of poisonous snakes are native to the United States: the pit vipers (cottonmouths, rattlesnakes, and copperheads) and the coral snake, a distant relative of the cobra. Pit viper venom contains hydrolytic enzymes capable of destroying most tissue components. They can produce hemolysis, destroy other tissue elements, and may affect the clotting ability of the blood. They produce tissue infarction and necrosis, especially at the site of the bite. A severe pit viper bite can produce death within 30 minutes. However, most fatalities occur from 6 to 30 hours after the bite, with 90 percent within the first 48 hours. Assessment findings for pit viper bites include fang marks (often little more than a scratch or abrasion); swelling and pain at wound site; continued oozing from wound; weakness, dizziness, or faintness; sweating and/or chills; thirst; nausea and vomiting; diarrhea; tachycardia and hypotension; bloody urine and GI hemorrhage (these are late); ecchymosis; necrosis; shallow respirations progressing to respiratory failure; and numbness and tingling around face and head. The first goal in treatment is to slow absorption of venom; remember that about 25 percent of bites are dry—that is, no venom is injected. Antivenin is available but should only be considered for severe cases as evidenced by marked systemic signs and symptoms. Routine treatment involves keeping the patient supine, immobilizing the affected limb with a splint, maintaining the extremity in a neutral position without any constricting bands, and giving supportive care with high-concentration oxygen, IV with crystalloid fluid, and rapid transport. Note: DO NOT apply ice, cold pack, or Freon spray to wound; DO NOT apply an arterial tourniquet; and DO NOT apply electrical stimulation from any source in an attempt to retard or reverse venom spread.

Coral snakes, which are small and have small fangs, are primarily found in the southwest. A mnemonic that you should remember is "Red touch yellow, kill a fellow; red touch black, venom lack." This indicates the stripe pattern of the coral snake: red-yellow-black-yellow-red. Coral snake venom contains some of the same enzymes as pit viper venom, but it additionally has a neurotoxin that will result in respiratory and skeletal muscle paralysis. Assessment findings include the following (noting that there may be no local or systemic effects for as long as 12 to 24 hours): localized numbness, weakness, drowsiness, ataxia, slurred speech and excessive salivation, paralysis of tongue and larynx producing difficulty in swallowing and breathing, drooping of eyelids, double vision, dilated pupils, abdominal pain, nausea and vomiting, loss of consciousness, seizures, respiratory failure, and hypotension. Treatment includes the following steps: (1) wash the wound with lots of water, (2) apply a compression bandage and keep extremity at the level of the heart, (3) immobilize the limb with a splint, (4) start an IV with crystalloid fluid, and (5) transport to the emergency department for antivenin. Note: DO NOT apply ice, cold pack, or freon spray to the wound; DO NOT incise the wound; and DO NOT apply electrical stimulation from any device in an attempt to retard or reverse venom spread.

Stings (injection injuries) can come from insects and marine animals. Many people die from allergic reactions to insect stings, particularly wasps, bees, hornets, and fire ants. Only the common honeybee leaves a stinger. Wasps, hornets, yellow jackets, and fire ants sting repeatedly until removed from contact. Assessment findings include localized pain, redness, swelling, and a skin wheal. Idiosyncratic reactions are not considered allergic if they respond well to antihistamines. Signs and symptoms of an allergic reaction include localized pain, swelling, redness, and skin wheal; itching or flushing of skin or rash; tachycardia; hypotension, bronchospasm, or laryngeal edema; facial edema; and uvular swelling. General management includes washing of the sting area, gentle removal of stinger if present (scrape, do not squeeze), application of cool compresses, and observation for allergic reaction or anaphylactic shock. Marine animal injection injuries are a threat in some coastal areas, especially in warmer, tropical waters. Toxin injection can be from jellyfish or coral stings or from punctures by the bony spines of animals such as sea urchins and stingrays. All marine venoms contain substances that produce pain that is disproportionate to the size of the injury. These toxins are unstable and heat sensitive, and heat will relieve the pain and inactivate the venom. Signs and symptoms of marine animal injection include intense local pain and swelling, weakness, nausea and vomiting, dyspnea, tachycardia, and hypotension or shock (in severe cases). In any case of suspected injection, treat by establishing and maintaining the airway, application of a constriction bandage between the wound and the heart no tighter than a watchband (to occlude lymphatic flow only), application of heat or hot water, and inactivation or removal or any stingers. Because both fresh and salt water contain considerable bacterial and viral pollution, you should always be alert to possible secondary infection of a wound. In cases of marine-acquired infections, be sure to consider *Vibrio* species.

t. **Commonly abused drugs**   **pp. 332–335**

The most commonly abused drugs include: (1) alcohol in its fermented and distilled forms; (2) barbiturates such as phenobarbital and thiopental; (3) cocaine (both crack and rock forms); (4) narcotics/opiates such as heroin, codeine, meperidine, morphine, hydromorphone, pentazocine, methadone, Darvon, and Darvocet; (5) marijuana and hashish (also called grass or weed on the street); (6) amphetamines such as Benzedrine, Dexedrine, and Ritalin (called speed on the street); (7) hallucinogens, including LSD, STP, mescaline, psilocybin, and PCP (also called angel dust); (8) sedatives from different chemical families, such as Seconal, Valium, Librium, Xanax, Halcion, Restoril, Dalmane, and phenobarbital; and (9) the benzodiazepines, Valium, Librium, Xanax, Halcion, Restoril, Dalmane, Centrax, Ativan, and Serax.

Many groups of drugs produce definable toxic syndromes. Knowledge of these syndromes is useful because it helps you cluster information for compounds that produce similar clinical pictures. (1) Anticholinergic toxidrome is caused by belladonna alkaloids, atropine, scopolamine, synthetic anticholinergics, and incidental anticholinergics such as antihistamines, tricyclic antidepressants, and phenothiazines. Signs and symptoms include dry skin/mucous membranes, blurred near vision, fixed dilated pupils, tachycardia, hyperthermia and flushing, lethargy, CNS signs, respiratory failure, and cardiovascular collapse. Management is as described for the tricyclics in objective 11. (2) Narcotic toxidrome is due to illicit drugs such as heroin and opium, prescription narcotics such as meperidine and methadone, and combination medications including narcotic agents such as hydromorphone, diphenoxylate (Lomotil), and oxycodone. Assessment findings include CNS depression, pinpoint pupils, slowed respirations, hypotension, and positive response to naloxone. Note that pupils may be dilated and excitement may predominate the clinical picture. (3) The sympathomimetic toxidrome is caused by aminophylline, amphetamines, caffeine, cocaine, ephedrine, dopamine, methylphenidate (Ritalin), and phencyclidine. Features include CNS excitation, hypertension, seizures, and tachycardia (hypotension with caffeine).

8. **Given a variety of scenarios, develop treatment plans for patients with toxicologic and substance abuse disorders.**   **pp. 302–337**

The priorities for someone who is clearly in urgent distress due to toxicologic and substance abuse disorders are the same as for a patient who is affected by a potentially life-threatening emergency of another origin. Remember that the basic assessment of a patient with a toxicological emergency includes careful scene size-up, protection of rescue personnel, and rapid response to any needs to support the ABCs. Ensure adequate airway, breathing (ventilation), and circulation. This is particularly important for someone whose emergency may be affecting the respiratory and cardiovascular systems. Treatment includes decontamination and use of antidotes, where available. Rapid transport is standard. Detailed specifics for many drugs, toxic substances, and animal bites and stings are given in other objectives for this chapter. Most toxicologic and substance abuse disorders in the prehospital setting will require a minimum of supportive measures, such as airway maintenance, oxygenation, ventilatory management, and hemodynamic and cardiac monitoring. You should always provide oxygen, allow a position of comfort, and initiate an IV. Timely communication to the receiving facility is also important so it can prepare for appropriate decontamination and establish specialty treatment plans.

Case Study Review

Reread the case study on pages 299–300 in Paramedic Care: Medicine; *then, read the following discussion.*

This case study demonstrates how paramedics react to a stressful emergency involving an unconscious person who proves to be someone familiar to them as a former patient. It demonstrates many of the general challenges involved in recognition and response to a life-threatening toxicological emergency.

©2013 Pearson Education, Inc.
Paramedic Care: Principles & Practice, Vol. 4, 4th Ed.

Kevin, Jake, and Shawn receive one of the briefest of calls, "unconscious person." Even before the team reaches the address, they realize that the address seems familiar to them; as they see the location, they remember that they have been called here before to care for a woman with a history of chronic depression and difficulty coping with stressful situations. The study does not state how Shawn knows that a team had been called here as recently as four days previously; it is possible that the team called for log information after realizing that the patient was well known in their service sector.

Initial scene size-up does not reveal any sign of toxicological threat to the team. The woman's boyfriend, who placed the 911 call, is apparently unharmed by any gas or other potentially invisible threat. There are a number of clues obvious to the team that indicate that the woman's unconsciousness is tied to an intentional toxicological emergency. They see an empty bottle of Tylenol (acetaminophen) and an empty bottle of nortriptyline, a tricyclic antidepressant. The nearby pharmacy receipt has the current day's date on it. In addition, the team can smell alcohol in the air and can see several empty bottles of wine. Even as one team member begins an initial assessment of the patient, the others can conclude that a multiple-ingestion overdose has occurred that involves acetaminophen, a tricyclic antidepressant, and alcohol. This is substantiated by the only history, a statement by the boyfriend that the patient had called him and said she "just couldn't take it anymore." The timing of the ingestion is unclear. Certainly the woman was able to make a telephone call and speak coherently 2 hours or so before the 911 call was made.

Initial assessment reveals that the woman is alive but in extremis: She is unresponsive, has slow, shallow respirations indicative of respiratory depression, and tachycardia with weak pulses. The team begins with the ABCs, intubating the patient and beginning mechanical ventilation. Although the study does not state that they are also giving supplemental oxygen, you should assume that they are doing so with high-concentration oxygen. They quickly establish IV access and place essential monitors; again, details are not given, but electrocardiogram (ECG) monitoring and pulse oximetry would be indicated. Continuous assessment of vitals is essential in this type of unstable situation.

The team checks for signs of trauma or other coexisting conditions and finds evidence of previous suicidal intent: multiple shallow scars across both wrists. Rapid transport is initiated, and the team remembers to bring all bottles of medicine found at the scene. Despite their intensive supportive care, the patient does not improve en route and has a generalized, grand mal seizure in the emergency department. Further care and transfer to the ICU are insufficient, and the patient dies in the ICU roughly 48 hours after admission due to cardiac dysrhythmias and liver failure. An autopsy, the results of which are pending, may provide further information on the details of her ingestion and her progressive organ failure.

This vignette contains many of the elements of common toxicological emergencies: a severely ill patient, little history of the immediate event besides clues apparent at the scene, and a struggle for the paramedic team to support the woman's vital functions while transporting her to the hospital for more definitive treatment. This case study also points out something else you will see with some toxicological emergencies: It isn't possible to save every patient. Whether the emergency is accidental or intentional, some patients cannot be saved, even when everything is done correctly and promptly by the paramedic team.

Content Self-Evaluation

MULTIPLE CHOICE

_____ 1. Which of the following statements about the epidemiology of toxicological emergencies is NOT true?

    A. The frequency of toxicological emergencies continues to increase both in number and severity.

    B. About 70 percent of accidental poisonings occur among children aged 6 years or younger.

    C. Toxicological emergencies account for about 5 percent of emergency department visits and EMS responses.

    D. More serious poisonings, especially in older children, may represent intentional poisoning by a parent or caregiver.

    E. Adult poisonings and overdoses account for 95 percent of the fatalities in this category.

_____ **2.** Immediate effects of toxins are often localized to the site of entry, whereas delayed effects are often systemic in nature.
   A. True
   B. False

_____ **3.** Many inhalation exposures are accidental, and leading agents include the following
   A. carbon dioxide, carbon tetrachloride, and ammonia.
   B. toxic vapors, plants, and chlorine.
   C. carbon monoxide, nitrous oxide, and petroleum-based products such as gasoline.
   D. carbon monoxide, ammonia, and toxic vapors.
   E. chlorine, cleaners (soaps and alkalis), and carbon monoxide.

_____ **4.** All of the following are guidelines to follow in cases of toxicological emergencies, EXCEPT
   A. maintaining a high index of suspicion for possible poisonings.
   B. recording everything you see or smell at the scene that might help determine cause.
   C. taking appropriate measures to protect all rescue personnel and any bystanders.
   D. centering general management on support of ABCs, decontamination of the patient, and use of an antidote, if there is one.
   E. removing the patient from a toxic environment as promptly as possible.

_____ **5.** Never delay supportive measures or transport due to a delay in contacting the poison control center.
   A. True
   B. False

_____ **6.** The most common route of entry for toxic substances is
   A. inhalation.   **D.** injection.
   B. ingestion.   **E.** adsorption.
   C. surface absorption.

_____ **7.** The three principles of decontamination are
   A. removal of patient from toxic environment, reduction in intake of toxin, and increase in elimination of toxin from body.
   B. removal of patient from toxic environment, removal of patient's clothing and washing of patient's body, increase in elimination of toxin from body.
   C. removal of patient from toxic environment, reduction in intake of toxin, and use of antidote, if one is available.
   D. removal of patient's clothing and washing of body, reduction in intake of toxin, and reduction in absorption of toxin already in body.
   E. reduction in intake of toxin into the body, reduction of absorption of toxin already in the body, and increase in elimination of toxin from the body.

_____ **8.** The most widely used means of reducing absorption of toxins in the body is
   A. gastric lavage (stomach pumping).   **D.** whole bowel irrigation.
   B. activated charcoal.   **E.** chelating agents.
   C. syrup of ipecac.

_____ **9.** Do not involve law enforcement in a possible suicide case until it is clear that suicide was intended.
   A. True
   B. False

_____ **10.** Which of the following is NOT a question commonly asked of a poisoning patient during the focused history?
   A. How much of the agent(s) did you ingest?
   B. How long ago did you ingest the agent(s)?
   C. Were any people with you when you ingested the agent(s)?
   D. What is your weight?
   E. Have you attempted to treat yourself in any way?

©2013 Pearson Education, Inc.
Paramedic Care: Principles & Practice, Vol. 4, 4th Ed.

_____ 11. The physical exam is crucial in toxicological emergencies, and it has two purposes: (1) identifying physical evidence of intoxication and (2) detecting any underlying illness or condition that might affect either the patient's symptoms or the outcome of exposure.
  A. True
  B. False

_____ 12. Which of the following statements is NOT correct when treating ingestion emergencies?
  A. Maintaining the ABCs is the top priority, along with monitoring of all vitals.
  B. Prevention of aspiration is a major objective, and intubation may be necessary.
  C. An IV at keep-vein-open rate is recommended for all potentially dangerous ingestion incidents.
  D. Induce vomiting unless it is against local protocol or you are told not to do so by the poison control center.
  E. Follow general treatment guidelines with decontamination procedures.

_____ 13. The priorty order for surface-absorption exposures are to remove the patient from the toxic environment, perform the initial assessment, and then ensure your safety.
  A. True
  B. False

_____ 14. The typical signs and symptoms of carbon monoxide poisoning include
  A. a burning sensation in the mouth and throat, headache, and confusion.
  B. headache, seizure or coma, and tachypnea.
  C. tachypnea, pulmonary edema, and a burning sensation in the mouth and throat.
  D. tachypnea, tachycardia, headache, and confusion.
  E. headache, nausea and vomiting, and confusion or other altered mental status.

_____ 15. The narcotic toxidrome is characterized by CNS depression, whereas the sympathomimetic toxidrome is characterized by CNS excitation.
  A. True
  B. False

_____ 16. Response to poisoning with one of the cardiac medications often involves bradycardia, which may require use of
  A. atropine.   D. digoxin.
  B. an external pacing device.   E. calcium.
  C. a beta blocker.

_____ 17. Common assessment findings for ingestion with a caustic include all of the following, EXCEPT
  A. chest and abdominal pain.   D. hoarseness and/or stridor.
  B. drooling and trouble swallowing. E. pain in the lips, tongue, throat, or
  C. facial burns.   gums.

_____ 18. Drugs with narrow therapeutic indexes are more likely to be involved in accidental toxicological emergencies. Two such drugs are
  A. lithium and the selective serotonin reuptake inhibitors (SSRIs).
  B. tricyclic antidepressants and salicylates.
  C. tricyclic antidepressants and lithium.
  D. tricyclic antidepressants and SSRIs.
  E. salicylates and lithium.

_____ 19. It is particularly important to know the time of ingestion when a blood test (timed properly) can predict degree of damage. Two drugs to which this statement especially applies are
  A. acetaminophen and tricyclics.
  B. SSRIs and tricyclics.
  C. acetaminophen and nonsteroidal anti-inflammatory drugs.
  D. salicylates and nonsteroidal anti-inflammatory drugs.
  E. salicylates and acetaminophen.

20. If you suspect mixed ingestion with tricyclics and benzodiazepines, do NOT use flumazenil because it may precipitate seizures.
    A. True
    B. False

21. Serotonin syndrome includes all of the following signs and symptoms, EXCEPT
    A. nausea, diarrhea, and abdominal cramps.
    B. hypotension.
    C. agitation and confusion.
    D. hyperthermia.
    E. rigidity, incoordination, and myoclonic jerks.

22. Chelating agents are often useful in cases of toxicity due to
    A. lithium.
    B. theophylline.
    C. some cardiac medications.
    D. heavy metals.
    E. salicylates.

23. Which of the following statements is NOT true about MAO inhibitors?
    A. Overdose cases may be very serious, even though initial signs/symptoms may appear hours after ingestion.
    B. MAO inhibitors have been used to treat depression and obsessive-compulsive disorder.
    C. MAO inhibitors as a group have a narrow therapeutic index.
    D. MAO inhibitors may interact negatively with foods containing tyramine, such as cheese and wine.
    E. In overdose, death usually follows the eventual signs of tachycardia, hypertension, and coma.

24. In cases of suspected food poisoning or poisoning involving plants and mushrooms, it is important to bring samples along with the patient, if possible.
    A. True
    B. False

25. In cases involving bites or stings, fatalities are most likely among patients who have an allergic reaction or anaphylaxis to insect stings.
    A. True
    B. False

26. In common toxic drug ingestions, the use of benzodiazepines is frequently recommended with
    A. alcohol, narcotics, and barbiturates.
    B. alcohol, hallucinogens, and barbiturates.
    C. cocaine, amphetamines, and hallucinogens.
    D. cocaine, alcohol, and amphetamines.
    E. cocaine, amphetamines, and barbiturates.

27. Which of the following statements about delirium tremens is NOT true?
    A. They usually develop two to three days after withdrawal of alcohol.
    B. They can occur in individuals who have experienced recent binge drinking.
    C. DTs are marked by decreased level of consciousness with hallucinations.
    D. Seizures and delirium tremens are ominous signs.
    E. DTs are associated with a significant mortality rate.

©2013 Pearson Education, Inc.
Paramedic Care: Principles & Practice, Vol. 4, 4th Ed.

MATCHING

Write the letter of the term in the space provided next to the definition to which it applies.

A. injection

B. tolerance

C. toxin

D. inhalation

E. poisoning

F. substance abuse

G. therapeutic index (or window)

H. ingestion

I. delirium tremens (DTs)

J. enterotoxin

K. decontamination

L. surface absorption

M. overdose

N. toxidrome

O. withdrawal

P. addiction

_____ 28. An exposure to a nonpharmacological toxic substance

_____ 29. Entry of a substance into the body via a break in the skin

_____ 30. Result of drug discontinuance in which body reacts severely to absence of drug

_____ 31. Group of clinical signs and symptoms consistently associated with exposure to a particular type of toxin

_____ 32. Dependence on a drug—physiological, psychological, or both

_____ 33. Potentially lethal syndrome found when alcohol is withdrawn from chronic abusers

_____ 34. Dosage range between effective and toxic dosages

_____ 35. Need to progressively increase dosage to achieve same effect

_____ 36. Process of minimizing toxicity by reducing amount of toxin absorbed into the body

_____ 37. Entry of a substance into the body via the skin or mucous membranes

_____ 38. Exposure to an amount of pharmacological substance greater than normally tolerated

_____ 39. Bacterial exotoxin that produces GI symptoms and diseases such as food poisoning

_____ 40. Entry of a substance into the body via the respiratory tract

_____ 41. Any chemical that causes adverse effects on an organism exposed to it

_____ 42. Use of pharmacological product for purposes other than those medically defined for it

_____ 43. Entry of a substance into the body via the GI tract

FILL IN THE BLANKS

Write the answers to the following questions in the spaces provided.

44. The four routes of entry into the body for toxins are _____, _____, _____, and _____.

45. The _____ are a chemical group often used as pesticides and frequently involved in surface-absorption emergencies.

Special Project

Analyzing an Emergency Scene

Use your experience and what you have learned in this chapter to answer the questions about the following scenario.

You are called to the apartment of an elderly gentleman after his son called 911 to report that when he called his father for a nightly check, his father had slurred speech and sounded confused. The son told dispatch that his father had felt "under the weather" with a cold recently but had otherwise been in his usual, somewhat fragile, state of health. No specifics were given.

You find the patient alone in his apartment. He is an unkempt, confused gentleman who repeatedly introduces himself and asks your names. He looks moderately uncomfortable, has nasal congestion and a mild cough, and says he has been "a bit ill" for several days. He states that he took a long nap, and then got up and took his pills. He says he doesn't need any help, and that he just needs to sit a bit to clear his head. When asked what pills he took, and how long ago, he says he "thinks" he just took the bedtime pills, but he may also have taken the afternoon ones because he might have slept through the normal time to take them. He doesn't know where the pharmacy bottles are because his visiting nurse makes up his pill case once a week. You note on the nightstand next to the bed a pill case, one of those that has the days of the week and several times per day marked on it with a compartment for each dosing time. You observe that several compartments for each day have tablets or capsules, often multiple.

1. What kind of toxicological emergency might this situation represent, and would you suspect accidental or intentional circumstances?

As you start your physical assessment, the patient says, "Oh, my, I'm dizzy," and sits awkwardly on the floor. His pulse is difficult to determine, but it is weak, slow, and possibly irregular.

2. What are your initial interventions?
3. What priorities do you give to calling the PCC, medical direction, and initiating transport?
4. What, if anything, do you take with you from the apartment?

©2013 Pearson Education, Inc.
Paramedic Care: Principles & Practice, Vol. 4, 4th Ed.

Hematology

Review of Chapter Objectives

After reading this chapter, you should be able to:

1. Define key terms introduced in this chapter.

Knowing and being able to apply the key terms in each chapter is critical to understanding chapter concepts. Write the list of key terms. Then write the definition of each one in your own words. Check your understanding by confirming the definitions in the text glossary. Correct any misunderstandings. Create a study aid by writing each key term on the front of an index card and the definition on the back. Use the cards to quiz yourself, or to have someone quiz you.

2. Describe the role of heredity in the risk for hematologic disorders.   **pp. 355, 357, 358**

Heredity plays a considerable role in several hematologic disorders, including hemophilia, sickle cell disease, Von Willebrand disease, and autoimmune diseases.

Hemophilia is a sex-linked disease that causes abnormally low levels of an essential blood-clotting protein (Factor VIII). It affects approximately 1–2 persons per 10,000 in the United States.

Sickle cell disease is inherited. It primarily affects African Americans, although other ethnic groups can be affected. These include Puerto Ricans and people of Spanish, French, Italian, Greek, and Turkish heritage. If both parents carry a gene for sickle cell anemia, the chances are one in four that the child will have normal hemoglobin. The chances are two in four that he will have both normal hemoglobin and sickle hemoglobin, which is referred to as sickle cell trait. The chances are one in four that he will have only sickle hemoglobin (no normal hemoglobin.) This condition is referred to as sickle cell disease.

In Von Willebrand's disease, factor VIII: vWF, a component of factor VIII, is deficient. It is produced by the endothelial cells and is necessary for normal platelet adhesion. Thus, in addition to the clotting problem, platelet function is abnormal in patients with von Willebrand's disease. Although the disease is inherited, it is not sex linked, equally affecting both females and males. A sign of this disease is excessive bleeding, primarily after surgery or injury. It is not associated with the deep muscle or joint bleeding of hemophilia, nor is it usually as serious, although nosebleeds, excessive menstruation, and gastrointestinal bleeds can occur. Von Willebrand's disease that causes abnormal platelet function is an inherited disease and causes excessive bleeding in patients.

Autoimmune diseases occur when the body makes antibodies against its own tissues. These antibodies may be limited to specific organs, such as the thyroid, as occurs in Hashimoto's thyroiditis. Or, they may involve virtually every tissue type, as in the antinuclear antibodies of systemic lupus erythematosis (SLE) that attack the body's cell nuclei. Several anemias result from autoimmunity and will be discussed later in this chapter.

3. **Relate the anatomy and physiology of the hematologic system to the pathophysiology and assessment of patients with hematologic disorders.** pp. 342–358

The components of the hematopoietic system include the blood, bone marrow, liver, spleen, and kidneys. The process of hematopoiesis forms the cellular components of blood. In the fetus, this first takes place outside the bone marrow in the liver, spleen, lymph nodes, and thymus. By the fourth month of gestation, the bone marrow begins to produce blood cells. After birth and across the span of life, bone marrow continues to fulfill this critical function, barring the development of some pathological process.

In hematopoiesis, the stem cell reproduces to maintain a constant population of cells. Some stem cells further differentiate into myeloid multipotent stem cells that, in turn, differentiate into unipotent progenitors, which ultimately mature into the formed elements of blood: red blood cells (RBCs), white blood cells (WBCs), and platelets. Pluripotent stem cells may also differentiate into common lymphoid stem cells, ultimately becoming lymphocytes. Erythropoietin, the hormone responsible for RBC production, is produced by the kidneys and, to a lesser extent, the liver. The liver also removes toxins from the blood and produces many of the clotting factors and proteins in plasma. The spleen plays an important role in the immune system, with its cells that scavenge abnormal blood cells and bacteria.

Disorders or problems of the WBCs (leukocytes) have a significant impact on the body's defense system. These problems include leukopenia (too few WBCs) and leukocytosis (too many WBCs). A variation of leukopenia is neutropenia, in which there are too few neutrophils; this is potentially dangerous, because the absolute count for neutrophils is an excellent indicator of the immune system's status. Improper white blood cell formation may also cause disorders such as leukemia (cancer of the hematopoietic cells) or lymphoma (cancer of the lymphatic system).

Many times hematological disorders are discovered and diagnosed when the patient seeks assistance for another medical condition, because the signs and symptoms associated with hematological problems may be quite varied. Fever often accompanies infection, WBC abnormalities (immunocompromised and prone to infection), and transfusion reactions. Acute hemodynamic compromise can be found in patients with anemia secondary to acute blood loss, coagulation disorders, or autoimmune disease. Confirmation of hematological disorders is usually dependent on laboratory analysis, but a complete history will go a long way toward developing an accurate diagnosis. Additional specific considerations include mental status, dizziness, vertigo, or syncope, all of which may be indicative of anemia. Visual problems should alert you to the possibility of autoimmune disorders or sickle cell disease.

Skin color may be another indicator of hematological problems. Jaundice may indicate liver disease or hemolysis of RBCs, whereas polycythemia is often associated with a florid (reddish) appearance, as pallor is with anemia. Observe for petechiae or purpura and bruising. Itching is commonly associated with hematological problems because of an excess of bilirubin as a result of liver disease or hemoglobin breakdown. Many patients report itching over a bruise. Look for evidence of prolonged bleeding, such as multiple bandages over a relatively minor wound.

Palpate the lymph nodes of the neck, clavicle, axilla, and groin. Enlarged lymph nodes are commonly seen in conjunction with hematopoietic disorders.

Gastrointestinal effects may be quite varied. Patients with clotting disorders may report epistaxis, bleeding gums, or melena. Many patients with clotting disorders report atraumatic bleeding of the gums. Ulcerations of the gums and oral mucosa as well as thrush (viral infection of the mouth) are often seen with immunocompromised patients. Abdominal pain is often seen in patients with hematological disorders. You may also be able to discern hepatic or splenic enlargement on your abdominal exam.

You should always ask about joint pain and examine the major joints closely in any patient in whom you suspect hematological problems. Minor trauma can cause significant hemarthrosis in patients with clotting disorders such as hemophilia. Many patients with autoimmune disorders frequently complain of arthralgia (joint pain) in all of their major joints.

You may also see a variety of cardiorespiratory presentations that are linked to hematological disorders. Signs of hypoxia, such as tachypnea, tachycardia, and even chest pain, may be indicative of anemia. Occasionally, patients with bleeding disorders may develop hemoptysis. As always, you should be alert to signs and symptoms of shock and be prepared to initiate prompt therapy.

©2013 Pearson Education, Inc.
Paramedic Care: Principles & Practice, Vol. 4, 4th Ed.

4. Recognize medications used to decrease the risk of thrombosis. pp. 348–349

Patients who lack certain clotting factors can have bleeding disorders that may complicate their assessment and treatment. Other patients take medications that decrease the effectiveness of platelets or the coagulation cascade.

Certain medications, such as aspirin, dipyridamole (Persantine), and ticlopidine (Ticlid), irreversibly alter the enzyme, thus decreasing the platelets' ability to aggregate and initiate the coagulation cascade. Other medications, such as heparin and warfarin (Coumadin), cause changes within the clotting cascade that prevent clot formation. Heparin, in conjunction with antithrombin III (a naturally occurring thrombin inactivator), rapidly inactivates thrombin, which then prevents formation of the fibrin clot. Warfarin (Coumadin) blocks vitamin K activity necessary to generate the activated forms of clotting factors II, VII, IX, and X, effectively interrupting the clotting cascade.

Glycoprotein IIb-IIIa receptors are present on the platelet membrane and are the major platelet surface receptor involved in the final common pathway of platelet aggregation. When platelets become activated, the glycoprotein IIb-IIIa receptor undergoes a conformational change and becomes able to crosslink fibrinogen, thereby serving as the final common pathway resulting in platelet aggregation. Glycoprotein IIb/IIIa inhibitors are medications used in the treatment of acute coronary syndrome, often in combination with angioplasty with or without stent placement. These agents are frequently given in combination with heparin or aspirin to prevent clotting before and during invasive heart procedures. Glycoprotein IIb/IIIa inhibitors are classified as potent platelet inhibitors. These agents are used to prevent platelets from binding together, which can occur in patients with heart attacks and after angioplasty with or without stent placement. The following are specific glycoprotein IIb/IIIa inhibitors and their brand names:

- Abciximab (ReoPro)
- Eptifibatide (Integrilin)
- Tirofiban (Aggrastat)

Vitamin K (AquaMEPHYTON) enhances clotting. Certain by-products of tobacco smoking (especially in females on birth control pills) also enhance clotting. Relative or complete immobility, trauma, polycythemia (high red blood cell count), and cancer may also lead to increased clotting, as blood becomes relatively stagnant. The stagnation of blood allows platelet activation to begin, which leads to clotting. To counteract the effects of decreased activity, many patients take aspirin or other antiplatelet inhibitors and wear compressive stockings to facilitate venous drainage from the lower extremities.

5. Adapt the scene size-up, primary assessment, patient history, secondary assessment, and use of monitoring technology to meet the needs of patients with complaints and presentations related to hematologic disorders. pp. 350–358

During the scene size-up, your general impression will be very important, as you will be looking for clues that can indicate the patient's condition. The causes of hematologic disorders are numerous. One of the first questions you will answer will be whether there is a history of hematologic disease, such as hemophilia, sickle cell disease, Von Willebrand's disease, or an autoimmune disease. Evaluate the patient's level of consciousness using the AVPU method, as well as speech, skin appearance, and posture. The patient's emotional status may also provide clues to the patient's developing condition that may be altered due to pain, hypoxemia, or hemorrhage.

Complete your primary ABCD assessment and recognize any findings that would indicate a hematologic emergency. Determine responsiveness and assess the airway, breathing, and circulation. Alterations in the hematologic system may present as life-threatening bleeds or overwhelming infections with septic shock. Do not spend time obtaining a complete set of vital signs during the primary assessment. Your secondary assessment should include a respiratory, cardiovascular, and skin assessment; accurate history; and physical exam with a full set of vital signs. Initiate all appropriate monitoring devices. For example, alterations in ventilatory function may be observed in a patient experiencing a hematologic emergency associated with severe anemia, hypoxemia, or hemorrhage. Capnography measures exhaled or end-tidal carbon dioxide (CO_2) and can assist the paramedic in evaluating the ventilation rate and quality, and perfusion, in such a patient. Pulse oximetry is used to monitor a patient's general state of oxygenation and perfusion. Be sure to get a complete set of baseline vital signs early in the process.

Changes in vitals along with alterations in mental status may indicate early shock due to hemorrhage or other processes. Critical or unstable patients should be considered candidates for expeditious transport.

6. **Use a process of clinical reasoning to guide and interpret the patient assessment and management process for patients with hematologic disorders.** pp. 350–358

As a paramedic, it is vital that you develop your clinical reasoning process to quickly recognize and treat hematologic emergencies to improve patient outcome. This is because diagnosis and treatment with many hematologic emergencies is time-sensitive. Develop an organized general impression to rapidly identify signs and symptoms of hematologic emergencies. This will include obtaining an accurate history.

Assessment includes initial size-up, SAMPLE focused history with attention to current complaint, medical history, and physical examination. History of present illness will reveal whether the condition is acute, chronic, or an acute flare-up of a chronic problem.

When performing the physical exam, evaluate each system methodically as you would in any other patient. If the history suggests a hematological problem, look for potential pathology during the physical exam that may confirm your working diagnosis and be a clue to developing complications. Physical exam findings that can indicate an underlying hematologic condition include:

- Feelings of dizziness or weakness, vertigo
- Numbness or motor deficits
- Syncope
- Visual disturbances or loss
- Jaundice (yellow skin), itching, pallor, petechiae, purpura, or bruises
- History of prolonged bleeding
- Hepatomegaly (enlarged liver) or splenomegaly (an enlarged spleen)
- Epistaxis (nosebleed), hematemesis, or melena (dark, tarry stool)
- Bleeding of the gums
- Dyspnea, abdominal pain, chest pain, or body aches

The primary treatment for hematologic emergencies is to rapidly identify signs and symptoms of hematologic emergencies that can lead to shock. In cases not associated with alarm symptoms and shock, pain management and supportive measures are appropriate. Management of patients presenting with signs and symptoms of shock can include oxygenation, ventilatory assistance, fluid resuscitation, suctioning, assisting ventilations, keeping the patient warm, and electrocardiogram (ECG) monitoring. Make a strong effort to make the patient comfortable, keep NPO, prevent aspiration, and be prepared for developing shock. Consider the following:

- *Airway and breathing.* Position any patient that you suspect has a hematologic emergency in the position most comfortable for the patient. Protect the airway. Because nausea and vomiting are common in patients with hematologic conditions, you should have an emesis container close and have suction ready. Keep the patient NPO.
- *Circulatory support.* Establish IV access. It is important to have an accessible route for fluid volume resuscitation and medications. Some patients may need an additional IV if rapid blood loss is possible, such as in patients with upper or lower GI bleeding.
- *Pharmacological interventions.* Medications are available to treat signs and symptoms in patients with hematologic emergencies. When calling for orders, consider that the initial dose may not sufficiently alleviate the patient's nausea or pain. Request an initial dose and a prn dose with your initial contact with medical direction. This will keep you from being unprepared or having to call again later. Medications vary, but can include antiemetics, non-narcotic analgesics, narcotic analgesics, H2 blockers, and proton-pump inhibitors, to name a few.
- *Psychological support.* Patients suffering from a hematologic emergency are likely also to suffer anxiety, depression, or anger. The experiences associated with hematologic emergencies are often frightening or frustrating for patients because the pain is often intense and frequent throughout their lives. Some of the associated gastrointestinal (GI) symptoms may be perceived as embarrassing to patients, such as lower GI bleeds that result in fecal incontinence. Provide the patient with effective therapeutic communication and emotional support and explain the treatment regimen. Careful explanation and emotional support will help allay anxiety and apprehension.

- *Transport considerations.* Assess, provide emergency care, and transport the patient as quickly and safely as possible. Rapidly transport any patient who is at risk for shock or is demonstrating signs of shock secondary to a hematologic emergency. Constantly reevaluate and monitor the patient's airway, breathing, circulation, and neurologic status. In addition, reevaluate the patient's nausea and pain scale. Provide additional antiemetics and analgesics as appropriate.

7. **Describe the pathophysiology of specific hematologic problems, including the following:**

   a. **Anemias**   p. 354

   The most common disease associated with RBCs is defined as a hematocrit of less than 37 percent in women and less than 40 percent in men. The majority of patients remain asymptomatic until their hematocrit drops below 30 percent. Anemia is due to either a reduction in the total number of RBCs or quality of hemoglobin; it may also be due to acute or chronic blood loss. Anemia is a sign of an underlying disease process that is either destroying RBCs and hemoglobin or decreasing their production. Anemias may be hereditary or acquired.

   The signs and symptoms associated with anemia are related to the associated hypoxia that results from the decrease in RBCs or hemoglobin. Depending on the rapidity of onset, signs and symptoms may be subtle or dramatic, depending in some degree on the patient's age and underlying state of health. Signs and symptoms may include fatigue, dizziness, headache, pallor, and tachycardia, or dyspnea with exertion. If the anemia develops rapidly, it may overwhelm the body's compensatory mechanisms, in which case you may observe postural or frank hypotension, tachycardia, peripheral vasoconstriction, and decreased mental status.

   Anemia may be self-limited or can be a lifelong illness requiring transfusions on a recurring and periodic basis. Confirmation of the illness and determination of its cause will be predictive of its prognosis.

   b. **Sickle cell disease**   pp. 354–355

   This disease is an inherited disorder of RBC production that causes hemoglobin to be produced in a "C" or sickle shape during low-oxygen states. These patients also have a hemolytic anemia as a result of destruction of abnormal RBCs. The average life span of sickled cells is about one-sixth that of a normal red cell, approximately 10 to 20 days versus 120 days. Additionally, the sickled shape increases the blood's viscosity, leading to sludging and obstruction of capillaries and small vessels. Blockage of blood flow to various tissues and organs is common, usually following periods of stress. The process, called a vasoocclusive crisis, is characteristic of the disease and over time leads to organ damage, particularly in the cardiovascular, renal, and neurologic systems.

   Sickle cell disease primarily affects African Americans, although other ethnic groups may also be affected, such as Puerto Ricans and people of Spanish, French, Italian, Greek, or Turkish heritage. If both parents carry the sickle cell gene, the chances are one in four that their child will have normal hemoglobin.

   Patients will develop three types of problems. Vasoocclusive crisis causes severe abdominal and joint pain, priapism, and renal or cerebrovascular infarcts. Hematological crises present with a drop in hemoglobin, sequestration of RBCs in the spleen, and problems with bone marrow function. Infectious crises mark the third type of problem, as the patients are functionally immunosuppressed and the loss of splenic function makes them vulnerable to infection. Infections become increasingly common and often are the cause of death.

   c. **Polycythemia**   pp. 355–356

   Polycythemia is an abnormally high hematocrit occurring due to excess production of RBCs. A relatively rare disorder, it typically occurs in people over the age of 50. It can occur secondary to dehydration. The increased RBC load increases the patient's risk of thrombosis. Most deaths from polycythemia are due to thrombosis.

   The signs and symptoms of polycythemia vary. The primary finding is a hematocrit of 50 percent or greater, which is usually accompanied by an increased number of WBCs and platelets. The large number of RBCs may cause platelet dysfunction, resulting in bleeding abnormalities such as epistaxis, spontaneous bruising, and gastrointestinal bleeding. Other complaints may include headache, dizziness, blurred vision, and itching. Severe cases can result in congestive heart failure.

d. Leukopenia/neutropenia   p. 356

The white blood cells (WBC) are the body's principal defense system. Problems with WBCs typically result from too few white blood cells (leukopenia). The neutrophil is the main blood component protecting against a bacterial or fungal infection. A reduction in the number of neutrophils (neutropenia) predisposes the patient to bacterial and fungal infections.

The status of the WBCs is easily determined by obtaining a complete blood count. A normal WBC count ranges from 5,000 to 9,000 per cubic millimeter of blood. A decrease in the number of WBCs indicates a problem with WBC production in the marrow or destruction of WBCs. Because bacterial infections pose a major risk to humans, an absolute neutrophil count is a better indicator of the immune system's status. The prehospital treatment of leukopenia/neutropenia is supportive. Pay special attention to preventing infection in the patient, as his immune system is overstressed or may be functioning inadequately.

e. Leukocytosis   p. 356

A condition resulting in too many WBCs or characterized by improper WBC function is called leukocytosis. This occurs when the body is exposed to an infectious agent or is particularly stressed. Following exposure, the immune system is stimulated and the marrow and spleen start releasing WBCs to help the body fight infection. A WBC count between 10,800 and 23,000 per cubic millimeter of blood is characteristic of a bacterial infection. During periods of stress, immature neutrophils may be released into the circulation. These differ from mature neutrophils in that they have a segmented nucleus. These cells are referred to as "bands" or "segs." An increase in the number of bands is indicative of a significant bacterial infection. Causes of leukocytosis include bacterial infection, rheumatoid arthritis, diabetic ketoacidosis (DKA), leukemia, pain, and exercise. Viral infections tend to have little effect on the WBC count or, in some cases, actually cause a decrease in the WBC count. A WBC count greater than 30,000 per cubic millimeter is called a *leukemoid reaction*. A WBC count this high indicates a problem with excess WBC production. Any patient with a significantly elevated WBC count should be evaluated for possible leukemia.

f. Leukemia   p. 356

Cancers of the hematopoietic cells occur when the precursors of WBCs in the bone marrow begin to replicate abnormally. Initially the proliferation of WBCs is confined to the bone marrow but then spreads to the peripheral circulation. Leukemia is classified by the type of cell involved and may be either acute or chronic. Examples include acute or chronic lymphocytic leukemia, acute or chronic myelogenous leukemia, or hairy cell leukemia. Although leukemias may occur across the life span, some are more commonly associated with specific age groups. For instance, acute lymphocytic leukemia (ALL) is seen predominately in children and young adults, whereas chronic lymphocytic leukemia (CLL) is most common in the sixth and seventh decades of life.

The signs and symptoms of leukemia are variable, although anemia and thrombocytopenia (decreased number of platelets) are common. These patients often appear acutely ill, complain of fatigue, and are febrile due to secondary infection. Lymph nodes will be enlarged. The history often includes weight loss and anorexia, as well as a feeling of abdominal fullness or pain that occurs as a result of liver and spleen enlargement.

The management of leukemia is a marvel of modern medicine, as treatments such as chemotherapy, radiation therapy, and bone marrow transplantation have resulted in cures of specific types. Where ALL was once a virtual death sentence, now more than 50 percent of the pediatric patients live a normal life with the disease cured or in remission.

g. Lymphoma   p. 357

Lymphomas are cancers of the lymphatic system. Malignant lymphoma is classified by the cell type involved, which indicates the stem cell from which the malignancy arises, as either Hodgkin's or non-Hodgkin's lymphoma. In the United States each year, approximately 40,000 people are diagnosed with non-Hodgkin's lymphoma, and 7,500 are diagnosed with Hodgkin's lymphoma.

The most common presenting sign of non-Hodgkin's lymphoma is painless swelling of the lymph nodes, whereas those with Hodgkin's lymphoma typically have no related symptoms. Some patients report fever, night sweats, anorexia, weight loss, and pruritus. The long-term survival rate is much better with Hodgkin's lymphoma. Many people with this disease who were treated with radiation, chemotherapy, or both are considered cured.

h. Thrombocytosis   p. 357

Thrombocytosis is an increase in the number of platelets, usually due to increased platelet production (essential thrombocytosis). It is also seen in polycythemia vera, where both red blood cells and platelets are increased. Thrombocytosis often complicates chronic myelogenous leukemia. Thrombocytosis can be secondary to other disorders, such as malignant diseases, hemolytic anemias, acute hemorrhage, and autoinflammatory diseases.

i. Thrombocytopenia   p. 357

Thrombocytopenia is an abnormal decrease in the number of platelets. It is due to decreased platelet production, sequestration of platelets in the spleen, destruction of platelets, or any combination of the three. Many drugs can induce thrombocytopenia. Acute idiopathic thrombocytopenia purpura (ITP) results from destruction of platelets by the immune system. It is most commonly seen in children following a viral infection. ITP is characterized by easy bruising, bleeding, and a falling platelet count. Chronic ITP usually occurs in adult women and is often associated with autoimmune disease.

j. Hemophilia and von Willebrand's disease   pp. 357–358

Hemophilia is a disorder in which one of the proteins necessary for blood clotting is missing or defective. A deficiency of factor VIII is called hemophilia A, which is the most common inherited disorder of hemostasis. The severity of the disease is related to the amount of available circulating factor VIII, and patients are classified as mild, moderate, or severe on that basis. A deficiency of factor IX is known as hemophilia B or Christmas disease, which is more rare but also more severe than hemophilia A.

Hemophilia is a sex-linked inherited bleeding disorder. The gene with the defective encoding is carried on the X chromosome; this means that if the mother is a carrier, her son will inherit this disorder. Conversely, female offspring who inherit the defective gene from their mother will be carriers, but will not exhibit the clotting defect. For a female to exhibit the defect, she must inherit the defect from both parents, that is, a mother who is a carrier and a father who has hemophilia. Hemophilia A affects 1 in 10,000 males. The signs and symptoms of hemophilia include prolonged bleeding, numerous bruises, deep muscle bleeding characterized as pain or a "pulled muscle," and bleeding in the joints known as hemarthrosis.

In von Willebrand's disease, factor VIII: vWF, a component of factor VIII, is deficient. It is produced by the endothelial cells and is necessary for normal platelet adhesion. Thus, in addition to the clotting problem, platelet function is abnormal in patients with von Willebrand's disease. Although the disease is inherited, it is not sex linked, equally affecting both females and males. A sign of this disease is excessive bleeding, primarily after surgery or injury. It is not associated with the deep muscle or joint bleeding of hemophilia, nor is it usually as serious, although nosebleeds, excessive menstruation, and gastrointestinal bleeds can occur.

k. Disseminated intravascular coagulation   p. 358

Disseminated intravascular coagulopathy (DIC), also called consumption coagulopathy, is a disorder of coagulation caused by the systemic activation of the coagulation cascade. Normally, inhibitory mechanisms localize coagulation to the affected area through a combination of rapid blood flow and absorption of the fibrin clot. In DIC, circulating thrombin cleaves fibrinogen to form fibrin clots throughout the circulation, causing widespread thrombosis and occasionally end-organ ischemia.

Bleeding, the most frequent sign of DIC, occurs as a result of the reduced fibrinogen level, consumption of coagulation factors, and thrombocytopenia. It most commonly results from sepsis, hypotension, obstetrical complications, severe tissue injury, brain injury, cancer, and major hemolytic transfusion reactions. The patient may exhibit a purpuric rash, often over the chest and abdomen. The disease is quite grave and has a poor prognosis.

l. Multiple myeloma   p. 358

Multiple myeloma is a cancerous disorder of plasma cells, the type of B cell responsible for producing immunoglobulins (antibodies). Rarely seen in patients under the age of 40, approximately 14,000 new cases are diagnosed each year. Usually, multiple myeloma begins with a change or mutation in a plasma cell in the bone marrow. These cancerous cells crowd out the normal healthy cells and lead to a reduction in blood cell production. The patient then becomes anemic and prone to infection. The first sign is often a pain in the back or ribs as the diseased marrow weakens the bones, and as a result, pathological fractures may occur. The resulting anemia leads to fatigue, and reduced platelet production places the patient at risk of bleeding. Calcium levels rise as a result of the bone destruction, and this often leads to renal failure.

8. **Given a variety of scenarios, develop treatment plans for patients with hematologic disorders.**   pp. 350–358

The priorities for someone who is clearly in urgent distress due to hematologic disorders are the same as for a patient who is affected by a potentially life-threatening emergency of another origin. Ensure adequate airway, breathing (ventilation), and circulation. This is particularly important for someone whose emergency may be affecting the respiratory and cardiovascular systems. Most hematologic disorders in the prehospital setting will require a minimum of supportive measures, such as airway maintenance, oxygenation, ventilatory management, and hemodynamic and cardiac monitoring. You should always provide oxygen, allow a position of comfort, initiate an IV, and treat nausea, vomiting, and pain.

You should always be prepared to treat shock. Cases that seem to represent progressive, nonhemorrhagic conditions such as sickle cell anemia and autoimmune diseases should also be monitored for stability.

Case Study Review

Reread the case study on page 341 in Paramedic Care: Medicine; *then, read the following discussion.*

This case study draws attention to the assessment, management, and transport of a patient with a hematological disorder. Further, it also underscores the fact that the "nature of the call" as based on dispatch information may not in fact be the primary problem for the patient. In this case, for example, Christian and Victoria are dispatched for what seems to be a minor fall in a shopping mall, but instead turns out to be a potentially life-threatening event for their patient.

Medic 102 is dispatched for what appears to be a minor fall on a short flight of stairs at a shopping mall. As you'll recall, although it is important to treat the injuries caused by accidental falls, it is equally important to determine what caused the fall; so as always, scene size-up is an important part of the call. In addition to gauging the situation in terms of your personal safety and that of your patient and other people who may be present, you should be observant for possible contributing factors for the fall, such as spills or poorly maintained or broken steps.

The initial impression of this patient escalates the gravity of the situation beyond that of a "minor fall." Although C. J. is conscious and able to localize his pain, it is readily apparent that he is unstable as evidenced by his confusion, tachypnea, and tachycardia, with a weakly palpable radial pulse and obvious profuse diaphoresis. Recognizing the severity of the situation, Christian and Victoria move quickly to expedite C. J.'s transport to the hospital; however, in doing so, they take appropriate concern for the potential for spinal injury by logrolling him onto a backboard and quickly initiating oxygen therapy and establishing vascular access.

Once en route to the hospital, Victoria performs a more complete assessment. In addition to the already noted large ecchymotic area on the right flank, she finds a large effusion of the right knee and, equally important, finds a Medic-Alert tag indicating that C. J. has hemophilia A. Victoria recalls from her training that hemophilia is a clotting deficiency disorder that requires the administration of clotting factors to formulate clots and makes even seemingly minor trauma a potential life threat. Although Victoria has observed an improvement in C. J.'s mental status since the administration of oxygen and fluids, she completes her assessment by obtaining vital signs. With a blood pressure of 90/60, pulse of 120, and respirations of 24, C. J. is currently stable but needs continued monitoring. Victoria applies a splint to C. J.'s right knee, knowing that immobilization will help alleviate some of his pain as well as prevent further injury.

She contacts the emergency department (ED), knowing that C. J.'s condition, injuries, and hemophilia will require more than a "routine trauma" response. On the basis of her radio report, the ED physician orders the needed clotting factor from the pharmacy and alerts the trauma team. Complete and concise reporting to the receiving facility allows it to adequately prepare and, ultimately, best meet the patient's physiological needs.

©2013 Pearson Education, Inc.
Paramedic Care: Principles & Practice, Vol. 4, 4th Ed.

Content Self-Evaluation

MULTIPLE CHOICE

_____ 1. All of the following are components of the adult hematopoietic system, EXCEPT the
   A. blood.
   B. bone marrow.
   C. thymus.
   D. liver.
   E. spleen.

_____ 2. The major determinants of blood volume are red cell mass and
   A. erythropoietin levels.
   B. plasma volume.
   C. total body water.
   D. stem cell percentage.
   E. bone marrow volume.

_____ 3. The component of the red blood cell that is responsible for transporting oxygen is the
   A. basophil.
   B. granulocyte.
   C. hemoglobin.
   D. neutrophil.
   E. lymphocyte.

_____ 4. The Bohr effect describes the relationship between pH and oxygen delivery in that the more acidic the blood, the more readily oxygen is released to the tissues.
   A. True
   B. False

_____ 5. All of the following will cause a right shift of the oxyhemoglobin dissociation curve and thus increase the rate that oxygen is released to the tissues, EXCEPT
   A. increased carbon dioxide.
   B. increased temperature.
   C. decreased pH.
   D. decreased activity.
   E. increased activity.

_____ 6. The term for the packed cell volume of red cells per unit of blood volume is
   A. hematocrit.
   B. hemoglobin.
   C. red blood cell count.
   D. blood type.
   E. white blood count.

_____ 7. White blood cells that primarily function in allergic reactions to release histamine are called
   A. lymphocytes.
   B. neutrophils.
   C. eosinophils.
   D. monocytes.
   E. basophils.

_____ 8. White blood cells that primarily function to fight infection are called
   A. lymphocytes.
   B. neutrophils.
   C. eosinophils.
   D. monocytes.
   E. basophils.

_____ 9. T cells and B cells, which play critical roles in immunity, are types of white blood cells called
   A. lymphocytes.
   B. neutrophils.
   C. eosinophils.
   D. monocytes.
   E. basophils.

_____ 10. The condition that occurs when the body develops antibodies against itself is called
   A. acquired immunodeficiency.
   B. autoimmune disease.
   C. rejection.
   D. chemotaxis.
   E. inherited immunodeficiency.

_____ **11.** Causes of the inflammatory process include all of the following, EXCEPT
    A. infectious agents.
    B. chemical agents.
    C. trauma.
    D. immunological agents.
    E. genetics.

_____ **12.** The formed blood cell components responsible for blood clotting are
    A. red blood cells.
    B. white blood cells.
    C. lymphocytes.
    D. platelets.
    E. monocytes.

_____ **13.** The protein on the surface of a blood cell that allows blood to be typed is known as a(n)
    A. antibody.
    B. antigen.
    C. thrombocyte.
    D. granulocyte.
    E. monocyte.

_____ **14.** The process of red blood cell destruction is known as
    A. sequestration.
    B. fibrinolysis.
    C. hemolysis.
    D. hematopoiesis.
    E. phagocytosis.

_____ **15.** Tiny red dots found on the skin that may be indicative of hematological disorders are called
    A. purpura.
    B. jaundice.
    C. ecchymosis.
    D. petechiae.
    E. bruises.

_____ **16.** An excess of bilirubin, either from liver disease or the breakdown of hemoglobin, can cause
    A. gingivitis.
    B. generalized sepsis.
    C. arthralgia.
    D. priapism.
    E. pruritus.

_____ **17.** Often, one of the earliest indications of hematological problems is
    A. gingivitis.
    B. generalized sepsis.
    C. arthralgia.
    D. priapism.
    E. pruritus.

_____ **18.** A hematocrit of 50 percent or greater is the principal finding in
    A. anemia.
    B. leukopenia.
    C. polycythemia.
    D. thrombocytopenia.
    E. non-Hodgkin's lymphoma.

_____ **19.** Painless swelling of the lymph nodes is the most common presenting sign of
    A. anemia.
    B. leukopenia.
    C. polycythemia.
    D. thrombocytopenia.
    E. non-Hodgkin's lymphoma.

_____ **20.** An abnormal decrease in the number of platelets, which can be induced by many drugs, is
    A. anemia.
    B. leukopenia.
    C. polycythemia.
    D. thrombocytopenia.
    E. non-Hodgkin's lymphoma.

©2013 Pearson Education, Inc.
Paramedic Care: Principles & Practice, Vol. 4, 4th Ed.

MATCHING

Write the letter of the term in the space provided next to the most appropriate description of it.

A. erythropoietin

B. leukopoiesis

C. hematocrit

D. polycythemia

E. anemia

F. hemostasis

G. sickle cell disease

H. fibrinolysis

I. bilirubin

J. thrombosis

K. leukemia

L. antigen

M. thrombocytopenia

N. purpura

O. multiple myeloma

_____ 21. The packed cell volume of red blood cells per unit of blood

_____ 22. Clot formation

_____ 23. Protein on the surface of a donor's red blood cells that the patient's body recognizes as "not self"

_____ 24. Reddish-purple blotches related to multiple hemorrhages into the skin

_____ 25. An abnormally high hematocrit due to an excess production of red blood cells

_____ 26. An inherited disorder of red blood cell production

_____ 27. By-product of the breakdown of hemoglobin that is converted from porphyrin

_____ 28. An inadequate number of red blood cells or inadequate hemoglobin within the red blood cells

_____ 29. Hormone responsible for red blood cell production

_____ 30. Cancer of the hematopoietic cells

_____ 31. The process through which stem cells differentiate into the white blood cells' immature forms

_____ 32. The process through which plasmin dismantles a blood clot

_____ 33. An abnormal decrease in the number of platelets

_____ 34. A cancerous disorder of plasma cells

_____ 35. The combined three mechanisms that work to prevent or control blood loss

Special Project

Completing a Table

Complete the following table by filling in the boxes.

Hematological Disorder	Common Signs and Symptoms	Prehospital Management
Anemia		
Hemophilia		
Leukemia		
Lymphoma		
Sickle cell anemia		

10

Infectious Diseases and Sepsis

Review of Chapter Objectives

After reading this chapter, you should be able to:

1. **Define key terms introduced in this chapter.**

   Knowing and being able to apply the key terms in each chapter is critical to understanding chapter concepts. Write the list of key terms. Then write the definition of each one in your own words. Check your understanding by confirming the definitions in the text glossary. Correct any misunderstandings. Create a study aid by writing each key term on the front of an index card and the definition on the back. Use the cards to quiz yourself, or to have someone quiz you.

2. **Explain public health principles related to infectious diseases.**   pp. 363–364

   The task of public health epidemiologists is to study how infectious diseases affect populations, as well as to predict and describe how disease moves from individuals to populations and determine what the impact of the disease is on the population. Paramedics must evaluate the host (patient), what they believe to be the infectious agent, and the environment. Based on that assessment, they may opt to use more aggressive personal protective equipment (PPE). They must also consider the patient, those in the patient's environment, and the environment where the patient is being transported all to be at risk for infection.

3. **Describe the roles of local, state, and federal agencies involved in infectious disease surveillance and outbreaks.**   p. 364

   Local agencies including hospitals, fire departments, and EMS agencies cooperate with state and local health departments to monitor and report the incidence and prevalence of disease. Additionally, numerous federal agencies are involved in tracking the morbidity and mortality of infectious disease, as well as setting standards for workplace disease prevention and control standards. These include: the U.S. Department of Health and Human Services (DHHS) Centers for Disease Control and Prevention (CDC), the National Institute for Occupational Safety and Health (NIOSH), and the U.S. Department of Labor's Occupational Safety and Health Administration (OSHA).

4. **Differentiate between the characteristics of bacteria, viruses, prions, fungi, protozoa, and parasites as causes of infectious diseases.** pp. 364–366

Bacteria—Microscopic single-celled organisms (1 to 20 micrometers in length) that can be differentiated by their reaction to a chemical staining process; classified by type as spheres (cocci), rods, and spirals.

Viruses—Disease-causing organisms that are much smaller than bacteria and are only visible with an electron microscope; obligate intracellular parasites, they can grow and reproduce only within a host cell.

Prions—a new classification of disease-producing agents that microbiologists used to refer to as "slow viruses." They are neither prokaryotes nor eukaryotes but particles of protein, folded in such a way that proteases (enzymes that break down proteins) cannot act on them.

Fungi—Plant-like microorganisms, most of which are not pathogenic.

Protozoans—Single-celled parasitic organisms with flexible membranes and ability to move; rarely a cause of disease in humans, but commonly considered opportunistic pathogens in those patients with compromised immune function.

Helminths (worms)—Parasitic organisms that live in or on another organism and are common causes of disease where sanitation is poor; various forms include pinworms, hookworms, and trichinella.

5. **Describe the interactions of the agent, host, and environment as determining factors in disease transmission.** pp. 366–368

The elements of disease transmission include the interactions of host, infectious agent, and environment. Infectious agents invade hosts by either direct or indirect transmission, and may be bloodborne, airborne, or transmitted by fecal–oral route. Factors that affect the likelihood that an exposed individual will become infected and then actually develop disease include correct mode of entry, virulence (strength), number of organisms transmitted, and host resistance.

6. **Describe the phases of the infectious process.** p. 368

Exposure to an infectious agent may result in contamination or penetration. Penetration implies that infection has occurred, but infection should never be equated with disease. Once infected, the host goes through a latent period when he cannot transmit an infectious agent to someone else. This is followed by the communicable period when the host may exhibit signs of clinical disease and can transmit the infectious agent to another host. The time between exposure and the appearance of symptoms is known as the incubation period, which may range from a few days to months or years. Most viruses and bacteria have antigens that stimulate the body to produce antibodies. The presence of these antibodies in the blood indicates exposure to the particular disease that they fight. This process is known as seroconversion. The window phase refers to the time between exposure and seroconversion. The disease period is the duration from the onset of signs and symptoms of disease until the resolution of symptoms or death.

7. **Describe the body's defenses against disease.** pp. 368–370

The immune system is the body's mechanism for defending against foreign invaders. The various cells involved in the immune response are sometimes collectively referred to as the reticuloendothelial system (RES) because their locations are so widely scattered throughout the body. *Reticulo* means network and *endothelial* refers to certain cells that line blood vessels, the heart, and various body cavities. Key to the immune system's response is the ability to differentiate "self" from "nonself." Once an invader is recognized as "nonself," a series of actions is initiated to eradicate the foreign material; this process is known as the inflammatory response. This response involves selected leukocytes (white blood cells) that attack the infectious agent in a process called phagocytosis. Neutrophils act first and then 12 to 24 hours later are followed by macrophages. The macrophages release chemotactic factors, which trigger additional immune system responses.

©2013 Pearson Education, Inc.
Paramedic Care: Principles & Practice, Vol. 4, 4th Ed.

The complement system provides an alternative pathway to deal with foreign invaders more quickly than is accomplished through cell-mediated or humoral immunity. This system of at least 20 proteins works with antibody formation and the inflammatory reaction to combat infection by starting a cascade of biochemical events triggered by tissue injury.

8. Explain the principles and practices of infection control in prehospital care, including your responsibilities as well your rights under the Ryan White Act.　　　　　　　　　　　　　　　　　　　**pp. 370–375**

Our first line of defense is our skin, so it is very important to keep your skin in good condition—free of cuts and abrasions. Because health care workers wash their hands frequently, consider using hand lotion after washing your hands to maintain skin integrity. PPE provides an additional barrier to exposure, thus minimizing the risk of infection from bloodborne and airborne organisms. Isolating all body substances and avoiding contact with them further reduces risk of exposure. Using disposable items for patient care also decreases risk, as does exercising caution around "sharps." Thorough and vigorous hand washing also goes a long way to reduce inadvertent contamination. Dispose of biohazard wastes as proscribed by local laws and regulations. Decontaminate and disinfect infected equipment according to local standard operating procedures (SOPs) and protocols.

Under the Ryan White Act, employers are required to provide a medical evaluation and treatment for any paramedic or other EMS provider exposed to an infectious disease. The nature of the exposure is assessed based on the route, dose, and nature of the infectious agent. As part of the medical evaluation, employees are entitled to receive counseling about alternatives for treatment, the risks of treatment, signs, symptoms, the possibility of developing disease, and preventing further spread of the potential infection. This includes the available medications, their potential side effects, and their contraindications. Treatment must be in line with current U.S. Public Health Service recommendations.

9. Identify patients with risk factors for infectious disease.　　　　　　　　　　　　**p. 375**

Infection is the presence of an agent within the host, without necessarily causing disease. Not all exposures result in transmission of microorganisms, nor are all infectious agents communicable. Risk of infection is considered theoretical if transmission is acknowledged to be possible but has not actually been reported. It is considered measurable if factors in the infectious agent's transmission and associated risks have been identified from reported data. Generally, the risk of disease transmission increases if a patient has open wounds, increased secretions, active coughing, or any ongoing invasive treatment where exposure to an infectious body fluid is likely.

10. Adapt the scene size-up, primary assessment, patient history, secondary assessment, and use of monitoring technology to meet the needs of patients with complaints and presentations related to infectious diseases.　　**pp. 375–402**

When assessing a patient, always maintain a high index of suspicion that an infectious agent may be involved. Consider the dispatch information, evaluate the environment for its suitability for transmitting infectious agents, and maintain appropriate Standard Precautions. Gloves are the mandatory minimum level of PPE required on every patient contact. Consider eye protection.

When approaching a patient with a possible infectious disease, look for general indicators of infection, such as unusual skin signs, fever, weakness, profuse sweating, malaise, anorexia, and unexplained worsening of existing disease states. If an infection is localized, signs of inflammation may include redness, swelling, tenderness to palpation, capillary streaking, and warmth in the affected area. A rash or other diagnostic skin signs may make identifying an infectious disease much easier.

Complete your primary ABCD assessment and recognize any findings that would indicate serious signs and symptoms associated with infectious disease. Always start with the least invasive step, visual inspection. This includes checking patient appearance and positioning as well as visually inspecting the skin, looking for any signs of infections. Your secondary assessment should include an accurate history and physical exam with a full set of vital signs. Obtain an oral temperature if the equipment is available. Initiate all appropriate monitoring devices. For example, alterations in ventilatory function may be observed in a patient experiencing serious signs and symptoms associated with infectious disease. Capnography measures exhaled or end-tidal carbon dioxide (CO_2) and can assist the paramedic in evaluating the ventilation rate and quality in such a patient. Pulse oximetry is used to monitor a patient's general state of perfusion. Be sure to get a complete set of baseline vital signs early in the process. Changes in vitals along with alterations in mental status may indicate early shock due to volume loss or other processes.

Patients with infection are at risk for vomiting, aspiration, and hypovolemic shock, so frequent assessment of the airway, breathing, and circulation is vital. Abdominal pain and nausea/vomiting are also commonly associated with infectious agents.

11. Use a process of clinical reasoning to guide and interpret the patient assessment and management process for patients with infectious diseases. pp. 375–402

As a paramedic, it is vital that you develop your clinical reasoning process to quickly recognize and treat emergent signs and symptoms associated with infectious disease to improve patient outcome. This is because diagnosis and treatment with many infectious diseases emergencies is time-sensitive. Develop an organized general impression to rapidly identify signs and symptoms of infectious disease. This will include obtaining an accurate history and identifying possible exposure to infectious agents.

When assessing any patient, you should maintain a high index of suspicion that an infectious agent may be involved. Evaluate every environment for its suitability to transmit infectious agents and always maintain appropriate Standard Precautions. Be alert to clues about the potential for infectious disease based on the patient's past medical history and medication use, as well as his chief complaint and the history of present illness. Look for general indicators of infection, such as unusual skin signs or rashes, fever, weakness, profuse sweating, malaise, or dehydration. Follow the standard format for assessing medical patients.

Infectious diseases are manifested in many different ways. Management of patients presenting with serious signs and symptoms can include oxygenation, ventilatory assistance, fluid resuscitation, suctioning, assisting ventilations, keeping the patient warm, and electrocardiogram (ECG) monitoring. Make a strong effort to make the patient comfortable, keep NPO, prevent aspiration, and be prepared for developing shock. Consider the following:

- *Airway and breathing.* Position the patient in the position most comfortable for the patient. Protect the airway. Because nausea and vomiting are common in patients with infectious agents, you should have an emesis container close and have suction ready. Keep the patient NPO.
- *Circulatory support.* Establish IV access based on your local protocols. It is important to have an accessible route for fluid volume resuscitation and medications. Some patients may need an IV if rapid volume loss from diaphoresis, vomiting, or diarrhea is present.
- *Pharmacological interventions.* Medications are available to treat signs and symptoms in patients suffering from infectious disease. When calling for orders, consider that the initial dose may not sufficiently alleviate the patient's nausea or pain. Request an initial dose and a prn dose with your initial contact with medical direction. This will keep you from being unprepared or having to call again later. Medications vary, but can include antiemetics, non-narcotic analgesics, H2 blockers, and proton-pump inhibitors, to name a few.
- *Psychological support.* Patients suffering from infectious disease, acute or chronic, are likely also to suffer anxiety, depression, or anger. The experiences associated with infection are often frightening for patients because they often can often blame themselves or hold themselves responsible for the infection. Some infectious diseases may be perceived as embarrassing to patients because of how they contracted the disease. Provide the patient with effective, nonjudgmental therapeutic communication and emotional support and explain the treatment regimen. In most cases, it is appropriate to explain to the patient what may be occurring and why. Careful explanation and emotional support will help allay anxiety and apprehension.
- *Transport considerations.* Assess, provide emergency care, and transport the patient as quickly and safely as possible. Rapidly transport any patient who is at risk for shock or is demonstrating signs of shock secondary to infectious disease. Constantly reevaluate and monitor the patient's airway, breathing, circulation, and neurologic status. In addition, reevaluate the patient's nausea and pain scale. Provide additional antiemetics and analgesics as appropriate. Be sure to maintain infection control procedures and complete appropriate decontamination/disinfection of the ambulance and equipement as needed.

12. **Describe the pathophysiology of infectious diseases of immediate concern to EMS providers.**   **pp. 376–402**

To summarize, the interactions between a host, an infectious agent, and the environment are the elements of disease transmission. Recognizing that infectious agents invade hosts through either direct or indirect transmission, you should generally be able to determine which is applicable given the patient presentation. Your role as an EMS provider is to interrupt disease transmission while providing safe and effective care for your patient, based on your recognition of signs and symptoms and your knowledge of the physiologic priorities for emergency care. There are several infectious diseases that are a concern to EMS. They are as follows:

Human immunodeficiency virus (HIV)

—HIV is a retrovirus with affinity for human T lymphocytes with the CDA marker.
—Transmitted via blood, blood products, and body fluids, HIV enters the body through breaks in the skin, mucous membranes, eyes, or by placental transmission (13 to 30 percent transmission rate).
—Destruction of the immune system leads to the development of opportunistic infections and cancers.
—There is no vaccine or cure, although postexposure prophylaxis with triple therapy (two reverse transcriptase inhibitors and one protease inhibitor) may be helpful.
—Practice Standard Precautions for all potential blood/body fluid exposures during patient care activities.

Hepatitis A (HAV)

—Hepatitis A virus is transmitted by fecal–oral route. It has an incubation period of three to five weeks, with greatest probability of transmission in the latter half of that period.
—The disease causes inflammation of the liver (also known as viral or infectious hepatitis) evidenced by general malaise, fever, anorexia, nausea and vomiting, and possibly jaundice, although many infections are asymptomatic.
—Vaccines (Havrix and Vaqta) provide effective active immunization.
—EMS workers should employ universal precautions against bloodborne or fecal–oral transmission.

Hepatitis B (HBV)

—Hepatitis B virus is transmitted by direct contact with contaminated blood or body fluids and is very highly infectious. There is a 1.9 to 40 percent transmission rate via cutaneous exposure and a rate of 5 to 35 percent via needle stick. The HBV incubation period is 8 to 24 weeks.
—HBV causes inflammation of the liver (also known as serum hepatitis) evidenced by general malaise, fever, anorexia, nausea and vomiting, and possibly jaundice, cirrhosis, and malignancies. Some 60 to 80 percent of infections, however, are asymptomatic.
—Vaccines (Recombivax HB, Engerix B) provide effective immunization after completion of series of three IM injections and follow-up antibody screening.
—Employ universal precautions against bloodborne transmission.

Hepatitis C (HCV)

—Hepatitis C virus is transmitted by direct contact with contaminated blood or body fluids.
—A majority of patients have chronic hepatitis C, which has the ability to cause active disease years later.
—HCV often causes liver fibrosis, which progresses over the years to cirrhosis.
—Effective vaccines do not yet exist, although there has been some success in treating disease with alpha interferon, often in combination with ribavirin.
—Employ universal precautions against bloodborne transmission.

Hepatitis D (HDV)

—Hepatitis D virus seems only to coexist with hepatitis B.
—HDV virus is transmitted by direct contact with contaminated blood or body fluids.

—HDV causes inflammation of the liver evidenced by general malaise, fever, anorexia, nausea and vomiting, and possibly jaundice, cirrhosis, and malignancies.

—Immunization against HBV confers immunity to HDV.

—Employ universal precautions against bloodborne transmission.

Hepatitis E

—Hepatitis E virus is transmitted, like hepatitis A, by the fecal–oral route; it is more commonly associated with contaminated drinking water.

—Hepatitis E causes inflammation of the liver evidenced by general malaise, fever, anorexia, nausea, and vomiting. It occurs primarily in young adults, with highest rates among pregnant women.

—Employ universal precautions against fecal–oral transmission.

Tuberculosis (TB)

—The causative bacteria of the disease is *Mycobacterium tuberculosis*.

—TB is commonly transmitted through airborne droplets but may also be contracted by direct inoculation through mucous membranes and broken skin or by drinking contaminated milk.

—The communicability of TB is variable, with an incubation period of 4 to 12 weeks, although disease usually develops from 6 to 12 months after infection.

—TB primarily affects the respiratory system, including a highly contagious form in the larynx, and may spread to other organ systems, causing extrapulmonary TB.

—No vaccine exists, although postexposure prophylaxis is helpful.

—Protect against disease transmission by practicing universal precautions, plus donning an N95 (or HEPA) respirator, as well as employing appropriate respiratory precautions while performing cardiopulmonary resuscitation (CPR) or intubation; masking the patient will also reduce exposure to droplet nuclei.

Meningococcal meningitis

—The causative organism for meningococcal meningitis is *Neisseria meningitidis*.

—The infection asymptomatically colonizes in the upper respiratory tract of healthy individuals and then is transmitted by respiratory droplets.

—Presentation includes fever, chills, headache, nuchal rigidity with flexion, arthralgia, lethargy, malaise, altered mental status, vomiting, and seizures; characteristic petechiae rash is common in pediatric cases.

—The incubation period is from 2 to 4 days, but potentially as long as 10 days.

—Meningococcal vaccines are available against some of the serotypes but are not routinely recommended for immunization of health care workers; postexposure drug prophylaxis is effective.

—Practice universal precautions and use masks on self and patient.

Tetanus

—*Clostridium tetani* bacillus is the causative organism.

—Tetanus is transmitted by exposure to *C. tetani* spores, which are present in the soil, street dust, and feces. The condition is often associated with puncture wounds, deep lacerations, or injections.

—Localized symptoms include rigidity of muscles in close proximity to the wound. Generalized symptoms include pain and stiffness of the jaw that may progress to cause muscle spasm and rigidity of the entire body; respiratory arrest may result.

—The incubation period is variable (usually 3 to 21 days, or 1 to 3 months); shorter periods are linked to more severe illness.

—Universal precautions should afford sufficient protection, although respiratory protection and goggles are advised for intubation.

—Vaccinations usually begin in childhood (DTP, or diphtheria-tetanus toxoid, pertussis) and every 10 years thereafter; postexposure prophylaxis is often recommended.

Chickenpox

—Chickenpox is caused by the varicella zoster virus (VZV) in the herpes virus family.

—It is transmitted by airborne droplet inhalation plus direct contact with weeping lesions or contaminated linens.

—Respiratory symptoms include malaise and low-grade fever, followed by a rash that starts on the face and trunk and progresses to the rest of the body, including the mucous membranes. The fluid-filled vesicles that form the rash rupture, leaving small ulcers that scab over within a week.

—The incubation period is from 10 to 21 days.

—An effective vaccine exists (Varivax) and is required in some states for admission to elementary school or day care; it is also recommended for susceptible health care workers.

—Employ universal precautions and place masks on patients. Extensive decontamination of the ambulance and any equipment used for the patient with chickenpox is strongly recommended.

Pertussis (whooping cough)

—Pertussis is caused by the bacterium *Bordetella pertussis*.

—It is transmitted via respiratory secretions or in an aerosolized form and is highly contagious.

—The disease has a three-phase clinical presentation. The catarrhal phase of one to two weeks resembles a common cold and fever. In the paroxysmal phase of one month or longer, fever subsides and the patient develops a mild cough that quickly becomes severe and violent. Rapid consecutive coughs are accompanied by deep high-pitched inspiration, and coughing produces copious thick mucus and may lead to increased intracranial pressure and, potentially, intracerebral hemorrhage. Finally, in the convalescent phase, the frequency and severity of the coughs decrease, and the patient is no longer contagious.

—The incubation period is 6 to 20 days.

—Mask the patient and observe Standard Precautions, including postexposure hand washing.

—Booster doses of DTP (diphtheria-tetanus toxoid, pertussis) should be considered.

Influenza

—Influenza is caused by viruses designated types A, B, C.

—It is transmitted by airborne droplet inhalation, direct contact, or autoinoculation.

—The disease is characterized by sudden onset of chills, fever (usually of three to five days' duration), malaise, muscle aches, nasal discharge, and cough that may be severe and of long duration.

—The incubation period is from one to three days.

—Immunization is available and recommended for the elderly, those who live in institutional settings, military recruits, and health care workers.

—Antiviral agents such as amantadine are available but are only effective against type A.

—Universal Standard Precautions and good hand washing are recommended.

Scabies

—Scabies is caused by infestation of a mite, *Sarcoptes scabiei*.

—The condition is contracted by exposure through close personal contact, from hand holding to sexual contact. Mites remain viable on clothing or bedding for up to 48 hours.

—Upon attaching to a new host, the female burrows into the epidermis to lay eggs within 2½ minutes. Larvae hatch shortly and are full-grown adults in 10 to 20 days. The primary symptom of the condition is intense itching.

—The incubation period is two to six weeks after infestation. It remains communicable until all mites and eggs are destroyed.

—No immunization is available.

—Bag and remove all linens immediately. Decontaminate stretcher and patient compartment as for lice. Remove and decontaminate any clothing that may have contacted the patient.

Lice (pediculosis)

—There are three varieties of infestation: *Pediculus humanus var. capitis* (head lice), *Pediculus humanus var. corporis* (body lice), and *Pthirus pubis* (pubic lice or crabs).
—Lice are transmitted by direct contact, which may or may not be associated with sexual activity.
—Eggs hatch within 7 to 10 days.
—Infestation results in parasitic infection of the skin of the scalp, trunk, or pubic area, which is primarily characterized by intense itching. Red macules, papules, and urticaria commonly appear on the shoulders, buttocks, abdomen, or genital areas.
—No immunization is available.
—Spray the ambulance interior close to the cot and the area by the patient's head with an insecticide, preferably one containing permethrin. Wipe and clean all surfaces to remove insecticide residues.

Lyme disease

—Lyme disease is caused by the tick-borne spirochete *Borrelia burgdorferi*.
—It is transmitted by the bite of an infected tick.
—A flat, painless red lesion may appear at the bite site (and may appear to resemble a bull's eye). This may be accompanied by malaise, headache, and muscle aches; then the spirochete spreads to the skin, nervous system, heart, and joints. Meningitis, cardiac conduction defects, and arthritis are common. Recurrence can appear months to years after initial exposure.
—The incubation period ranges from 3 to 32 days.
—Immunization is available (LYMErix) as a series of three vaccinations.
—Employ universal precautions. Also, when responding in wooded areas, check for ticks, and spray the ambulance compartment with an arthropod-effective insecticide.

Gastroenteritis

—Causative organisms for the condition may be viruses, bacteria, and parasites.
—It is highly contagious via the fecal–oral route, including the ingestion of contaminated food or water.
—Prolonged vomiting and diarrhea may cause dehydration and electrolyte disturbances.
—No immunization is available.
—Follow universal precautions and use aggressive hand washing.

13. **Describe the actions to take if you are exposed to an infectious disease.**   pp. 374–375

Understanding the mechanism for disease transmission, as well as the relationship between infectious agent, host, and environment, will allow the EMS provider to make appropriate decisions regarding personal protection against disease. To supplement the body's natural defenses against disease, EMS providers must protect themselves against infectious exposures. Prevention is the most effective approach to infectious disease. All body fluids are possibly infectious, and universal precautions should be followed at all times.

All exposures to blood, blood products, or any potentially infectious material should be immediately reported to the designated infectious disease control officer (IDCO). The nature of the exposure is assessed based on route (percutaneous, mucosal, or cutaneous), dose, and nature of the infectious agent. For instance, in the case of HIV, the highest risk exposure involves percutaneous exposure with a large volume of blood, a high antibody titer against a retrovirus in the source patient, deep percutaneous injury, or actual intramuscular injection.

14. **Given a variety of scenarios, develop treatment plans for patients with suspected infectious disease.**   pp. 375–402

The priorities for someone who is clearly in urgent distress due to infectious disease are the same as for a patient who is affected by a potentially life-threatening emergency of another origin. Ensure adequate airway, breathing (ventilation), and circulation. This is particularly important for someone whose infectious process may be affecting the respiratory and cardiovascular systems. Intractable nausea and vomiting can cause respiratory distress. This is especially true for the patient with an underlying pulmonary disease. Also, persistent vomiting can cause alterations in heart rate and blood pressure, produce dramatic volume losses, and place the patient at risk for aspiration. Most infectious diseases in

©2013 Pearson Education, Inc.
Paramedic Care: Principles & Practice, Vol. 4, 4th Ed.

the prehospital setting will require a minimum of supportive measures, such as airway maintenance, oxygenation, ventilatory management, and hemodynamic and cardiac monitoring. You should always provide oxygen, allow a position of comfort, initiate an IV as appropriate, and treat nausea, vomiting, and pain.

Remember that prevention is the best approach and, for that reason, you should presume that every patient is potentially infectious and take appropriate precautions to minimize your exposure. Your own personal accountability in the area of infection control is equally important: Do not go to work if you have any signs or symptoms of illness, keep your immunizations up to date, and always practice effective hand hygiene.

15. **Describe EMS providers' roles in patient education and preventing disease transmission.** pp. 399–400

Paramedics have an opportunity to assume a leadership role in the area of disease prevention and education. As patient advocates, EMS professionals are often active in public and community education and are ideally positioned to influence the public's behavior. CPR and first-aid classes offer a platform to also introduce and discuss issues related to disease transmission. Leading by example is extremely important. Paramedics, especially those working in rural and suburban areas, reflect the general community. They are in close contact with the people they serve, and are well respected in their communities. Taking an active part in public disease-prevention education will be among your most important roles as a paramedic.

16. **Explain the pathophysiology, risk factors, assessment, and prehospital management of sepsis/systemic inflammatory response syndrome (SIRS).** pp. 401–402

Sepsis is the 10th most common cause of death in the world and the most common cause of death in debilitated patients in hospital intensive care units. Sepsis, sometimes called septicemia, is a life-threatening medical condition caused by a whole-body inflammatory state called systemic inflammatory response syndrome (SIRS). It occurs in response to a known or suspected infection (usually bacterial). The original site of infection can be anywhere in the body and the infection usually spreads to the vascular system or other sterile areas. Common sites of SIRS origin include the gastrointestinal system (peritonitis, pancreatitis), the genitourinary system (pyelonephritis, urinary tract infection [UTI]), the neurologic system (meningitis), the hepatobiliary system (liver, gallbladder), the respiratory system (pneumonia), or the skin (cellulitis). Sepsis can also result from medical interventions and devices, including IV lines, surgical wounds and drains, decubitus ulcers, urinary catheters, and others.
Those most at risk of developing sepsis are:

• People with immunosuppression (e.g., from AIDS, chemotherapy, steroids)
• Patients who are hospitalized (e.g., with surgery, pneumonia)
• People with preexisting infections or medical conditions (e.g., diabetes, pancreatitis)
• People with severe trauma (e.g., burns, polytrauma)
• People with a genetic tendency for sepsis
• The very old or very young

The diagnosis of sepsis is made when the patient has an infection (documented or suspected) and at least two of the following signs and symptoms:

• Heart rate > 90 beats per minute
• Abnormal body temperature (>100.4°F [>38.°C] or < 96.8°F [<36°C])
• Tachypnea (>20 breaths per minute or a $PaCO_2$ < 32 mmHg)
• Abnormal white blood cell count (<4,000 or > 12,000 cells/microliter) on a complete blood count (CBC).

Severe sepsis includes the presence of sepsis (as defined in the previous section) and evidence of hypoperfusion:

• Mottled skin
• Delayed capillary refill (>3 seconds)
• Decreased urine output (<0.5 mL/kg/hr)

- Lactate > 1 mmol/L
- Altered mental status
- Abnormal findings in electroencephalogram (EEG)
- Platelet count less than 100,000 cells/mL
- Disseminated intravascular coagulation (DIC)
- Acute lung injury or acute respiratory distress syndrome (ARDS)
- Cardiac dysfunction, shown on echocardiography or direct measurement of cardiac output

Early recognition and aggressive treatment for sepsis is necessary for the best outcome. The early signs and symptoms of sepsis/SIRS can be subtle. Many septic patients are initially cared for by EMS. Hospitals and physicians have developed specific treatment strategies for sepsis referred to as Early Goal-Directed Therapy (EGDT). This includes:

- Supplemental oxygen with or without intubation and mechanical ventilation
- Central venous line placement
- Fluid resuscitation
- Maintenance of blood pressure > 90 mmHg with vasopressors
- Administration of broad-spectrum antibiotics.

In the prehospital setting, management includes oxygenation, ventilation, fluid resuscitation, and vasopressor support as needed.

Case Study Review

Reread the case study on pages 362–363 in Paramedic Care: Medicine; *then, read the following discussion.*
This case study draws attention to the potential for EMS personnel to be exposed to infectious and communicable disease when in the course of routine delivery of emergency care.

Elizabeth and Stuart are dispatched on a routine call for a person complaining of difficulty breathing. The patient looks acutely ill and the observed signs and symptoms indicate a pulmonary infection. The report of prolonged respiratory problems, recent weight loss, night sweats, and hemoptysis should raise the index of suspicion for tuberculosis. Appropriately, they administer oxygen via nonrebreather mask and establish vascular access at a keep-open rate.

Although not specified in this scenario, it is hoped that Elizabeth and Stuart practiced universal precautions while caring for this patient, just as with any other. It is reasonable and appropriate to adopt a high-index-of-suspicion-driven response to potential exposures to any infectious agent. Fortunately, their exposure to this patient did not result in their becoming infected with tuberculosis.

Content Self-Evaluation

MULTIPLE CHOICE

_____ 1. Microscopic single-celled organisms that can be differentiated by their reaction to a chemical staining process are called
  A. helminths.
  B. bacteria.
  C. viruses.
  D. fungi.
  E. protozoans.

_____ 2. Single-celled parasitic organisms that are a common cause of opportunistic infection are called
  A. helminths.
  B. bacteria.
  C. viruses.
  D. fungi.
  E. protozoans.

©2013 Pearson Education, Inc.
Paramedic Care: Principles & Practice, Vol. 4, 4th Ed.

_____ 3. All microorganisms that reside in our bodies are pathogenic.
   A. True
   B. False

_____ 4. Visible only by electron microscope, obligate intracellular parasites that resist antibiotic treatment are called
   A. helminths.
   B. bacteria.
   C. viruses.
   D. fungi.
   E. protozoans.

_____ 5. All of the following are airborne diseases, EXCEPT
   A. meningitis.
   B. tuberculosis.
   C. measles.
   D. syphilis.
   E. influenza.

_____ 6. The presence of an infectious agent within the host, without necessarily causing disease, is referred to as
   A. infection.
   B. contamination.
   C. communicable.
   D. exposure.
   E. virulence.

_____ 7. All of the following are factors that affect disease transmission, EXCEPT
   A. mode of entry.
   B. virulence.
   C. dose of organism.
   D. host resistance.
   E. type of organism.

_____ 8. Surface proteins on viruses and bacteria that stimulate the production of antibodies are called
   A. pathogens.
   B. prokaryotes.
   C. antigens.
   D. prions.
   E. eukaryotes.

_____ 9. The creation of antibodies following an exposure to a disease is called
   A. incubation.
   B. seroconversion.
   C. latency.
   D. infection.
   E. contamination.

_____ 10. All of the following are agents for the body's general immune response, EXCEPT
   A. neutrophils.
   B. monocytes.
   C. macrophages.
   D. lymphocytes.
   E. antigens.

_____ 11. Cellular-mediated immunity does not result in the formation of antibodies against foreign antigens.
   A. True
   B. False

_____ 12. The principal immunoglobulin in human serum and the major class of immunoglobulin in the immune response is
   A. IgA.
   B. IgD.
   C. IgE.
   D. IgG.
   E. IgM.

_____ 13. The body's formation of antibodies against itself is known as
   A. autoinoculation.
   B. contamination.
   C. autoimmunity.
   D. phagocytosis.
   E. cellular-mediated immunity.

14. Antibodies, B lymphocytes, and T lymphocytes are produced by the
    A. thymus.
    B. spleen.
    C. complement system.
    D. bone marrow.
    E. lymph nodes.

15. Sterilization is the recommended level of decontamination for all equipment used by EMS personnel.
    A. True
    B. False

16. At the scene of a motor vehicle collision, all of the following are appropriate infection control measures, EXCEPT
    A. wearing gloves and changing them between patients.
    B. using protective eyewear or face shields to limit splash exposures.
    C. recapping needles to reduce risk of needle stick to others.
    D. decontaminating all reusable equipment.
    E. putting all contaminated dressings in a leak-proof biohazard bag.

17. Risk factors for developing infectious disease include
    A. immunosuppression.
    B. diabetes.
    C. artificial heart valves.
    D. alcoholism.
    E. all of the above.

18. Which of these infectious diseases poses the greatest risk to EMS personnel as a result of work-related exposures?
    A. AIDS
    B. Tuberculosis
    C. Hepatitis A
    D. Hepatitis B
    E. Hantavirus

19. The most significant problem associated with HIV is
    A. opportunistic infection.
    B. hemorrhage.
    C. dementia.
    D. blindness.
    E. splenomegaly.

20. The most common form of hepatitis transmitted by the fecal–oral route is
    A. hepatitis A.
    B. hepatitis B.
    C. hepatitis C.
    D. hepatitis D.
    E. hepatitis E.

21. Primarily a respiratory disorder, the most common preventable adult infectious disease in the world is
    A. hepatitis A.
    B. tuberculosis.
    C. HIV.
    D. pneumonia.
    E. influenza.

22. Your 60-year-old patient reports an acute onset of high fever, chills, dyspnea, pleuritic chest pain, and a productive cough. You suspect
    A. hantavirus.
    B. tuberculosis.
    C. HIV.
    D. pneumonia.
    E. influenza.

23. Your patient has a low-grade fever and malaise and is covered from head to toe with fluid-filled vesicles and small ulcers. You suspect
    A. measles.
    B. rubella.
    C. chickenpox.
    D. meningitis.
    E. scabies.

©2013 Pearson Education, Inc.
Paramedic Care: Principles & Practice, Vol. 4, 4th Ed.

_____ **24.** Your patient reports an acute onset of high fever, stiff neck, and severe headache. You suspect
   A. measles.   **D.** meningitis.
   B. rubella.   **E.** scabies.
   C. chickenpox.

_____ **25.** All of the following are viral infections that may be contracted in the EMS setting, EXCEPT
   A. measles.   **D.** meningitis.
   B. rubella.   **E.** scabies.
   C. chickenpox.

_____ **26.** The most important personal precaution against disease transmission is
   A. effective hand washing.
   B. up-to-date immunizations.
   C. postexposure prophylaxis.
   D. disinfection of equipment.
   E. compliance with infection control policies.

_____ **27.** Your partner reports a sudden onset of fever, chills, malaise, muscle aches, nasal discharge, and a cough. You suspect
   A. hantavirus.   **D.** pneumonia.
   B. tuberculosis.   **E.** influenza.
   C. HIV.

_____ **28.** All of the following are causative organisms for food poisoning, EXCEPT
   A. _Escherichia coli._   **D.** _Salmonella._
   B. _Haemophilus influenzae._   **E.** _Shigella._
   C. _Campylobacter._

_____ **29.** The clinical presentation of encephalitis often mimics that of meningitis.
   A. True
   B. False

_____ **30.** All of the following are sexually transmitted diseases, EXCEPT
   A. HSV-2.   **D.** HPV.
   B. chlamydia.   **E.** gonorrhea.
   C. HAV.

Special Project

Decontamination Procedures

Complete the following table regarding decontamination procedures.

Method and Cleaning Agent	Indication	Effectiveness
Low-level disinfection		
Agent:		
Intermediate-level disinfection		
Agent:		
High-level disinfection		
Agent:		
Sterilization		
Agent:		

Psychiatric and Behavioral Disorders

Review of Chapter Objectives

After reading this chapter, you should be able to:

1. Define key terms introduced in this chapter.

Knowing and being able to apply the key terms in each chapter is critical to understanding chapter concepts. Write the list of key terms. Then write the definition of each one in your own words. Check your understanding by confirming the definitions in the text glossary. Correct any misunderstandings. Create a study aid by writing each key term on the front of an index card and the definition on the back. Use the cards to quiz yourself, or to have someone quiz you.

2. Describe special considerations for your safety and the safety of your crew, the patient, and bystanders when responding to calls for behavioral and psychiatric disorders.
pp. 407, 408

The safety of EMS personnel is paramount, and it is appropriate for paramedics to withdraw from a violent situation until law enforcement or other additional resources arrive. Whenever you receive or assess information that would put safety at risk, you must contact dispatch so that all responders are notified of safety concerns. Sometimes bystanders are at risk as well. Bystanders may attempt to enter the scene or intervene not knowing about safety concerns, being only guided by their desire to help or care for a loved one, neighbor, or friend. Sources of safety concerns not only come from the patient, but also from family and bystanders. Occasionally family and bystanders may be convinced of their observations and not understand the patient's intent or underlying behavioral health issue. Effective therapeutic communication and interpersonal skills are vital to diffusing and resolving misunderstandings that affect safety on scene.

3. Describe the biological, psychosocial, and sociocultural influences on psychiatric and behavioral disorders.
p. 408

The general causes of behavioral and psychiatric disorders are biological (organic), psychosocial, and sociocultural. Biological (organic) causes are related to disease processes or structural changes in the brain. Psychosocial causes are related to the patient's personality, dynamics of unresolved conflict, or crisis management methods. Sociocultural causes are related to the patient's actions and interactions within society. It should be noted that many psychiatric disorders are due to altered brain chemistry.

Remember that you cannot be sure that a patient is suffering from a purely psychological condition until you have completely ruled out medical conditions, such as hypoglycemia, traumatic injury, and substance abuse. Failure to comply with the prescribed medication regimen may cause exacerbation of a patient's psychiatric condition and lead to the development of a behavioral emergency. Societal events (rape, assault, and acts of violence) may contribute to alterations in someone's emotional status, as can interpersonal events, such as death of a loved one or loss of a relationship.

4. Adapt the scene size-up, primary assessment, patient history, secondary assessment, and use of monitoring technology to meet the needs of patients with complaints and presentations related to psychiatric and behavioral disorders. pp. 408–422

During the scene size-up, your general impression will be very important, as you will be looking for clues that can indicate the patient's condition. The causes of behavioral health disorders are numerous. One of the first questions you will answer will be whether there is a history of behavioral health disorders, such as anxiety/depression, bipolar disorder, schizophrenia, or phobias. Evaluate the patient's level of consciousness using the AVPU method, as well as speech, skin appearance, and posture. The patient's emotional status and affect may also provide clues to the patient's developing condition that may be altered due to perception, impaired thinking, delusions, or hallucinations.

Complete your primary ABCD assessment and recognize any findings that would indicate a behavioral health emergency. Always start with the least invasive step, visual inspection. This includes evaluating the patient's affect, appearance, and position as well as visually inspecting the patient's environment. Your secondary assessment should include a mental status assessment, accurate history, and physical exam with a full set of vital signs. Initiate all appropriate monitoring devices. For example, alterations in ventilatory function may be observed in a patient experiencing a behavioral health disorder associated with hyperventilation or suicidal ideation. Capnography measures exhaled or end-tidal carbon dioxide (CO_2) and can assist the paramedic in evaluating the ventilation rate and quality in such a patient. Pulse oximetry is used to monitor a patient's general state of perfusion. Be sure to get a complete set of baseline vital signs early in the process if the patient allows. Some behavioral health patients may not be cooperative with vital signs or monitoring technology. Changes in vitals along with alterations in mental status may indicate early shock due to hemorrhage or other processes.

5. Explain the application and importance of the mental status examination in patients with psychiatric and behavioral disorders. p. 410

One of the most important objectives of your secondary assessment is to perform a mental status exam (MSE). The MSE allows the prehospital professional to rapidly recognize patients who could be suicidal, homicidal, or experiencing symptoms of a progressively developing behavioral health disorder. The elements of an MSE include:

- *General appearance.* The patient's appearance can provide important information when looking at his "big picture." Observe hygiene, clothing, and overall appearance.
- *Behavioral observations.* Observe verbal or nonverbal behavior, strange or threatening appearance, and facial expressions. Note tone of voice, rate, volume, and quality.
- *Orientation.* Does the patient know who he is and who others are? Is he oriented to current events? Can he concentrate on simple questions and answer them?
- *Memory.* Is the patient's memory intact for recent and long-term events?
- *Sensorium.* Is the patient focused? Paying attention? What is his level of awareness?
- *Perceptual processes.* Are the patient's thought patterns ordered? Does he appear to have any hallucinations, delusions, or phobias?
- *Mood and affect.* Observe for indicators of the patient's mood. Is it appropriate? What is his prevailing emotion? Depression, elation, anxiety, or agitation? Other?
- *Intelligence.* Evaluate the patient's speech. What is his level of vocabulary? His ability to formulate an idea?
- *Thought processes.* What is the patient's apparent form of thought? Are his thoughts logical and coherent?
- *Insight.* Does the patient have insight into his own problem? Does he recognize that a problem exists? Does he deny or blame others for his problem?

- *Judgment.* Does the patient base his life decisions on sound, reasonable judgments? Does he approach problems thoughtfully, carefully, and rationally?
- *Psychomotor.* Does the patient exhibit an unusual posture or is he making unusual movements? Patients with hallucinations may react to them. For example, a patient who believes he is covered with insects may be picking at his skin to remove the "bugs."

6. **Use a process of clinical reasoning to guide and interpret the patient assessment and management process for patients with psychiatric and behavioral disorders.**   **pp. 408–422**

As a paramedic, it is vital that you develop your clinical reasoning process to quickly recognize patients with serious signs and symptoms associated with behavioral health disorders. Develop an organized general impression to rapidly identify signs and symptoms indicating suicidal ideation or homicidal thoughts. An accurate history includes:

- Does the patient have any current suicidal or homicidal thoughts?
- Did the patient have a plan?
- Did the patient act on the plan or any of those suicidal or homicidal thoughts?
- Does the patient have a history of attempting suicide before or have a history of homicidal tendencies?

Your interpersonal skills are crucial to your success as an EMS professional, and never more so than when you are caring for a patient who is having a behavioral emergency. Limit environmental distractions at the scene. Introduce yourself and note how the patient responds to you, altering your approach if the patient becomes agitated. Establish eye contact and place yourself at the patient's level. Listen carefully and do not physically threaten the patient. Ask open-ended questions while being truthful with the patient, and never play along with hallucinations or delusions. Focus your questioning and assessment on the immediate problem.

Generally, the examination of a behavioral emergency patient is largely conversational. If you need to perform hands-on assessment activities, defer their completion until you have had the opportunity to establish rapport and, even then, do not make any sudden moves that may startle the patient. If a patient is restrained, be sure to monitor the patient frequently and carefully to ensure that the airway is patent and that he is not experiencing positional asphyxia.

7. **Describe the characteristics of and general approach to the following general classifications of psychiatric disorders:**

a. **Cognitive disorders**   **p. 411**

Cognitive disorders are psychiatric disorders with organic causes such as brain injury or disease. These types of disorders include conditions caused by metabolic disease, infections, neoplasm, endocrine disease, degenerative neurologic disease, and cardiovascular disease. They might also be caused by physical or chemical injuries due to trauma, drug abuse, or reactions to prescribed drugs. The specific brain pathology will differ based on the type of disease. Two types of cognitive disorders are delirium and dementia.

Delirium is characterized by a relatively rapid onset of widespread disorganized thought. These patients suffer from inattention, memory impairment, disorientation, and a general clouding of consciousness. In some cases, individuals may experience vivid visual hallucinations. Delirium is characterized by a fairly acute onset (hours or days) and may be reversible. Delirium may be due to a medical condition, substance intoxication, substance withdrawal, or multiple etiologies. Confusion is a hallmark of delirium.

Dementia may be due to several medical problems. Included among the more common causes of dementia are Alzheimer's disease (both early and late onset), vascular problems, AIDS, head trauma, Parkinson's disease, and substance abuse. Regardless of its cause, dementia involves memory impairment, cognitive disturbance, and pervasive impairment of abstract thinking and judgment. Unlike delirium, dementia usually develops over months and, in many cases, is irreversible.

b. Schizophrenia   p. 411

Schizophrenia is a common mental health problem, affecting an estimated 1 percent of the U.S. population. Its hallmark is a significant change in behavior and a loss of contact with reality. Signs and symptoms often include hallucinations, delusions, and depression. The schizophrenic patient may live in his "own world" and be preoccupied with inner fantasies. Although several biological and psychosocial theories attempt to explain the condition and its manifestations, its definitive cause is unknown.

c. Anxiety disorders   pp. 411–412

The group of illnesses known as anxiety disorders is characterized by dominating apprehension and fear. These disorders affect approximately 2 to 4 percent of the population. Broadly defined, anxiety is a state of uneasiness, discomfort, apprehension, and restlessness. More specifically, anxiety disorders fall into three categories: panic disorder, phobia, and post-traumatic stress syndrome.

The *DSM-IV* does not list panic attacks in themselves as a disease. Characterized by recurrent, extreme periods of anxiety resulting in great emotional distress, they are symptoms of disease and are included among the criteria for other disorders (panic disorder, agoraphobia). Panic attacks differ from generalized feelings of anxiety in their acute nature. They are usually unprovoked, peaking within 10 minutes of their onset and dissipating in less than 1 hour. All people have some source of fear or anxiety that they consciously avoid.

When this fear becomes excessive and interferes with functioning, it is called a phobia. A phobia, generally considered an intense, irrational fear, may be due to animals, the sight of blood (or injection or injury), situational factors (elevators, enclosed spaces), or environmental conditions (heights or water). Exposure to the situation or item will induce anxiety or a panic attack. Some patients experience extreme phobias that prevent or limit their normal daily activities. For example, a patient suffering from agoraphobia (fear of crowds) may confine himself to his home and avoid ever venturing outdoors. In most patients, however, the phobia is less severe; the patient realizes that his fear is unreasonable, and the anxiety dissipates.

d. Mood disorders   pp. 412–413

The *DSM-IV* defines mood as "a pervasive and sustained emotion that colors a person's perception of the world." Common examples of mood alterations include depression, elation, anger, and anxiety. The main mood disorders are depression and bipolar disorder. Depression is characterized by a profound sadness or feeling of melancholy. It is common in everyday life and is to be expected following the breakup of a relationship or the loss of a loved one. Most of us have experienced some sort of depression, at least in its mildest form. It is one of the most prevalent psychiatric conditions, affecting from 10 to 15 percent of the population. When depression becomes prolonged or severe, however, it is diagnosed as a *major depressive episode.*

Bipolar disorder is characterized by one or more manic episodes (periods of elation), with or without subsequent or alternating periods of depression. In the past, the term *manic-depressive* was used to describe this condition. Bipolar disorder is not particularly common, affecting approximately less than 1 percent of the population.

e. Substance-related disorders   pp. 413–414

Substance abuse is a common disorder. Many patients you will encounter in EMS will be under the influence of one or a myriad of substances. Any patient exhibiting symptoms of a psychiatric or behavioral disorder should be screened for substance use and/or abuse. Substance abuse patients may present as being depressed, psychotic, or delirious, and their signs and symptoms may mimic those of many behavioral disorders. The *DSM-IV* lists substance abuse as a psychiatric disorder; you should consider it a serious condition. Any mood-altering chemical has the potential for abuse. Alcohol is a common part of our culture, but can be abused. The user of a substance may be intoxicated from the effects of the chemical or may be ill from addiction or withdrawal of the chemical. Intoxication, in and of itself, may cause behavioral problems.

f. Somatoform disorders   p. 414

Somatoform disorders are characterized by physical symptoms that have no apparent physiological cause. They are believed to be attributable to psychological factors. People who suffer from somatoform disorders believe their symptoms are serious and real.

©2013 Pearson Education, Inc.
Paramedic Care: Principles & Practice, Vol. 4, 4th Ed.

g. Factitious disorders
p. 414

Factitious disorders are sometimes confused with somatoform disorders. They are characterized by the following three criteria:

- An intentional production of physical or psychological signs or symptoms
- Motivation for the behavior is to assume the "sick role"
- External incentives for the behavior (e.g., economic gain, avoiding work, avoiding police) are absent

Although patients suffering from factitious disorders essentially feign their illnesses, that does not preclude the possibility of true physical or psychological symptoms. The disorder is apparently more common in males than in females. In severe cases, patients will go to great lengths to obtain medical or psychological treatment.

h. Dissociative disorders
pp. 414–415

Like somatoform disorders, dissociative disorders are attempts to avoid stressful situations while still gratifying needs. In a manner, they permit the person to deny personal responsibility for unacceptable behavior. The individual avoids stress by *dissociating* from his core personality. These behavior patterns can be complex but are quite rare. The disorders include:

Psychogenic Amnesia: Amnesia is a partial or total *inability* to recall or identify past events, and psychogenic amnesia is a *failure* to recall. The "forgotten" material is present but "hidden" beneath the level of consciousness.

Fugue State: An amnesic individual may withdraw even further by retreating into what is known as a fugue state. A patient in a fugue state actually flees as a defense mechanism and may travel hundreds of miles from home.

Multiple Personality Disorder: In multiple personality disorder, sometimes called *dissociative identity disorder*, the patient reacts to an identifiable stress by manifesting two or more complete systems of personality. Although such disorders have received a great deal of attention in television, film, and novels, they are actually quite rare.

Depersonalization: Depersonalization is a relatively more frequent dissociative disorder that occurs predominantly in young adults. Patients experience a loss of the sense of one's self. These individuals suddenly feel "different"—that they are someone else or that their bodies have taken on a different form. The disorder is often precipitated by acute stress.

i. Eating disorders
p. 415

Anorexia Nervosa. Anorexia is the loss of appetite. Anorexia nervosa is a disorder marked by excessive fasting. Individuals with this disorder have an intense fear of obesity and often complain of being fat even though their body weight is low. They suffer from weight loss (25 percent of body weight or more), refusal to maintain body weight, and often a cessation of menstruation from severe malnutrition.

Bulimia Nervosa. Recurrent episodes of seemingly uncontrollable binge eating with compensatory self-induced vomiting or diarrhea, excessive exercise, or dieting and with a full awareness of the behavior's abnormality characterize bulimia nervosa. Individuals often display personality traits of perfectionism, low self-esteem, and social withdrawal.

j. Personality disorders
p. 415

Most adults' personalities are attuned to social demands. Some individuals, however, often seem ill equipped to function adequately in society. These people might be suffering from a personality disorder. Stemming largely from immature and distorted personality development, these personality, or character, disorders result in persistently maladaptive ways of perceiving, thinking, and relating to the world.

The broad category of personality disorder includes problems that vary greatly in form and severity. Although others might describe them as "eccentric" or "troublesome," some patients with personality disorders function adequately. In extreme cases, patients act out against or attempt to manipulate society.

k. Impulse control disorders
pp. 415–416

Related to the personality disorders are the *impulse control disorders*. Recurrent impulses and the patient's failure to control them characterize these disorders. Disorders of impulse control may be harmful to the patient and others. Prior to committing the act, the patient will have an increasing sense of tension. After the act, he will either have pleasure gratification or release.

8. **Describe the epidemiology, including risk factors, of suicide.** p. 416

It is estimated that 20 percent of the population has some type of mental health problem and that as many as one in seven will require treatment for an emotional disturbance.

All of the following are considered to be risk factors for suicide: previously attempted suicide, depression, age (15 to 24 years of age or over age 40), substance abuse, social isolation, major separation, trauma, major physical stresses, loss of independence, suicide of a parent. Also significant is having possession of a mechanism for suicide and having a specific plan and/or expressing it. Women attempt suicide more than men, but men—especially those over 55 years of age—are more likely to succeed. Statistically, suicide successes and methods vary widely by race, sex, and culture.

9. **Describe special considerations for assessment and management of psychiatric and behavioral disorders in geriatric and pediatric populations.** pp. 416–417

Some behavioral disorders are particularly common among patients at the ends of the age spectrum—the young and the elderly. Your awareness of age-related conditions will help you to assess and interact with these patients.

Common physical problems among the elderly include dementia, chronic illness, and diminished eyesight and hearing. The elderly also experience depression that is often mistaken for dementia.

Behavioral emergencies are not limited to adults. Children also have behavioral crises. Although the child's developmental stage will affect his behavior, general guidelines will assist you when confronting an emotionally distraught or disruptive child.

10. **Explain the characteristics and management of excited delirium syndrome.** p. 417

Excited delirium syndrome, also called *agitated delirium*, appears to be a factor in sudden death associated with restraint situations. Excited delirium is both a mental state and physiological arousal that appears to result from increased dopamine levels in the brain. Excited delirium can be caused by drug intoxication (including alcohol) or psychiatric illness or a combination of both. Cocaine and other stimulants are well-known causes of drug-induced excited delirium.

It may become apparent that a patient is suffering from excited delirium only when he suddenly collapses. Beware of the patient who becomes suddenly tranquil after frenzied activity. This is often followed by cardiac collapse and death. Many deaths from excited delirium cannot be prevented. However, excited delirium must always be suspected when a patient is restrained. Paramedics should have a low threshold for using chemical restraint in the patient with possible excited delirium. Allowing the patient to struggle (i.e., against restraints) is a risk factor for sudden death.

11. **Describe special considerations in the assessment and management of TASERed patients.** pp. 417–418

As a paramedic, you may be summoned to evaluate a patient who has been subdued with a TASER. In many instances, the TASER darts may still be in place. First, before you approach any patient who has been subdued by a TASER or other less lethal weapon, you should assure that the scene is safe. Most patients who have been subdued by these devices will have no injury. In most instances, they can be observed for approximately 15 minutes and then allowed to go with law enforcement if no further problems occur. Patients should have the following findings before being released to law enforcement:

- Glasgow Coma Score of 15
- Heart rate less < 110 per minute
- Respiratory rate > 12 per minute
- Normal SpO_2 (> 94 percent)
- Systolic blood pressure > 100 mmHg
- The dart must not have penetrated the eye, face, neck, breast (females), axilla, or genitalia.
- The patient has no other acute medical condition, including trauma, hypoglycemia, and/or acute psychiatric disturbances such as excited delirium syndrome.

If the subject meets the criteria above, the TASER darts can be removed. The procedure is as follows:

- Ensure that the TASER is no longer active and has been secured.
- Use scissors to cut the wire at the base of each dart, thus disconnecting it from the device.
- While wearing gloves, grasp the cylinder of the TASER dart between your thumb and index finger and remove the dart with a quick, firm hold directed perpendicular to the skin surface. Dispose of the dart in a sharps container, being careful not to sustain an injury with the device.
- Clean each dart wound with an appropriate antiseptic solution.
- Cover each dart wound with a Band-Aid or other sterile dressing. The Band-Aid or dressing can be removed in 24 to 48 hours if there are no problems.
- Offer the patient transport to the hospital, if necessary. Document your findings and obtain appropriate releases. Encourage the subject/patient to seek follow-up care if he develops signs of infection around one or both of the punctures. These include fever, increasing pain, erythema, warmth, swelling, and/or purulent drainage.

Your local protocols may vary somewhat. Always follow local protocols in this regard. If you encounter any other issues such as arrhythmias or other abnormalities, treat the patient accordingly. When in doubt, err on the side of safety and transport the patient to the emergency department for subsequent evaluation. Remember, patients with excited delirium syndrome are at high risk for sudden death. These patients should be treated aggressively and transported emergently to a hospital.

12. **Describe the indications, procedures, precautions, and necessary documentation associated with the use of physical and chemical restraint to manage violent patients.**   pp. 419–422

The application of physical and chemical restraints to a patient must be performed with the understanding that overstepping the boundaries of proper restraint may be perceived as battery, assault, or false imprisonment. Restraint of an individual may even lead to serious allegations of civil rights violations. For these reasons, the EMS service should always review patient restraint policies with appropriate legal counsel.

If a patient is known to be violent, EMS personnel should ensure that law enforcement personnel secure the scene before EMS enters. However, this is not always possible, and paramedics should always be alert for unexpectedly agitated patients or those with escalating emotions. The safety of EMS personnel is paramount, and it is appropriate for paramedics to withdraw from a violent situation until law enforcement or other additional resources arrive. Paramedics should also anticipate the potential for exposure to blood and body fluids during patient restraint. Restraint procedures can expose EMS providers to blood, saliva, urine, or feces. Based on the situation, appropriate barrier protection should be worn during patient restraint.

Methods of restraint include verbal de-escalation, physical restraint, and chemical restraint. The chosen method should always be the least restrictive method that ensures the safety of the patient and EMS personnel. These methods of restraint may often be applied in a stepwise fashion, but with extremely violent individuals immediate physical restraint may be indicated to ensure the safety of the patient, EMS personnel, and bystanders.

The application of verbal techniques to calm the patient is usually the first method paramedics should employ. This method is safest because it does not require any physical contact with the patient. The conversation must be honest and straightforward, with a friendly tone. Avoid direct eye contact and encroachment on the patient's "personal space," which may create added stress and anxiety. Always attempt to have equally open escape routes for both paramedics and the patient should it become necessary. Always assess the patient for suicidal and/or homicidal ideation. Verbal intervention sometimes defuses the situation or at least prevents further escalation and may avert the need for further restraint tactics.

When physically restraining a patient, paramedics must make every effort to avoid injuring the patient. Patient restraint policies must therefore recommend restraint devices that are associated with the least chance of inflicting injury. Physical restraint is accomplished with materials and techniques that will restrict the movement of a person who is considered to be a danger to himself or others. Examples include both soft restraints (sheets, wristlets, and chest Posey) and hard restraints (plastic ties, handcuffs, and leathers).

Chemical restraint is defined as the administration of specific pharmacological agents to decrease agitation and increase the cooperation of patients who require medical care and transportation. EMS systems may use a variety of agents for chemical restraint of the agitated or combative patient. The goal is to subdue excessive agitation and struggling against physical restraints. Ideally, this pharmacological sedation will change the patient's behavior without reaching the point of amnesia or altering the patient's level of consciousness.

13. **Given a variety of scenarios, develop treatment plans for patients with psychiatric and behavioral disorders.** pp. 408–422

Throughout your training, you will encounter a variety of real and simulated patients with behavioral or psychiatric emergencies. Use the information in the text, as well as the application of this information as demonstrated by your instructors, preceptors, and mentors, to enhance your ability to assess, manage, and transport patients with behavioral emergencies. Every emergency call has an element of behavioral emergency in it; your patience and professionalism will help minimize the emotional component for everyone involved.

The priorities for someone who is clearly in urgent distress due to psychiatric and behavioral health disorders are similar to those who are affected by a potentially life-threatening emergency of another origin. This is especially true in the case of suicidal ideation, suicidal attempts, or intentional drug overdose. Ensure the safety of yourself, your crew, and your patient. Many behavioral emergencies for which you are dispatched will also warrant mutual response by law enforcement personnel. Gain control of the scene. Remove anyone who agitates the patient or adds confusion to the scene. Examine the environment for signs of violence and potential weapons. Approach every situation cautiously and, when feasible, observe the patient from a distance first before approaching. Avoid invading the patient's personal space.

Maintain adequate airway, breathing (ventilation), and circulation. This is particularly important for someone whose suicide attempt may be affecting the respiratory and cardiovascular systems. Most psychiatric and behavioral health disorders in the prehospital setting will require a minimum of supportive measures, such as airway maintenance, oxygenation, ventilatory management, and hemodynamic and cardiac monitoring. You should always provide oxygen, allow a position of comfort, initiate an IV when indicated, and treat the patient as appropriate. Be aware that not all patients will cooperate with your interventions and some may continue to be a danger to you, your crew, and even themselves. Watch for signs of aggression. If a patient becomes violent, use of restraint may become necessary; in such cases, carefully follow your service's protocols for such circumstances and be sure to document your actions thoroughly.

The key to dealing with the emotionally disturbed patient is to listen carefully. Place yourself at the patient's level, but keep a safe and proper distance, not invading the patient's personal space. Ask open-ended questions that require your patient to respond in detail. Be comfortable with silence and take whatever time is necessary to get the whole story of the situation. Do not lie to or make fun of the patient. Be nonjudgmental.

The laws of consent specify that any competent person has the right to refuse to consent to treatment. Further, no competent person may be transported against his will. Any person who is in imminent danger of harming himself or others is not considered competent to refuse treatment and transport. Most states have laws that allow persons fitting this criterion to be transported against their will to a hospital or approved psychiatric facility for evaluation.

Case Study Review

Reread the case study on pages 406–407 in Paramedic Care: Medicine; *then, read the following discussion.*

   This case study draws attention to the assessment and management of a commonly encountered patient presentation, in which an individual is exhibiting bizarre behavior in a public setting.

The paramedics arrive on the scene and obtain information about the situation from the store manager who has placed the 911 call. When the patient notices their arrival and becomes more agitated, they retreat to the ambulance and request assistance from law enforcement personnel.

   As is often the case, the police officers recognize the patient from previous interactions with him. Before approaching the patient, the paramedics and police officers coordinate their plans and anticipate the potential need for restraint. The use of a team approach to subdue and restrain the patient minimizes the risk of injury for all involved. Once the patient is safely restrained, a thorough assessment is performed to rule out possible medical or traumatic causes for the patient's altered mental status and agitation. En route to the hospital the patient is carefully monitored to ensure his well-being.

Content Self-Evaluation

MULTIPLE CHOICE

_____ 1. Organic causes for behavioral emergencies include all of the following, EXCEPT
   A. tumor.
   B. depression.
   C. substance abuse.
   D. infection.
   E. hypoglycemia.

_____ 2. It is always safe to assume that a patient exhibiting bizarre behavior is suffering from a psychological problem or disease.
   A. True
   B. False

_____ 3. The term that describes the state of a patient's cerebral functioning is
   A. affect.
   B. mood.
   C. mental status.
   D. orientation.
   E. sensorium.

_____ 4. The best approach for gaining information from a behavioral emergency patient is to
   A. ask questions requiring yes-or-no answers.
   B. talk loudly to establish control.
   C. ask open-ended questions.
   D. physically restrain the patient before questioning.
   E. move quickly to expedite transport and then question.

_____ 5. The structured exam designed to quickly evaluate a patient's level of mental functioning is the
   A. neurological exam.
   B. mental status exam.
   C. psychiatric evaluation.
   D. Glasgow coma score.
   E. stroke assessment scale.

_____ 6. The most likely way to provoke violence or aggression in a behavioral emergency patient is to
   A. listen carefully to his responses.
   B. appear patient and unhurried.
   C. ask open-ended questions.
   D. invade his personal space.
   E. avoid rapid or sudden movements.

7. Panic attack, phobias, and post-traumatic stress syndrome are classified as
   A. types of schizophrenia.
   B. personality disorders.
   C. variants of depression.
   D. bipolar disorders.
   E. anxiety disorders.

8. The most prevalent form of psychiatric problem is
   A. schizophrenia.
   B. personality disorder.
   C. depression.
   D. bipolar disorder.
   E. anxiety disorder.

9. Profound sadness, diminished ability to concentrate, and feelings of worthlessness are commonly associated with
   A. schizophrenia.
   B. personality disorders.
   C. depression.
   D. bipolar disorders.
   E. anxiety disorders.

10. Medications commonly used in the management of schizophrenia are
    A. antipsychotics.
    B. sedatives.
    C. antihistamines.
    D. antipsychotics and sedatives.
    E. sedatives and antihistamines.

11. Common causes of dementia include all of the following, EXCEPT
    A. Alzheimer's disease.
    B. head trauma.
    C. cardiac seizure.
    D. Parkinson's disease.
    E. AIDS.

12. Hallucinations, delusions, and disorganized thought, speech, and behavior are commonly associated with
    A. schizophrenia.
    B. personality disorders.
    C. depression.
    D. bipolar disorders.
    E. anxiety disorders.

13. The compelling desire to use a substance, inability to reduce use of a substance, and repeated unsuccessful efforts to quit using that substance are indicators of
    A. psychological dependence.
    B. physical dependence.
    C. substance tolerance.
    D. factitious disorder.
    E. somatoform disorder.

14. The primary objective in patient restraint is to
    A. initiate punitive response.
    B. stop dangerous behaviors.
    C. limit patient strength.
    D. reduce legal liability.
    E. assure patient and rescuer safety.

15. When a pediatric or geriatric patient is experiencing a behavioral emergency, the paramedic should always consider using chemical restraints.
    A. True
    B. False

©2013 Pearson Education, Inc.
Paramedic Care: Principles & Practice, Vol. 4, 4th Ed.

MATCHING

Write the letter of the word or phrase in the space provided next to its definition.

A. delirium

B. dementia

C. schizophrenia

D. delusions

E. hallucinations

F. catatonia

G. paranoid

H. bipolar disorder

I. personality disorder

J. depersonalization

_____ **16.** Feeling detached from oneself

_____ **17.** Condition characterized by relatively rapid onset of widespread disorganized thought

_____ **18.** Fixed false beliefs

_____ **19.** Condition that results in persistently maladaptive behavior

_____ **20.** Sensory perceptions with no basis in reality

_____ **21.** Condition characterized by one or more manic episodes, with or without subsequent or alternating periods of depression

_____ **22.** Condition characterized by immobility, rigidity, and stupor

_____ **23.** Common disorder involving significant behavioral changes and disorganized thought

_____ **24.** Preoccupation with feelings of persecution

_____ **25.** Condition involving gradual development of memory impairment and cognitive disturbance

Special Project

Crossword Puzzle

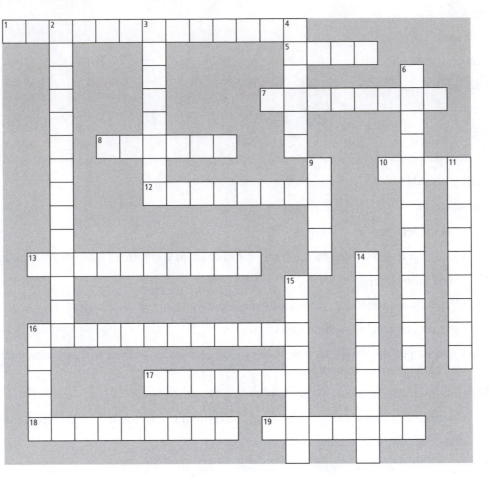

Across

1. Common mental health problem associated with significant behavioral change and a loss of contact with reality

5. Feeling of alarm in expectations of danger

7. Person's observable conduct and activity

8. Excessive fear that interferes with functioning

10. Pervasive emotion that colors a person's perception of the world

12. Condition involving gradual development of memory impairment and cognitive disturbance

13. One of the three general causes of behavioral emergencies, related to disease processes or structural changes

16. Another of the three general causes of behavioral emergencies, related to the person's personality style, unresolved conflicts, or crisis management methods

17. Sometimes known as a manic-depressive mood disorder

18. Displays of rigidity, immobility, and stupor often associated with schizophrenia

19. Intentional taking of one's own life commonly seen in association with depression

Down

2. Sensory perception with no basis in reality

3. Preoccupation with a feeling of persecution

4. Visible indicators of mood

6. Another of the three general causes of behavioral emergencies, related to the patient's actions and interactions with society

9. Excessive excitement or activity

11. Fixed false beliefs that are not widely held within the context of the individual's cultural or religious group

14. Extreme response to stress characterized by impaired ability to deal with reality

15. Condition characterized by a relatively rapid onset of widespread disorganized thought

16. Extreme anxiety resulting in great emotional distress

Chapter

12

Diseases of the Eyes, Ears, Nose, and Throat

Review of Chapter Objectives

After reading this chapter, you should be able to:

1. **Define key terms introduced in this chapter.**

   Knowing and being able to apply the key terms in each chapter is critical to understanding chapter concepts. Write the list of key terms. Then write the definition of each one in your own words. Check your understanding by confirming the definitions in the text glossary. Correct any misunderstandings. Create a study aid by writing each key term on the front of an index card and the definition on the back. Use the cards to quiz yourself, or to have someone quiz you.

2. **Relate the anatomy and physiology of the eyes, ears, nose, and throat to the pathophysiology and assessment of patients with diseases of the eyes, ears, nose, and throat.** pp. 428–440

   The eyes are well protected by a group of bones that form the ocular orbit. The orbit is padded with subcutaneous tissue that cushions and protects the eye from injury. Movement of the eyes is controlled by six extraocular muscles that allow us to look in various directions. Two movable folds of skin, the eyelids, protect the eyes from the environment. The eyelashes function as sensors to cause rapid closure of the eyelids when a foreign substance approaches the eyes. Several accessory glands secrete an oily substance called sebum onto the eyelids to keep them soft and pliable.

   A membrane called the conjunctiva covers and protects the exposed surface of the eye. Each eye has a lacrimal apparatus that manufactures and stores tears. The tears are manufactured in the lacrimal glands and then spread across the eye laterally to medially, where they then drain through the lacrimal ducts into the nose.

   The globe of the eye contains two distinct fluid-filled cavities. The posterior cavity, the portion of the eye behind the lens, contains the vitreous humor. The vitreous humor is a clear, jellylike fluid that fills the entire vitreous cavity. The anterior cavity, the portion of the eye in front of the lens, contains the aqueous humor. The aqueous humor is a waterlike fluid that surrounds the iris, pupil, and lens. The anterior cavity is divided into the anterior chamber and the posterior chamber. Both chambers are filled with aqueous humor.

The eye comprises three layers. The innermost layer is the retina. The middle layer is the choroid. The outermost layer is the sclera or conjunctiva. Conjunctivitis is an infection or inflammation of the conjunctiva. The sclera is a tough, fibrous, protective tissue. It is also referred to as the "whites of the eyes." The anterior, transparent portion of the sclera is the cornea. The cornea allows light to pass into the eye and onto the retina. The cornea is curved, which allows it to focus the incoming image onto the curved surface of the retina.

A sty (alternative spelling: *stye*), also referred to as an external hordeolum, is an infection of the eyelid that results from blockage of the oil glands associated with an eyelash. It is typically located at the lash line and has the appearance of a small pustule or lump. The lump can point externally or internally. There is often associated swelling of the lid. The sty typically resolves when the gland blockage is relieved. This can be facilitated by the use of warm soaks. Occasionally, topical antibiotics are needed.

The external ear is the part of the ear that we can readily see on physical examination. The major portion of the external ear is called the pinna or auricle. The pinna collects sound waves and directs them into the external auditory canal through the external auditory meatus to contact the tympanic membrane. The external auditory canal extends to the tympanic membrane. The canal contains a protective substance called cerumen (earwax) that is secreted by specialized glands within the canal.

The middle ear is the portion of the ear that contains the auditory ossicles. The auditory ossicles are three small bones that are joined together and function to amplify sound waves received by the tympanic membrane. These three bones, called the malleus, incus, and stapes, are well protected within the tympanic cavity. The middle ear is connected to the pharynx by the Eustachian (auditory) tube. This connection to the pharynx enables equalization of pressure between the middle ear and the environment.

The inner ear is separated from the middle ear by the oval window. Hearing and equilibrium are provided by specialized receptors within the inner ear. These receptors are well protected by the bony labyrinth. The bony labyrinth is surrounded by a collection of tubes and chambers called the membranous labyrinth. The membranous labyrinth is filled with a fluid called endolymph.

Although the ear is vulnerable to trauma, there are multiple medical conditions that also can affect the ear. These include foreign bodies, infections, impacted cerumen, mastoiditis, and perforated tympanic membrane.

The nose has numerous functions. From the standpoint of sensory function, the nose is the organ of smell. The sense of smell originates from receptors in the olfactory region of the upper part of the nasal cavity. The nerves that arise from the olfactory receptors are a part of first cranial nerve (the olfactory nerve) and enter the brain through the cribriform plate. When the brain processes the incoming signals, we smell. The senses of smell and taste are closely related. The warming, cleansing, and humidification of air are also important functions of the nose.

The structures of the nose are highly vascular. A specific area, called Kiesselbach's plexus, is a network of four arteries located in the anteroinferior region of the nasal septum. It is the region where approximately 90 percent of nosebleeds occur.

Common nontraumatic conditions related to the nose and sinuses include epistaxis, foreign bodies, rhinitis, and sinusitis.

The mouth is the opening to the oral cavity and is the entrance to the gastrointestinal tract. These structures also serve as a conduit for the respiratory gases entering and leaving the respiratory system. The oral cavity senses and analyzes substances before swallowing, mechanically processes food, and enhances digestion through the introduction of lubrication and digestive enzymes. Structures within the oral cavity include the labia, palate, tongue, pharynx, uvula, tonsils and andenoids, teeth, salivary glands, esophagus, larynx, and epiglottis.

Medical conditions of the mouth and throat are common. They include pharyngitis, tonsillitis, oral candidiasis, peritonsillar abscess, oral cellulitis, foreign bodies, dental abscesses, epiglottitis, and tracheitis.

©2013 Pearson Education, Inc.
Paramedic Care: Principles & Practice, Vol. 4, 4th Ed.

3. **Adapt the scene size-up, primary assessment, patient history, secondary assessment, and use of monitoring technology to meet the needs of patients with complaints and presentations related to diseases of the eyes, ears, nose, and throat.** pp. 428–440

During the scene size-up, your general impression will be very important, as you will be looking for clues that can indicate the patient's condition. The causes of eyes, ears, nose, and throat (EENT) disorders are numerous. One of the first questions you will answer will be whether there is a history of EENT disease, such as seasonal allergies, herpes simplex virus, HIV, herpes zoster, cataracts, ear infections, dental abscesses, throat infections, and swallowing disorders. You will also inquire about contributing diseases, such as diabetes, hypertension, stroke, vertigo, A-fib, or renal failure. Evaluate the patient's level of consciousness using the AVPU method, as well as speech, skin appearance, and posture. The patient's emotional status may also provide clues to the patient's developing condition that may be altered due to pain, fever, or hemorrhage.

Complete your primary ABCD assessment and recognize any findings that would indicate an EENT emergency. Always start with the least invasive step, visual inspection. This includes checking patient appearance and positioning as well as visually inspecting the affected area. Your secondary assessment should include a detailed exam of the affected area, accurate history, and physical exam with a full set of vital signs. Initiate all appropriate monitoring devices. For example, alterations in ventilatory function may be observed in a patient experiencing an EENT emergency associated with severe infection, fever, or hemorrhage. Capnography measures exhaled or end-tidal carbon dioxide (CO_2) and can assist the paramedic in evaluating the ventilation rate and quality in such a patient. Pulse oximetry is used to monitor a patient's general state of perfusion. Be sure to get a complete set of baseline vital signs early in the process. Changes in vitals along with alterations in mental status may indicate early shock due to hemorrhage or other processes.

Patients with EENT conditions are at risk for nausea, vomiting, choking and aspiration, and hypovolemic shock, so frequent assessment of the airway, breathing, and circulation is vital.

4. **Use a process of clinical reasoning to guide and interpret the patient assessment and management process for patients with complaints and presentations related to diseases of the eyes, ears, nose, and throat.** pp. 428–440

As a paramedic, it is vital that you develop your clinical reasoning process to quickly recognize and treat acute EENT emergencies to improve patient outcome. This is because diagnosis and treatment with many acute EENT emergencies is time-sensitive. Develop an organized general impression to rapidly identify signs and symptoms EENT emergencies. This will include obtaining an accurate history. Patients who are especially at risk for EENT emergencies include post-surgical patients and patients with a history of hypertension, allergic reactions, or HIV, as well as patients on anticoagulants.

The primary assessment of patients with eyes, ears, nose, and throat problems is directed at identifying any life-threatening injuries or illnesses that may require immediate intervention. Immediate problems that must be corrected involve the following:

- Compromise to airway and ventilation
- Compromise of circulation due to traumatic injuries resulting in hemorrhage
- Penetrations to the head and neck
- Patient complaints of difficulty speaking, swallowing, significant throat pain, or throat tightness
- Inflammation and swelling of the epiglottis or foreign bodies can obstruct the airway
- Victims of inhalation burns
- Allergic reactions with angioedema
- Nosebleeds that cannot be controlled with pressure

The primary treatment for EENT emergencies is to rapidly identify signs and symptoms that affect the patient's airway, breathing, and circulation. Consider the following:

- *Airway and breathing.* Patients with suspected airway compromise who are breathing spontaneously should be allowed to maintain the position of comfort that enables them to maintain their airway. This is especially true in patients with epistaxis who, if not positioned appropriately, can swallow large amounts of blood. Because nausea and vomiting are common in patients with EENT disorders, you should have an emesis container close and have suction ready. Keep the patient NPO.
- *Circulatory support.* Establish at least one IV based on your local protocols. It is important to have an accessible route for fluid volume resuscitation and medications. Some patients may need an additional IV if rapid blood loss is possible, such as in patients with uncontrollable epistaxis. In patients with epistaxis, control bleeding by applying pressure for at least 10 minutes to the fleshy part of the nostrils.

5.   **Given a variety of scenarios, develop treatment plans for patients with complaints and presentations related to diseases of the eyes, ears, nose, and throat.**   **pp. 428–440**

The priorities for someone who is clearly in urgent distress due to EENT disorders are the same as for a patient who is affected by a potentially life-threatening emergency of another origin. Ensure adequate airway, breathing (ventilation), and circulation. This is particularly important for someone whose emergency may be affecting the airway as well as the respiratory and cardiovascular systems. Swelling of the airway can cause obstruction and difficulty breathing. Intractable nausea and vomiting can cause respiratory distress. This is especially true for the patient with an underlying pulmonary disease. Also, persistent vomiting can cause alterations in heart rate and blood pressure, produce dramatic volume losses, and place the patient to be at risk for aspiration. Most EENT disorders in the prehospital setting will require a minimum of supportive measures, such as airway maintenance, oxygenation, ventilatory management, and hemodynamic and cardiac monitoring. You should always provide oxygen, allow a position of comfort, initiate an IV, and treat nausea, vomiting, and pain.

Case Study Review

Reread the case study on page 425 in Paramedic Care: Medicine; *then, read the following discussion.*

This case study draws attention to the assessment and management of a commonly encountered patient presentation, in which an individual is experiencing complications of an EENT disorder.

The paramedics place the patient in a semi-Fowler's position and start a saline lock. They administer 4 mg of ondansetron and 50 mcg of fentanyl. They place a commercial nose clip onto the nose, administer humidified oxygen, and transport the patient to University Medical Center. The trip to the hospital is uneventful.

Examination by the emergency physician reveals multiple bleeding sites. Laboratory studies obtained in the emergency department reveal that the patient's prothrombin time, as measured by the International Normalized Ratio (INR), is six times normal. Based on this, an ear, nose, and throat (ENT) physician is consulted, and the patient is admitted to the hospital.

The patient receives vitamin K, to reverse the effects of the Coumadin, as well as fresh frozen plasma. Although he is anemic, he does not require transfusion. The emergency physician placed nasal packing that controlled the bleeding. The ear, nose, and throat physician evaluates the patient and determines that no further care is warranted. Following discharge, the patient is referred back to the Veterans Administration clinic for social care and monitoring of his prothrombin levels and Coumadin dose.

Content Self-Evaluation

MULTIPLE CHOICE

_____ 1. The tough, fibrous, protective tissue also referred to as the "whites of the eyes" is called the
- **A.** pupil.
- **B.** choroid.
- **C.** retina.
- **D.** sclera.
- **E.** iris.

_____ 2. The highly vascular tissue that provides essential nutrients to the tissues of the eye is the
- **A.** choroid.
- **B.** sclera.
- **C.** iris.
- **D.** pupil.
- **E.** retina.

_____ 3. A condition of infection and inflammation of the cornea that can cause a corneal ulcer is
- **A.** gonorrhea.
- **B.** herpes zoster.
- **C.** herpes simplex virus.
- **D.** HIV.
- **E.** pertussis.

_____ 4. Clouding of the lens of the eye associated with aging is called
- **A.** a cataract.
- **B.** hyphema.
- **C.** papilledema.
- **D.** optic neuritis.
- **E.** diabetes.

_____ 5. A chronic condition that commonly affects the eyes is
- **A.** neuritis.
- **B.** emphysema.
- **C.** diabetes.
- **D.** COPD.
- **E.** urethritis.

_____ 6. Separation of the retina from its supporting structures is called
- **A.** retinal detachment.
- **B.** optic lymphoma.
- **C.** retinal occlusion.
- **D.** optic neuritis.
- **E.** conjunctivitis.

_____ 7. The external auditory canal contains a protective substance called
- **A.** auditory ossicle.
- **B.** equilibrium.
- **C.** malleus.
- **D.** otitis media.
- **E.** cerumen.

_____ 8. A common infectious condition of the ear often seen in children is
- **A.** otitis intima.
- **B.** otitis media.
- **C.** otitis minima.
- **D.** external auditory.
- **E.** incusitis.

_____ 9. Functions of the nose include all of the following, EXCEPT
- **A.** filtering air.
- **B.** warming air.
- **C.** humidifying air.
- **D.** making mucus.

_____ 10. The clinical term for nosebleed is
- **A.** epistaxis.
- **B.** eustacia.
- **C.** pharynx.
- **D.** larynx.
- **E.** rhinitis.

_____ 11. The upper portion (roof) of the oral cavity is the
   A. adenoids.
   B. uvula.
   C. labia.
   D. tongue.
   E. palate.

_____ 12. Inflammation of the posterior aspect of the oral cavity is called
   A. pharyngitis.
   B. adenoiditis.
   C. otitis.
   D. gingivitis.
   E. abscess.

_____ 13. A common fungal (yeast) condition of the mouth is
   A. encephalitis.
   B. gingivitis.
   C. thrush.
   D. meningitis.
   E. otitis.

_____ 14. A type of oral bacterial cellulitis and inflammation is
   A. thrush.
   B. pharyngitis
   C. laryngitis.
   D. otitis media.
   E. Ludwig's angina.

_____ 15. Acute inflammation and infection of the epiglottis that is considered a life-threatening emergency is
   A. epiglottitis.
   B. thrush.
   C. rhinitis.
   D. meningitis.
   E. gingivitis.

©2013 Pearson Education, Inc.
Paramedic Care: Principles & Practice, Vol. 4, 4th Ed.

Nontraumatic Musculoskeletal Disorders

Review of Chapter Objectives

After reading this chapter, you should be able to:

1. **Define key terms introduced in this chapter.**

   Knowing and being able to apply the key terms in each chapter is critical to understanding chapter concepts. Write the list of key terms. Then write the definition of each one in your own words. Check your understanding by confirming the definitions in the text glossary. Correct any misunderstandings. Create a study aid by writing each key term on the front of an index card and the definition on the back. Use the cards to quiz yourself, or to have someone quiz you.

2. **Relate the anatomy and physiology of the musculoskeletal system to the pathophysiology and assessment of patients with nontraumatic musculoskeletal disorders.**   **pp. 445–456**

   The musculoskeletal system is made up of the muscular system and the skeletal system. It provides the body with form, support, stability, and the ability to move about the environment. The skeletal system consists of the body's bones, joints, ligaments, and associated connective tissues. The muscular system consists of the muscles, tendons, and associated connective tissues. The tendons are located at the end of the muscle and form a fibrous bundle that connects the muscle to bone. The tendon fibers are interwoven into the periosteum of the bone, forming a firm attachment. The skeletal muscles are controlled by the voluntary nervous system via the neuromuscular junctions. Nontraumatic medical conditions can affect any of these structures. Other body systems, such as the nervous system, also play a major role in nontraumatic medical conditions.

   The muscular system, because of its size and demands, is a significant user of energy. It is subject to fatigue and injury. Muscular complaints are common, and can be a source of significant disability for some patients.

   Most patients with nontraumatic musculoskeletal disorders will present with pain or tenderness. The physical examination findings you encounter will be as varied as the patients. As already stated, the patient will often complain of pain and tenderness that is much worse than usual or typical for the condition. Patients may complain of associated swelling or other abnormality. In some cases, specifically with the inflammatory disorders, there will be some loss of movement of the affected joints and associated structures. This can be due to pain or due to abnormalities in the structure of the joint itself.

With some of these conditions the neurologic and vascular systems may be affected as well. As many of these diseases progress, deformity, either temporary or permanent, can occur.

Common conditions that affect the muscular system include repetitive-motion disorders such as tendinitis, bursitis, myalgias, and carpal tunnel syndrome, to name a few. Osteoarthritis, osteoporosis, degenerative disc disease, inflammatory joint diseases, and rheumatoid arthritis represent common diseases of the skeletal system.

3. **Adapt the scene size-up, primary assessment, patient history, secondary assessment, and use of monitoring technology to meet the needs of patients with complaints and presentations related to nontraumatic musculoskeletal disorders.**   pp. 445–446

During the scene size-up, your general impression will be very important, as you will be looking for clues that can indicate the patient's condition. The causes of nontraumatic musculoskeletal disorders are numerous. Fortunately, most nontraumatic musculoskeletal disorders, although often painful, are not life threatening. One of the first questions you will answer will be whether there is a history of nontraumatic musculoskeletal disorders, such as rheumatoid arthritis, osteoarthritis, osteoporosis, degenerative joint and disc disease, gout, or systemic lupus erythematous, and any recent muscle strains. Discuss with the patient how the chronic disease has affected the patient's activities of daily living (ADLs). Many chronic nontraumatic musculoskeletal diseases contribute to falls and decreased mobility, such as rheumatoid arthritis, osteoarthritis, osteoporosis, degenerative joint and disc disease, and gout. Remaining systematic, evaluate the patient's level of consciousness using the AVPU method, as well as speech, skin appearance, and posture. The patient's emotional status and living conditions may also provide clues to the patient's developing condition.

Complete your primary ABCD assessment and recognize any findings that would indicate an emergency. Always start with the least invasive step, visual inspection. This includes checking patient appearance and positioning as well as visually inspecting the affected area. Your secondary assessment should include a detailed exam of the affected area, accurate history, and physical exam with a full set of vital signs. Initiate all appropriate monitoring devices. For example, alterations in ventilatory function may be observed in a patient experiencing severe pain associated with nontraumatic musculoskeletal disorders. Capnography measures exhaled or end-tidal carbon dioxide (CO_2) and can assist the paramedic in evaluating the ventilation rate and quality in such a patient. Pulse oximetry is used to monitor a patient's general state of perfusion. Be sure to get a complete set of baseline vital signs in your secondary assessment.

4. **Use a process of clinical reasoning to guide and interpret the patient assessment and management process for patients with nontraumatic musculoskeletal disorders.**   pp. 445–446

Your assessment of the patient with a nontraumatic musculoskeletal disorder will employ the same techniques and strategies as for a patient with any other complaint. This includes the primary assessment and ensuring the adequacy of the airway, breathing, and circulation. The secondary assessment should include a fairly focused and detailed history of the illness. It is often helpful to review the patient's medications for additional information regarding the condition and the level of pain the patient is suffering.

You should pay particular attention to the body region about which the patient is complaining. If your patient has joint pain, examine the joint for tenderness, swelling, erythema, and restriction in the range of motion. For muscle disorders, look for restrictions in the range of motion as well as for particular tender points and muscle spasm. For patients who are complaining of back pain, a more detailed exam is necessary to exclude conditions that require emergency treatment, such as cauda equina syndrome. The examination of the patient with back pain should include examination of the affected area and a neurologic exam including deep tendon reflexes (knee and ankle) as well as the search for sensory or motor deficits. Look particularly for signs of urinary or fecal incontinence as well as saddle anesthesia (numbness in the crotch and perineum). Many patients with chronic back pain have discogenic disease and will present with radicular symptoms (e.g., sciatica). These should be noted and considered as you formulate a treatment plan.

©2013 Pearson Education, Inc.
Paramedic Care: Principles & Practice, Vol. 4, 4th Ed.

For the most part, treatment of these conditions is supportive and symptomatic. Pain management can be provided with opiate analgesics as well as with nonsteroidal anti-inflammatory drugs (NSAIDs). In some cases, nonpharmacological treatments such as splinting, application of cold or heat packs, and similar strategies may be beneficial. In certain conditions, such as ankylosing spondylitis, the patient may present a challenge in terms of packaging and preparing for transport. Because many of these conditions include chronic pain, some patients will have an overlay of depression, anxiety, or both. Communication, empathy, and quality care will help to alleviate some of this. In many cases, the complaints related to these conditions may seem trivial. However, the patient knows his body and his disease and may summon EMS during a severe exacerbation of the illness.

5. **Describe the pathophysiology of general classifications of nontraumatic musculoskeletal disorders, including problems in the following classifications:**

   a. **Overuse/repetitive-motion disorders** pp. 449–450

   Repetitive motions, such as repeatedly lifting a patient or using a computer keyboard, can, over time, injure or inflame the tissues and structures that are being used. Technically speaking, overuse and repetitive-motion disorders are a form of trauma. However, because they tend to be chronic, they are often considered medical conditions. Despite the clinical similarities between overuse/repetitive-motion injuries and other types of musculoskeletal trauma, the pathophysiology is somewhat different. Although most injuries result from a single recognizable event, overuse and repetitive-motion disorders occur from repetitive events that ultimately lead to signs and symptoms that are similar to those associated with acute trauma.

   Repetitive-motion injuries are quite common and are due to microscopic tears of the affected tendons or muscles. However, unlike what occurs with acute trauma, the body is unable to repair the affected tissues because of continued use. Most repetitive-motion disorders are related to a vocation or avocation, and the patient often must or will continue to use the affected body part. In addition to repetitive movements, causes of repetitive-motion disorders include trauma, crystal deposits within the joint (e.g., gout), friction, and as a result of systemic diseases. Most patients with repetitive-motion disorders will complain of pain or tenderness in the affected area. Range of motion may be restricted because of swelling and/or pain. Examples of repetitive-motion injuries include tendinitis, bursitis, myalgias, carpal tunnel syndrome, and similar conditions.

   b. **Degenerative conditions** pp. 450–451

   A degenerative condition or disorder is one that results from a disturbance in normal functioning of the affected tissues or organ system. In some cases, the degeneration is due to age and simple wear and tear. Degenerative conditions can affect virtually any body system, and are not limited to those that affect the musculoskeletal system. Some of the most common degenerative musculoskeletal conditions are osteoarthritis, osteoporosis, and degenerative disc disease.

   c. **Inflammatory conditions** pp. 451–453

   Inflammatory joint diseases are group of rheumatologic conditions that result from inflammation within the joint. Inflammatory joint diseases are typically characterized by pain, stiffness, erythema, warmth, and swelling of the joint. The presence of increased fluid within the joint, called an effusion, is also common. In some cases the inflammation can be so severe that range of motion of the joint is lost. There are several inflammatory musculoskeletal disorders. These include rheumatoid arthritis, ankylosing spondylitis, and gout, to name a few.

   d. **Infectious conditions** pp. 453–455

   Soft tissue infections are infections that involve the skin, the underlying tissues, the fascia, as well as tendons and even muscle. The tissues of the muscular and skeletal system (and surrounding structures) are vulnerable to infection by various pathogens—primarily bacteria. Although soft-tissue infections are fairly common, infections of the bones and joints are less so. Because bone and joint infections tend to involve deeper structures, infection is relatively uncommon—but also more difficult to treat. An infection of the bone is referred to as osteomyelitis. Joints can also become infected, a condition called septic arthritis.

e. **Neoplastic processes** p. 455

A neoplasm is an abnormal growth of body tissue and is often called a tumor. Tumors can arise from bone and muscle tissue. A primary musculoskeletal tumor is one that arises from muscle, bone, or one of the associated tissues (e.g., synovium). A secondary musculoskeletal tumor is one that spreads to the muscle or bone from another site or tissue type (e.g., breast cancer, prostate cancer). Bone tumors can be benign or malignant (cancerous). The most common benign bone tumors are the osteochondromas. Most malignant bone tumors are sarcomas. Sarcomas arise from bone, cartilage, muscle, fat, and similar tissues.

f. **Chronic pain syndrome** p. 458

Pain is the most common reason people seek medical care. In some individuals, pain will persist longer than typically seen in others who have the same condition. This is referred to as chronic pain syndrome (CPS). CPS is a poorly defined condition, but generally includes ongoing pain that lasts anywhere in excess of three to six months. It typically includes multiple symptoms and complaints and has multiple causes, although these causes are complex and poorly understood. Chronic pain is somewhat more common in women. There are often associated psychological syndromes, including depression, anxiety, and hypochondriasis. CPS is often characterized by the presence of the six D's:

- Dramatization of complaints
- Drug misuse
- Dysfunction/disuse
- Dependency
- Depression
- Disability

g. **Pediatric conditions** p. 456

Although most nontraumatic musculoskeletal disorders occur in adults, some such conditions occur in children. For example, juvenile rheumatoid arthritis is a debilitating condition of children. There are other nontraumatic musculoskeletal disorders that can affect children. Among these are Osgood-Schlatter disease and slipped capital femoral epiphysis.

6. **Given a variety of scenarios, develop treatment plans for patients with nontraumatic musculoskeletal disorders.** pp. 445–456

The priorities for someone who is clearly in urgent distress due to nontraumatic musculoskeletal disorders are the same as for a patient who is affected by a potentially life-threatening emergency of another origin. Ensure adequate airway, breathing (ventilation), and circulation. This is particularly important for someone whose emergency may be affecting the airway as well as the respiratory and cardiovascular systems. Severe pain can affect the patient's vital signs. This is especially true for the patient with an underlying autoimmune disease. Most nontraumatic musculoskeletal disorders in the prehospital setting will require a minimum of care. However, some may require supportive measures such as airway maintenance, oxygenation, ventilatory management, and cardiac monitoring. Based on your clinical judgment, you should provide oxygen as appropriate, allow a position of comfort, and initiate an IV for the treatment of nausea, vomiting, and pain.

Case Study Review

Reread the case study on page 444 in Paramedic Care: Medicine; *then, read the following discussion.*

This case study draws attention to the assessment and management of a commonly encountered patient presentation, in which an individual is experiencing complications of a nontraumatic musculoskeletal disorder.

The paramedics remove the towel and inspect the wound. It is an approximately 5-cm linear laceration to the right side of his head. It will require sutures or staples. They place a dressing and bandage before turning their attention to preparing Bill for transport. The crew knows that Bill's ankylosing spondylitis has made his spinal column rigid and permanently curved. Because he has so much neck pain, they're assuming he has a potential fracture or injury to the spine. The crew is able to place a rigid cervical collar, but they know that Bill will not be able to lie flat and be placed on the long spine board. In anticipation of transport, Chris retrieves several blankets and towels from the ambulance. The crew members carefully move Bill to the ambulance stretcher and fill the void areas behind his neck and back with the towels to maintain his neck and back in a neutral position. Because of the excessive pain Bill is feeling, Larry places a saline lock and administers 50 mcg of fentanyl. This provides significant pain relief, and they move Bill to the ambulance for transport to the hospital.

The transport is uneventful, and the crew delivers Bill to the emergency apartment in improved condition. At the hospital, CT imaging of Bill's head, neck, and thoracic spine reveals no fractures, and the emergency department staff repairs the laceration with staples. Bill remains in the emergency department for several hours and is later discharged home in good condition.

Content Self-Evaluation

MULTIPLE CHOICE

_____ 1. Bones are joined together by
   A. ligaments.
   B. tendons.
   C. cartilage.
   D. fascia.
   E. osteocytes.

_____ 2. A form of flexible connective tissue that provides support and structure for joints is
   A. tendons.
   B. cartilage.
   C. fascia.
   D. tendons.
   E. osteoblasts.

_____ 3. An oily, straw-colored fluid that fills the joint space and serves to reduce friction is
   A. serum.
   B. saliva.
   C. gastric acid.
   D. synovial fluid.
   E. mucus.

_____ 4. Muscles are attached to bone by
   A. ligaments.
   B. tendons.
   C. cartilage.
   D. fascia.
   E. osteocytes.

_____ 5. Skeletal muscles are controlled by the
   A. periosteums.
   B. unmyelinated fibers.
   C. endocrine system.
   D. autonomic nervous system.
   E. somatic nervous system.

_____ 6. Injuries that are due to microscopic tears in tendons or muscles are called
   A. repetitive-motion injuries.
   B. lymphomas.
   C. friction injuries.
   D. osteoporosis.
   E. arthritis.

_____ 7. Inflammation of a tendon is called
   A. bursitis.
   B. carpal spasm.
   C. anemia.
   D. tendonitis.
   E. osteoporosis.

_____ 8. The most common form of bone disease characterized by a thinning of bone tissue and loss of bone density is
   A. osteomalacia.
   B. osteoporosis.
   C. osteoarthritis.
   D. avascular necrosis.
   E. ankylosing spondylitis.

_____ 9. A chronic autoimmune disease that leads to inflammation of the joints is
   A. osteoporosis.
   B. erythema.
   C. rheumatoid arthritis.
   D. spinal stenosis.
   E. scoliosis.

_____ 10. The most common cause of nontraumatic low back pain is
   A. epistaxis.
   B. osteomalacia.
   C. ankylosing spondylitis.
   D. degenerative disc disease.
   E. rheumatoid arthritis.

_____ 11. A chronic autoimmune disease that can affect the skin, joints, kidneys, and other organs is
   A. systemic lupus erythematosus.
   B. rheumatoid arthritis.
   C. osteoarthritis.
   D. osteoporosis.
   E. erythroblastosis fetalis.

_____ 12. Gout is a form of inflammatory arthritis that occurs when
   A. histamine is released by mast cells.
   B. prostaglandins are released locally.
   C. uric acid accumulates in the joints.
   D. epinephrine is released.
   E. bradykinin is released.

_____ 13. An infection of the soft tissues is
   A. encephalitis.
   B. cellulitis.
   C. pancreatitis.
   D. meningitis.
   E. otitis media.

_____ 14. An infection of the bone is
   A. cellulitis.
   B. pharyngitis.
   C. laryngitis.
   D. otitis media.
   E. osteomyelitis.

_____ 15. An abnormal growth of body tissue, such as a tumor, is called a(n):
   A. astrocyte.
   B. myalgia.
   C. neoplasm.
   D. sarcoma.
   E. tunic.

©2013 Pearson Education, Inc.
Paramedic Care: Principles & Practice, Vol. 4, 4th Ed.

MEDICINE
Content Review
Content Self-Evaluation

Chapter 1: Pulmonology

_____ 1. Place the structures of the respiratory system in order of inspiration.

    1. alveoli
    2. bronchi
    3. nasal cavity
    4. pharynx
    5. larynx
    6. trachea
    7. lungs

    A. 1, 7, 2, 6, 5, 4, 3   **D.** 3, 4, 5, 6, 2, 7, 1
    B. 3, 5, 4, 2, 6, 7, 1   **E.** 7, 2, 4, 5, 6, 1, 3
    C. 3, 4, 5, 2, 6, 7, 1

_____ 2. How long is the trachea?
    A. 11 cm   **D.** 8 inches
    B. 8 cm   **E.** 7 cm
    C. 11 inches

_____ 3. The carina is located in (at) the
    A. pharynx.   **D.** thyroid cartilage.
    B. larynx.   **E.** division of the bronchi.
    C. soft palate.

_____ 4. Aspirated material may pass into the right lung due to
    A. a straighter right mainstem bronchus.   **D.** peristalsis that occurs in the esophagus.
    B. an ineffective gag reflex.   **E.** the pleura.
    C. atelectasis.

_____ 5. The bronchioles are approximately 1 mm thick and contain primarily which type of muscle?
    A. Cardiac   **D.** Voluntary
    B. Smooth   **E.** Contractile
    C. Striated

_____ 6. Which pleura surrounds the lungs and does not contain nerve fibers?
    A. Alveolar   **D.** Pulmonary
    B. Bronchial-lobar   **E.** Visceral
    C. Parietal

_____ 7. The _____ pleura lines the thoracic cavity and contains nerve fibers.
    A. alveolar   **D.** pulmonary
    B. bronchial-lobar   **E.** visceral
    C. parietal

_____ 8. The _____ muscles aid in respiration and connect each rib.
   A. accessory
   B. diaphragmatic
   C. intercostal
   D. tracheal
   E. sternal

_____ 9. Which nerve innervates the diaphragm?
   A. Cardiac plexus
   B. Iliac
   C. Phrenic
   D. Vagus
   E. Thoracic

_____ 10. The chest's relative ease by which it expands during ventilation is known as
   A. airway resistance.
   B. rebound.
   C. transthoracic resistance.
   D. visceral pleura elasticity.
   E. compliance.

_____ 11. Which of the following conditions most likely is occurring in an emphysema patient who is experiencing dyspnea?
   A. Increased lung compliance
   B. Decreased lung compliance
   C. Increased airway resistance
   D. Decreased airway resistance
   E. Bronchospasm

_____ 12. Decreasing lung compliance in the elderly is best attributed to
   A. a decrease in nerve cells.
   B. a loss of elasticity of intercostal muscles.
   C. enlargement of the chest wall.
   D. weight loss.
   E. weight gain.

_____ 13. The air that remains in the alveoli at all times is referred to as
   A. expiratory reserve volume.
   B. functional reserve capacity.
   C. vital capacity.
   D. residual volume.
   E. inspiratory reserve volume.

_____ 14. Average residual volume is approximately
   A. 500 mL.
   B. 1,200 mL.
   C. 2,000 mL.
   D. 3,000 mL.
   E. 3,600 mL.

_____ 15. Average vital capacity is approximately
   A. 2,400 mL.
   B. 3,600 mL.
   C. 4,800 mL.
   D. 5,200 mL.
   E. 6,000 mL.

_____ 16. The primary portion of the brain that controls ventilation is the
   A. cerebellum.
   B. frontal lobe.
   C. medulla.
   D. vagus nerve.
   E. pons.

_____ 17. The medulla transmits impulses to the primary muscles of respiration through the _____ nerves.
   A. brachial plexus
   B. phrenic
   C. vagus
   D. vestibulocochlear
   E. cranial

_____ 18. The normal pH for the body is
   A. 7.15 to 7.25.
   B. 7.25 to 7.35.
   C. 7.35 to 7.45.
   D. 7.45 to 7.55.
   E. 7.55 to 7.60.

©2013 Pearson Education, Inc.
Paramedic Care: Principles & Practice, Vol. 4, 4th Ed.

_____ **19.** Elevated CO_2 in the bloodstream results in
  A. acidosis.
  B. alkalosis.
  C. hypernatremia.
  D. hyponatremia.
  E. glycolosis.

_____ **20.** Scenario: You are called to the scene of a 64-year-old male with a history of bronchitis and pneumonia. He takes Theodur, Atrovent, Solu-Medrol, and Lasix on a daily basis. He is breathing at a rate of 42, shallow and regular, and is complaining of shortness of breath. Most likely the patient's PCO_2 is
  A. 35 to 45 mmHg.
  B. less than 35 mmHg.
  C. greater than 45 mmHg.
  D. 80 to 100 mmHg.
  E. greater than 100 mmHg.

_____ **21.** One of the factors on which lung perfusion depends is
  A. adequate blood volume.
  B. adequate supply of carbon dioxide.
  C. homeostasis.
  D. intact cerebral capillaries.
  E. hyperventilation.

_____ **22.** Under NORMAL conditions, how much oxygen is transported dissolved in plasma?
  A. 2 percent
  B. 30 percent
  C. 40 percent
  D. 65 percent
  E. 98 percent

_____ **23.** The greatest amount of carbon dioxide is transported in the body to the lungs in the form of
  A. bicarbonate ions.
  B. water molecules.
  C. plasma.
  D. carboxyhemoglobins.
  E. erythrocytes.

_____ **24.** For inhalation to occur, the
  A. bronchi must dilate.
  B. chest cavity must create a negative pressure.
  C. diaphragm must relax.
  D. intercostal muscles must contract down and inward.
  E. chest cavity must create a positive pressure.

_____ **25.** The respiratory pattern with deep rapid breaths that result as a corrective measure from a metabolic acidosis condition is known as
  A. apneustic.
  B. Biot's.
  C. central neurogenic hyperventilation.
  D. Cheyne-Stokes.
  E. Kussmaul's.

_____ **26.** The respiratory pattern with deep, rapid respirations caused by a stroke or brain stem lesion and that may result in respiratory alkalosis is known as
  A. apneustic.
  B. Biot's.
  C. central neurogenic hyperventilation.
  D. Cheyne-Stokes.
  E. Kussmaul's.

_____ **27.** The respiratory pattern characterized by repeated episodes of irregular gasping ventilations separated by periods of apnea is known as
  A. apneustic.
  B. Biot's.
  C. Cheyne-Stokes breathing.
  D. Cheyne-Stokes.
  E. Kussmaul's.

_____ **28.** Which of the following is an alveoli perfusion disorder?
  A. Hypernatremia
  B. Hyponatremia
  C. Hypovolemia
  D. Hypoxemia
  E. Hyperkalemia

_____ 29. All of the following clues at the scene would indicate that the patient has an underlying respiratory disorder, EXCEPT a(n)
  A. cigarette pack.
  B. bronchodilation inhaler.
  C. oxygen tank.
  D. prescription bottle of Prozac.
  E. nebulizer.

_____ 30. Vibration felt in the chest during speaking is known as
  A. crepitus.
  B. pleurisy.
  C. subcutaneous emphysema.
  D. tactile fremitus.
  E. crackles.

_____ 31. Which of the following conditions would you expect to discover with a hollow sound when percussing the chest?
  A. Emphysema
  B. Hemothorax
  C. Pneumonia
  D. Pulmonary edema
  E. Bronchitis

_____ 32. A dull sound when percussing the chest indicates
  A. ascites.
  B. emphysema.
  C. hemothorax.
  D. pneumothorax.
  E. bronchitis.

_____ 33. A high-pitched whistling sound due to bronchoconstriction is known as
  A. pleural friction rub.
  B. crackles (rales).
  C. rhonchi.
  D. wheezing.
  E. stridor.

_____ 34. A harsh, high-pitched sound heard on inspiration and characteristic of an upper-airway obstruction is
  A. crackles (rales).
  B. snoring.
  C. pleural friction rub.
  D. wheezing.
  E. stridor.

_____ 35. A patient in respiratory distress has clubbing of the fingers. This condition's most likely pathophysiology is
  A. carbon monoxide poisoning.
  B. carpopedal spasms.
  C. persistent hypoxemia.
  D. respiratory alkalosis.
  E. pneumonia.

_____ 36. Scenario: Your patient is breathing at 32 times per minute. This is known as
  A. bradypnea.
  B. eupnea.
  C. hyperventilation.
  D. tachypnea.
  E. Kussmaul's respirations.

_____ 37. Which of the following conditions will have an inaccurate pulse oximetry reading?
  A. Carbon monoxide poisoning
  B. Hyperventilation syndrome
  C. Hypothermia
  D. Shock
  E. Sepsis

_____ 38. Capnography evaluates the amount of
  A. carbon dioxide expired in relation to inspired.
  B. carbon dioxide inspired in relation to expired.
  C. oxygen expired in relation to inspired.
  D. oxygen inspired in relation to expired.
  E. oxygen in relation to carbon dioxide.

©2013 Pearson Education, Inc.
Paramedic Care: Principles & Practice, Vol. 4, 4th Ed.

_____ **39.** A patient developing ARDS may have all of the following conditions, EXCEPT
  A. hyperthermia.
  B. pancreatitis.
  C. respiratory burns.
  D. sepsis.
  E. hypothermia.

_____ **40.** An excellent means to maintain patency of the alveoli in a patient who has adult respiratory distress syndrome is
  A. endotracheal intubation.
  B. furosemide.
  C. peak expiratory flow rate device.
  D. positive end expiratory pressure.
  E. use of digoxin.

_____ **41.** Patients with COPD have a _____ chance of dying within 10 years of diagnosis.
  A. 28 percent
  B. 42 percent
  C. 50 percent
  D. 65 percent
  E. 80 percent

_____ **42.** Approximately _____ of patients who die from asthma do so before reaching the hospital.
  A. 50 percent
  B. 45 percent
  C. 40 percent
  D. 35 percent
  E. 30 percent

_____ **43.** With which other symptoms of emphysema is significant smoking history best associated?
  A. Atrophy of the respiratory accessory muscles
  B. Obesity
  C. Pulmonary hypertension
  D. Pulmonary edema
  E. Hyperkinesia

_____ **44.** Which of the following diseases has a normal to decreased residual volume and a decreased vital capacity?
  A. Asthma
  B. Bronchitis
  C. Emphysema
  D. Pneumonia
  E. ARDS

_____ **45.** An initial and most dependable sign of an asthma attack is
  A. coughing.
  B. dyspnea.
  C. stridor.
  D. wheezing.
  E. crackles.

_____ **46.** An early sign of respiratory problems is
  A. agitation.
  B. an increased respiratory rate.
  C. cyanosis.
  D. dyspnea.
  E. a decreased respiratory rate.

_____ **47.** In patients who are experiencing status asthmaticus, the EMS provider should recognize that respiratory arrest is imminent and
  A. be prepared for endotracheal intubation.
  B. immediately administer a beta-agonist inhaled medication.
  C. encourage the patient to cough forcefully to avoid alveolar collapse.
  D. remember that quiet breathing is a sign that the patient is improving.
  E. immediately establish IV access.

_____ **48.** Upper respiratory infections include all of the following, EXCEPT
  A. bronchiolitis.
  B. epiglottitis.
  C. otitis media.
  D. pharyngitis.
  E. rhinitis.

____ **49.** Carbon monoxide poisoning is dangerous because
  A. carbon dioxide binds to hemoglobin more readily than oxygen.
  B. it leads to cellular alkalosis.
  C. it causes the overabsorption of oxygen into the blood plasma.
  D. it causes respiratory alkalosis.
  E. it causes respiratory alkalemia.

____ **50.** Risk factors associated with pulmonary embolisms include all of the following, EXCEPT
  A. pneumonia.
  B. recent surgery.
  C. sickle cell anemia.
  D. venous pooling during pregnancy.
  E. long-bone fractures.

Chapter 2: Cardiology

____ **51.** The single largest killer of Americans is
  A. adult respiratory distress syndrome.
  B. cancer.
  C. coronary heart disease.
  D. diabetes.
  E. hypotension.

____ **52.** The apex of the heart is located at the
  A. inferior aspect.
  B. left atrium.
  C. right atrium.
  D. superior aspect.
  E. hilum.

____ **53.** Pericardial fluid reduces friction as the heart beats and is encased between the parietal pericardium and the
  A. endocardium.
  B. epicardium.
  C. mesentery.
  D. myocardium.
  E. exocardium.

____ **54.** The innermost layer of the cardiac muscle is the
  A. endocardium.
  B. epicardium.
  C. myocardium.
  D. pericardium.
  E. mesentery.

____ **55.** Which chamber of the heart receives blood from the pulmonary circulation?
  A. Left atrium
  B. Left ventricle
  C. Right atrium
  D. Right ventricle
  E. None of the above

____ **56.** Identify in order the flow of blood through the heart, beginning with the superior vena cava.

  1. aortic semilunar valve
  2. mitral valve
  3. right ventricle
  4. pulmonary artery
  5. left atrium
  6. ascending aorta

  A. 1, 4, 5, 3, 2, 6
  B. 2, 3, 4, 5, 1, 6
  C. 3, 4, 5, 2, 1, 6
  D. 5, 2, 3, 4, 1, 6
  E. 1, 3, 5, 2, 4, 6

©2013 Pearson Education, Inc.
Paramedic Care: Principles & Practice, Vol. 4, 4th Ed.

_____ 57. The structure that provides blood supply to the right atrium, right ventricle, and part of the cardiac conduction system is the
  A. anterior descending artery.
  B. circumflex artery.
  C. left coronary artery.
  D. right coronary artery.
  E. sternal artery.

_____ 58. During diastole, which of the following valves is open?
  A. Aortic semilunar
  B. Heimlich's
  C. Pulmonary semilunar
  D. Tricuspid
  E. Einthoven's

_____ 59. The resistance against which the ventricles contract is known as
  A. afterload.
  B. end-diastolic volume.
  C. preload.
  D. pulse pressure.
  E. cardioinhibitory pressure.

_____ 60. Calculate cardiac output if the average stroke volume is 70 mL and the heart rate is 80 beats per minute.
  A. 2,800 mL/min
  B. 2,800 mL/hr
  C. 5,600 mL/min
  D. 5,600 mL/hr
  E. none of the above

_____ 61. An increase in peripheral vascular resistance results in
  A. decreased afterload.
  B. increased cardiac output.
  C. increased preload.
  D. increased stroke volume.
  E. decreased stroke volume.

_____ 62. The sympathetic nervous system innervates the heart through the
  A. brachial plexus.
  B. cardiac plexus.
  C. cervical plexus.
  D. vagus nerve.
  E. median nerve.

_____ 63. Hypokalemia in the myocardium results in
  A. increased automaticity and conduction.
  B. increased conduction.
  C. increased contractility.
  D. increased irritability.
  E. increased elasticity.

_____ 64. The group of cardiac muscle cells that contract simultaneously is known as
  A. the action potential.
  B. depolarization.
  C. dromotropy.
  D. transference.
  E. the syncytium.

_____ 65. The term that pertains to the speed of impulse transmission through the myocardium is
  A. chronotropy.
  B. dromotropy.
  C. inotropy.
  D. syncytium.
  E. entropy.

_____ 66. The normal electrical state of cardiac cells is
  A. the action potential.
  B. depolarization.
  C. repolarization.
  D. the resting potential.
  E. stasis.

_____ 67. For the cardiac cell to repolarize, which ion is pumped out of the cell?
  A. Calcium
  B. Magnesium
  C. Potassium
  D. Sodium
  E. Chromium

_____ 68. The ability of muscle cells to shorten is termed
    A. automaticity.
    B. conductivity.
    C. contractility.
    D. excitability.
    E. intercalatability.

_____ 69. The ability of cardiac cells to respond to an electrical stimulus is termed
    A. automaticity.
    B. conductivity.
    C. contractility.
    D. excitability.
    E. intercalatability.

_____ 70. The _____ has an intrinsic rate of 15 to 40 beats per minute.
    A. AV node
    B. bundle of His
    C. Purkinje system
    D. SA node
    E. left bundle branch

_____ 71. For lead I, placement of the leads is on the
    A. left arm and left leg.
    B. left arm and right leg.
    C. right arm and left arm.
    D. right arm and left leg.
    E. right arm and right leg.

_____ 72. The ECG component that represents atrial depolarization is the
    A. P wave.
    B. QRS complex.
    C. T wave.
    D. U wave.
    E. ST segment.

_____ 73. Ventricular repolarization is indicated on the ECG tracing by the
    A. P wave.
    B. QRS complex.
    C. T wave.
    D. U wave.
    E. ST segment.

_____ 74. The time necessary for ventricular depolarization is represented by the
    A. P-R interval.
    B. QRS interval.
    C. QT interval.
    D. ST segment.
    E. QRS complex.

_____ 75. An abnormal and prolonged delay in the AV node is indicated by a P-R interval
    A. between 0.12 and 0.20 second.
    B. between 0.04 and 0.12 second.
    C. greater than 0.40 second.
    D. less than 0.12 second.
    E. greater than 0.20 second.

_____ 76. The total duration of ventricular depolarization is represented by the
    A. P-R interval.
    B. QRS duration.
    C. QT interval.
    D. ST segment.
    E. QRS interval.

_____ 77. With a heart rate of 180 beats per minute, you would expect the QT interval to be
    A. approximately 0.40 second.
    B. between 0.33 and 0.42 second.
    C. greater than 0.42 second.
    D. less than 0.33 second.
    E. none of the above.

_____ 78. The duration from the beginning of the P wave to the beginning of the QRS complex is the
    A. P-R interval.
    B. QRS duration.
    C. absolute refractory period.
    D. relative refractory period.
    E. U wave.

_____ 79. The first half of the T wave is also called the
    A. absolute refractory period.
    B. relative refractory period.
    C. P-R interval.
    D. QT interval.
    E. P wave.

©2013 Pearson Education, Inc.
Paramedic Care: Principles & Practice, Vol. 4, 4th Ed.

_____ 80. A significant Q wave has a
   A. duration of at least 0.02 second.
   B. duration of at least 0.04 second.
   C. negative deflection at least one-fourth the height of the QRS complex.
   D. positive deflection at least one-half the height of the QRS complex.
   E. deflection equal to the height of the P wave.

_____ 81. Which of the following ECG lead combinations can be used to evaluate the anterior and lateral walls of the left ventricle?
   A. aVR and V_1
   B. V_1 and V_2
   C. V_3 and V_4
   D. V_5 and V_6
   E. V_1 and V_6

_____ 82. The _____ method of calculating heart rate counts the number of complexes in a 6-second strip.
   A. P-P interval
   B. R-R interval
   C. 6-second
   D. triplicate
   E. hexagonal

_____ 83. Which of the following is characteristic of an abnormal sinus rhythm?
   A. Irregular rhythm
   B. P-R interval of 0.16 second
   C. QRS duration of 0.08 second
   D. Rate of 60 to 100
   E. P wave before the QRS complex

_____ 84. The passive transfer of pacemaker sites from the SA node to other latent pacemaker sites in the atria or AV junction is
   A. wandering atrial pacemaker.
   B. premature atrial contraction.
   C. premature junctional contraction.
   D. premature ventricular contraction.
   E. atrial fibrillation.

_____ 85. Scenario: A 24-year-old female is complaining of chest pain and difficulty breathing. She has been up for three days studying for finals and has been taking ephedrine supplements to help her stay awake and alert. She also admits to drinking 12 Mountain Dew sodas in the past day. Vitals are BP 90/50, pulse 180, and respirations 42. Placing her on the ECG monitor, you notice a wave preceding the normal QRS complex, but you cannot discern P or T waves. You interpret this ECG as
   A. accelerated junctional rhythm.
   B. atrial fibrillation.
   C. sinus tachycardia.
   D. supraventricular tachycardia.
   E. first-degree AV block.

_____ 86. Scenario: Your patient is complaining of shortness of breath with a respiratory rate of 36, pulse of 76, and blood pressure of 118/64. The ECG in lead II shows P-P intervals of 0.20 second and R-R intervals of 0.80 second. The rhythm is regular, and conduction appears to be 4:1. The BEST treatment for this patient is
   A. cardioversion at 50 joules.
   B. diltiazem.
   C. oxygen via nonrebreather.
   D. procainamide.
   E. dextrose.

_____ 87. Scenario: A patient experiencing atrial fibrillation is being transported for a hip fracture. The patient has no complaints of chest pain or shortness of breath and is hemodynamically stable. You establish an IV and administer nitrous oxide for pain relief. Your management for her atrial fibrillation should include
   A. cardioversion at 50 joules.
   B. Cardizem.
   C. no further treatment.
   D. verapamil.
   E. a precordial thump.

_____ 88. The cardiac rhythm that is characterized by an irregularly irregular rhythm with an atrial rate of 350 to 750 and normal QRS complexes is
   A. atrial fibrillation.
   B. atrial flutter.
   C. sinus dysrhythmia.
   D. ventricular fibrillation.
   E. right bundle branch block.

_____ 89. The ECG that presents with a regular rhythm, no P waves, and a normal QRS duration at a rate of 50 is
   A. atrial fibrillation.
   B. accelerated idioventricular rhythm.
   C. supraventricular tachycardia.
   D. ventricular tachycardia.
   E. junctional escape rhythm.

_____ 90. A rhythm in which every third beat is a PVC is known as
   A. galloping.
   B. triplication.
   C. salvos.
   D. trigeminy.
   E. palpitation.

_____ 91. Which of the following antidysrhythmic agents is indicated in recurrent ventricular fibrillation and hemodynamically unstable ventricular tachycardia, and is contraindicated in cardiogenic shock and high-degree heart blocks?
   A. Adenosine
   B. Bretylium
   C. Amiodarone
   D. Verapamil
   E. Azithromycin

_____ 92. Which of the following antidysrhythmics is a calcium channel blocker?
   A. Adenosine
   B. Epinephrine
   C. Amiodarone
   D. Diltiazem
   E. Azithromycin

_____ 93. Which of the following is an adrenergic medication?
   A. Atropine
   B. Diltiazem
   C. Epinephrine
   D. Morphine sulfate
   E. Aztemizole

_____ 94. All of the following occur with beta-receptor stimulation, EXCEPT
   A. bronchodilation.
   B. negative dromotropic effects.
   C. positive chronotropic effects.
   D. positive inotropic effects.
   E. all occur with beta-receptor stimulation.

_____ 95. Scenario: You are managing a 100-kg semiconscious patient with a heart rate of 120, blood pressure of 80/40, and respirations of 12. He called EMS because of chest pain. Which of the following medications and dosages is correct for this patient?
   A. 4 mg of norepinephrine in 1,000 mL infused at 1 mL/min
   B. 4 mg of norepinephrine in 1,000 mL infused at 100 mL/hr
   C. 800 mg of dopamine in 500 mL of D_5W infused at 7.5 drop/min
   D. 800 mg of dopamine in 250 mL infused at 7.5 mL/hr
   E. 200 mg of amiodarone slow IV

_____ 96. Which of the following fibrinolytic agents is given over 2 minutes and repeated 30 minutes later?
   A. Activase
   B. Alteplase
   C. Aspirin
   D. Retavase
   E. Nubain

_____ 97. Which formula is used to calculate joules?
   A. Amperage (resistance × duration)
   B. Resistance × watts × time delivered
   C. Watts × amperage
   D. Watts × duration
   E. Resistance × watts

_____ **98.** Which of the following disorders is NOT cardiac related but may mimic the signs and symptoms of angina?
  A. Pneumonia   **D.** Costochondritis
  B. Dyspepsia   **E.** All of the above
  C. Pancreatitis

_____ **99.** Scenario: A patient is experiencing dyspnea, blood-tinged sputum, crackles (rales), and cyanosis. The most likely cause is
  A. cor pulmonale.   **D.** right ventricular failure.
  B. left ventricular failure. **E.** aneurysm.
  C. pulmonary embolism.

_____ **100.** Depriving the cardiac muscle of oxygen and other nutrients results in
  A. myocardial infarction.   **D.** subendocardial infarction.
  B. myocardial injury.   **E.** myocardial contractility.
  C. myocardial ischemia.

Chapter 3: Neurology

_____ **101.** The somatic nervous system primarily innervates
  A. cardiac muscle.   **D.** smooth muscle.
  B. glands.   **E.** the respiratory system.
  C. skeletal muscle.

_____ **102.** The _____ nervous system is mediated by epinephrine and norepinephrine.
  A. afferent   **D.** sympathetic
  B. parasympathetic   **E.** central
  C. somatic

_____ **103.** Acetylcholine is the neurotransmitter of which nervous system?
  A. Adrenergic   **D.** Sympathetic
  B. Afferent   **E.** Central
  C. Parasympathetic

_____ **104.** The space between the pia mater and the arachnoid membrane is the
  A. epiarachnoid space.   **D.** subdural space.
  B. epidural space.   **E.** cerebral space.
  C. subarachnoid space.

_____ **105.** The portion of the brain that connects the two hemispheres of the cerebrum is the
  A. cerebellum.   **D.** midbrain.
  B. cerebral cortex.   **E.** diencephalon.
  C. corpus callosum.

_____ **106.** The area of the brain responsible for emotions, hormone production, and autonomic functions is the
  A. hypothalamus.   **D.** thalamus.
  B. pituitary gland.   **E.** medulla oblongata.
  C. pons.

_____ **107.** The area of the brain that relays sensory information to the cerebellum and controls involuntary somatic and visceral functions is the
  A. cerebrum.   **D.** pons.
  B. midbrain.   **E.** medulla oblongata.
  C. pituitary gland.

_____108. The portion of the brain that regulates cardiovascular, respiratory, and digestive system activities is the
   A. cerebellum.
   B. hypothalamus.
   C. pons.
   D. thalamus.
   E. medulla oblongata.

_____109. The _____ lobe of the brain is responsible for speech.
   A. frontal
   B. occipital
   C. parietal
   D. temporal
   E. semiparietal

_____110. The _____ system is responsible for consciousness and stimuli response.
   A. carotid
   B. limbic
   C. vertebrobasilar
   D. reticular activating
   E. cephalic

_____111. Which efferent fibers carry impulses to the skeletal muscles?
   A. Somatic motor
   B. Somatic sensory
   C. Visceral motor
   D. Visceral sensory
   E. Visceral lymphatic

_____112. Which cranial nerve controls movement of the tongue?
   A. I
   B. III
   C. VI
   D. X
   E. XII

_____113. Which afferent cranial nerve is responsible for equilibrium?
   A. II
   B. IV
   C. VI
   D. VIII
   E. IX

_____114. If the patient is able to smile, frown, and wrinkle his forehead muscles, which cranial nerve is intact?
   A. I
   B. V
   C. VII
   D. XI
   E. XII

_____115. The first "I" in AEIOU-TIPS means
   A. infarction.
   B. impairment.
   C. insulin.
   D. infection.
   E. irritability.

_____116. A condition characterized by loss of memory and disorientation that is associated with chronic alcohol intake and a diet deficient in thiamine is
   A. Korsakoff's psychosis.
   B. Wernicke's syndrome.
   C. Lein's psychosis.
   D. Esselstyne's syndrome.
   E. Makynen seizure.

_____117. The type of stroke caused by a ruptured cerebral artery is
   A. occlusive.
   B. embolic.
   C. thrombotic.
   D. hemorrhagic.
   E. aneural.

_____118. The phase of a seizure in which a patient experiences alternating contraction and relaxation of the muscles is
   A. tonic.
   B. clonic.
   C. aural.
   D. hypertonic.
   E. postictal.

©2013 Pearson Education, Inc.
Paramedic Care: Principles & Practice, Vol. 4, 4th Ed.

_____119. All of the following are characteristics of a complex partial seizure, EXCEPT
  A. auditory hallucinations.
  B. a sense of déjà vu.
  C. localized tonic-clonic movement of one extremity.
  D. unusual odors.
  E. strange tastes.

_____120. A disease that is chronic and is characterized by progressive motor disorder with tremor, rigidity, bradykinesia, and postural instability is
  A. Alzheimer's.   D. Lou Gehrig's.
  B. Reed-Sternberg's.   E. Bell's palsy.
  C. Parkinson's.

Chapter 4: Endocrinology

_____121. An _____ gland secretes chemical substances to nearby tissues through a duct.
  A. endocrine   D. exocyte
  B. endocyte   E. exophyll
  C. exocrine

_____122. The tendency of the body to keep the internal environment and metabolism steady and normal is
  A. homeostasis.   D. steady state.
  B. glucogenesis.   E. culdocentesis.
  C. metabolism.

_____123. All of the following are endocrine glands, EXCEPT the
  A. adrenal.   D. salivary.
  B. hypothalamus.   E. gonads.
  C. pineal.

_____124. The posterior pituitary responds to nerve impulses from the
  A. hypothalamus.   D. thyroid.
  B. pancreas.   E. salivary.
  C. thalamus.

_____125. Which of the following is a major hormone effect of the hypothalamus?
  A. Stimulates the increased reabsorption of water
  B. Stimulates production and release of milk
  C. Stimulates the release of thyroid-stimulating hormone
  D. Stimulates vasoconstriction
  E. Stimulates blood cell production

_____126. Which endocrine gland's target tissues are muscle, the liver, and the cardiovascular system?
  A. Adrenal cortex   D. Pineal gland
  B. Adrenal medulla   E. Parathyroid
  C. Ovaries

_____127. All of the following are androgenic hormones, EXCEPT
  A. epinephrine.   D. testosterone.
  B. estrogen.   E. None of the above are androgenic
  C. progesterone.   hormones.

_____128. The endocrine gland that is located in the neck on either side and anterior-inferior of the laryngeal cartilage at the level of the cricoid cartilage is the
  A. adrenal gland.   D. thyroid gland.
  B. pituitary gland.   E. thymus gland.
  C. thalamus gland.

____129. The area of the pancreas that is considered endocrine tissue is the
  A. adrenal cortex.
  B. islets of Langerhans.
  C. Langerhans medulla.
  D. pancreatic medulla.
  E. bundle of His.

____130. The hormone _____ is responsible for increasing blood glucose.
  A. epinephrine
  B. glucagon
  C. glycogen
  D. insulin
  E. prolactin

____131. The conversion of protein and fat to form glucose is
  A. glucogenolysis.
  B. gluconeogenesis.
  C. glycogenolysis.
  D. glyconeogenesis.
  E. glucogenesis.

____132. The hormone _____ is secreted from delta cells in the pancreas and inhibits the secretion of glucagon and insulin.
  A. epinephrine
  B. glycogen
  C. insulinlytic
  D. melatonin
  E. somatostatin

____133. The disease marked by inadequate insulin activity in the body is
  A. "thyroid storm."
  B. myxedema.
  C. diabetes mellitus.
  D. thyrotoxicosis.
  E. nephritis.

____134. The normal blood glucose level is
  A. 60 to 100 mg/dL.
  B. 70 to 120 mg/dL.
  C. 80 to 140 mg/dL.
  D. 90 to 160 mg/dL.
  E. 100 to 180 mg/dL.

____135. Scenario: A diabetic patient presents with excessive urination. This condition is best attributed to
  A. decreased insulin.
  B. decreased serum glucose.
  C. elevated serum glucose.
  D. elevated insulin.
  E. elevated thymosin.

____136. The process of excessive urination in the diabetic patient is known as
  A. anabolism.
  B. glycosuria.
  C. ketosis.
  D. anuria.
  E. polyuria.

____137. Which of the following is a sign or symptom of a patient experiencing diabetic ketoacidosis?
  A. Acetone breath odor
  B. Apathy
  C. Diplopia
  D. Drooling
  E. Diaphoresis

____138. Kussmaul's respirations are seen in which of the following conditions?
  A. Diabetic ketoacidosis
  B. Hyperglycemic hyperosmolar nonketotic coma
  C. Hypoglycemia
  D. Insulin shock
  E. Thyrotoxicosis

____139. This disorder's signs and symptoms include prominent weight gain in the trunk, face, and neck, with accumulation of fat on the upper back and easily bruised, translucent skin.
  A. Addison's disease
  B. Cushing's syndrome
  C. Graves' disease
  D. Myxedema
  E. "Thyroid storm"

©2013 Pearson Education, Inc.
Paramedic Care: Principles & Practice, Vol. 4, 4th Ed.

_____**140.** This disorder's signs and symptoms include progressive weakness, fatigue, decreased appetite, and weight loss.
   A. Addison's disease
   B. Cushing's syndrome
   C. Graves' disease
   D. Myxedema
   E. "Thyroid storm"

Chapter 5: Immunology

_____**141.** _____ is another name for a disease-producing agent or invading substance.
   A. Antigen
   B. Antibody
   C. Pathogen
   D. Toxin
   E. Endotoxin

_____**142.** The immune response in which the body's immunoglobulins (Igs) attack pathogens is
   A. cellular immunity.
   B. humoral immunity.
   C. primary response.
   D. secondary response.
   E. tertiary response.

_____**143.** Place in order the sequence for a humoral response to an invading pathogen or antigen.

   1. secondary response
   2. release of IgG and IgM
   3. development of specific antibodies
   4. acquired immunity

   A. 1, 4, 3, 2
   B. 2, 1, 3, 4
   C. 3, 2, 4, 1
   D. 4, 2, 3, 1
   E. 1, 3, 2, 4

_____**144.** A young child is vaccinated against chickenpox. This type of immunity is known as
   A. acquired immunity.
   B. induced active immunity.
   C. natural immunity.
   D. passive immunity.
   E. induced immunity.

_____**145.** An unexpected and exaggerated reaction to a particular antigen is termed
   A. allergic reaction.
   B. anaphylaxis.
   C. hypersensitivity.
   D. sensitization.
   E. hyperallergenic crisis.

_____**146.** Scenario: Upon returning home after hiking in the woods for three days, Bill discovers he has a rash on both of his forearms. This is an example of
   A. anaphylaxis.
   B. repressed hypersensitivity.
   C. immediate hypersensitivity.
   D. sensitization.
   E. delayed hypersensitivity.

_____**147.** This substance is released when an allergen binds to IgE attached to basophils and mast cells.
   A. Dopamine
   B. Epinephrine
   C. Histamine
   D. Norepinephrine
   E. Pheromone

_____**148.** Which of the following occurs with the release of histamine during an allergic reaction?
   A. Bronchodilation
   B. Increased intestinal motility
   C. Decreased vascular permeability
   D. Vasoconstriction
   E. Increased red blood cell production

149. All of the following insects are of the order *Hymenoptera*, EXCEPT
    A. fire ants.
    B. honeybees.
    C. scorpions.
    D. wasps.
    E. yellow jackets.

150. Which of the following do the H_2 receptors mediate when they are stimulated?
    A. Decreased secretion of gastric acids
    B. Bronchoconstriction
    C. Intestinal contraction
    D. Peripheral vasodilation
    E. Bronchodilation

151. Which principal body system is NOT affected during anaphylaxis?
    A. Auditory
    B. Cardiovascular
    C. Gastrointestinal
    D. Respiratory
    E. All are affected

152. All of the following findings are common in anaphylaxis, EXCEPT
    A. facial edema.
    B. laryngeal edema.
    C. neck edema.
    D. pedal edema.
    E. pharyngeal edema.

153. Scenario: A patient is experiencing anaphylaxis. You might administer all of the following medications, EXCEPT
    A. diphenhydramine.
    B. epinephrine.
    C. furosemide.
    D. Solu-Medrol.
    E. Benadryl.

154. Which of the following antihistamine medications is the most potent for reducing symptoms due to excessive histamine release?
    A. Atarax
    B. Diphenhydramine
    C. Promethazine
    D. Vistaril
    E. Cromolyn sodium

155. For allergic reaction, the recommended concentration of subcutaneous epinephrine is
    A. 1:100.
    B. 1:1,000.
    C. 1:10,000.
    D. 1:100,000.
    E. none of the above.

Chapter 6: Gastroenterology

156. Dull and poorly localized pain that originates in the walls of hollow organs is
    A. parietal pain.
    B. referred pain.
    C. somatic pain.
    D. visceral pain.
    E. parenteral pain.

157. All of the following mechanisms are known to cause pain, EXCEPT
    A. distention.
    B. inspiration.
    C. inflammation.
    D. ischemia.
    E. All of the above cause pain.

158. Inflammation of the peritoneum is
    A. peritoneal abscess.
    B. peritonism.
    C. peritonitis.
    D. peritonomy.
    E. periocentesis.

159. The acronym OPQRST-ASPN is useful when evaluating the history of a patient complaining of abdominal pain. The "T" stands for
    A. temporary.
    B. time.
    C. transient.
    D. Trendelenburg.
    E. trending.

©2013 Pearson Education, Inc.
Paramedic Care: Principles & Practice, Vol. 4, 4th Ed.

_____ **160.** The terms _dull, sharp, constant,_ and _intermittent_ are used in which of the following components of history gathering?

    A. Associated symptoms   **D.** Region

    B. Palliation   **E.** Severity

    C. Quality

_____ **161.** Scenario: A 16-year-old male patient was thrown from a vehicle during a motor vehicle accident. He has Grey Turner's sign, which indicates

    A. abdominal fluid loss internally.   **D.** renal calculi.

    B. colon impaction.   **E.** esophageal tearing.

    C. diaphragmatic rupture.

_____ **162.** Which of the following organs is a component of the lower GI tract?

    A. Colon   **D.** Stomach

    B. Duodenum   **E.** Mouth

    C. Esophagus

_____ **163.** One reason for the high mortality rate associated with upper GI bleeding is

    A. a change in eating habits from red meat to vegetables.

    B. an active lifestyle—jogging and aerobic exercise, for example.

    C. patients treating themselves with over-the-counter remedies.

    D. middle-aged patients developing GI distress.

    E. lack of exercise.

_____ **164.** Irritation or erosion of the lining of this organ accounts for more than 75 percent of upper GI hemorrhage.

    A. Colon   **D.** Stomach

    B. Duodenum   **E.** Esophagus

    C. Ileum

_____ **165.** Mallory-Weiss syndrome is caused by

    A. colon cancer.   **D.** stomach ulcers.

    B. ischemia.   **E.** esophageal laceration.

    C. pancreatitis.

_____ **166.** Vomiting bright red blood is known as

    A. hematochezia.   **D.** melenin.

    B. hematemesis.   **E.** epistaxis.

    C. melena.

_____ **167.** Melena, which is dark, tarry, and foul-smelling stool, indicates partially digested

    A. bile.   **D.** protein.

    B. blood.   **E.** carbohydrates.

    C. fat.

_____ **168.** Which of the following medications can break down mucosal surfaces of the stomach and GI tract?

    A. Aspirin   **D.** Valium

    B. Erythromycin   **E.** Promethazine

    C. Lasix

_____ **169.** How many liters of fluid normally move through the GI tract in 24 hours?

    A. 2 to 5   **D.** 7 to 9

    B. 3 to 6   **E.** 10 to 12

    C. 4 to 8

_____170. Scenario: A 16-month-old female has experienced nausea and diarrhea for two days. She appears pale and clammy. Which of the following signs or symptoms would you also expect?
  A. Bradycardia
  B. Bradypnea
  C. Hypotension
  D. Hypothermia
  E. Hypertension

_____171. A blocked pancreatic duct can result in duodenal ulcers. This is because the pancreas secretes _____, which neutralizes chyme.
  A. bicarbonate ions
  B. glucagon
  C. glycol
  D. insulin
  E. oxytocin

_____172. Chronic and nonexsanguinating hematochezia is due to bleeding in the
  A. kidneys.
  B. lower GI tract.
  C. pancreas.
  D. upper GI tract.
  E. stomach.

_____173. The pathogenesis of appendicitis is best attributed to
  A. distal colitis.
  B. diverticulosis.
  C. obstruction of the appendiceal lumen by fecal material.
  D. proximal intestinal volvulus.
  E. inflamed varices.

_____174. Early appendicitis usually presents with nausea, vomiting, a low-grade fever, and
  A. Murphy's sign.
  B. Cullen's sign.
  C. Kerr's sign.
  D. periumbilical pain.
  E. Battle's sign.

_____175. Pain associated with appendicitis is usually located in the _____ quadrant.
  A. left lower
  B. left upper
  C. right lower
  D. right upper
  E. all of the above

_____176. The cause of cholecystitis is calculi lodged in the
  A. islets of Langerhans.
  B. duodenum.
  C. sphincter of Oddi.
  D. pancreatic duct.
  E. common bile duct.

_____177. Pain associated with cholecystitis is often acute and located in the _____ abdominal quadrant.
  A. left lower
  B. left upper
  C. right lower
  D. right upper
  E. all of the above

_____178. All of the following are categories of causation of pancreatitis, EXCEPT
  A. systemic.
  B. infectious.
  C. mechanical.
  D. metabolic.
  E. vascular.

_____179. Which of the following is known as infectious hepatitis?
  A. HAV
  B. HBV
  C. HCV
  D. HDV
  E. HEV

_____180. Which of the following pathogens is spread by the oral–fecal route?
  A. HAV
  B. HBV
  C. HCV
  D. HDV
  E. HEV

©2013 Pearson Education, Inc.
Paramedic Care: Principles & Practice, Vol. 4, 4th Ed.

Chapter 7: Urology and Nephrology

____181. More than 250,000 Americans suffer from which disease?
   A. Colitis
   B. Prostatic hypertrophy
   C. End-stage renal failure
   D. Pancreatitis

____182. The group of organs that is responsible for maintaining fluid and electrolyte balance for the body is the
   A. cardiovascular system.
   B. gastrointestinal system.
   C. integumentary system.
   D. urinary system.
   E. vascular system.

____183. A primary compound secreted in urine is
   A. bile.
   B. chyme.
   C. glucose.
   D. urea.
   E. sebum.

____184. A common acute disorder of the urinary system that affects over 500,000 Americans is
   A. dialysis.
   B. osmotic diuresis.
   C. prostatitis.
   D. renal calculi.
   E. prostatic hypertrophy.

____185. The urinary system is comprised of the kidneys, ureters, urinary bladder, and the
   A. bulbourethral glands.
   B. ovaries.
   C. prostate.
   D. urethra.
   E. fallopian tubes.

____186. The inner tissue of the kidney is the
   A. glomerulus.
   B. hilum.
   C. medulla.
   D. papilla.
   E. nephron.

____187. Which of the following processes is (are) involved in urine formation?
   A. Glomerular assemblage
   B. Reabsorption
   C. Retention
   D. Diaphoresis
   E. All of the above

____188. As blood passes through the glomerular capillaries, water and chemical materials are filtered out of the blood and into the
   A. Bowman's capsule.
   B. collecting duct.
   C. loop of Henle.
   D. pyramidal tracts.
   E. bundle of His.

____189. The random movement of molecules from an area of high concentration to an area of lower concentration is
   A. active transport.
   B. facilitated diffusion.
   C. osmosis.
   D. simple diffusion.
   E. facilitated osmosis.

____190. A solution whose concentration is higher than that of a second substance is
   A. hyperosmolar.
   B. hypoosmolar.
   C. isotonic.
   D. ultraosmolar.
   E. none of the above.

_____191. The movement of a molecule through a cell from an area of lower concentration to an area of higher concentration that requires cellular energy is
  A. facilitated osmosis.
  B. diuresis.
  C. facilitated diffusion.
  D. osmosis.
  E. active transport.

_____192. The dominant cation in intracellular fluid is
  A. Cl^-.
  B. H^+.
  C. K^+.
  D. Na^+.
  E. Fe^+.

_____193. The release of antidiuretic hormone results in
  A. decreased reabsorption of Cl^-.
  B. increased reabsorption of Na^+.
  C. increased reabsorption of water.
  D. increased secretion of H^+.
  E. none of the above.

_____194. A waste product of metabolism within muscle cells is
  A. creatinine.
  B. myoglobin.
  C. plasminogen.
  D. troponin.
  E. plasmin.

_____195. Angiotensin II is produced by the interaction of angiotensin-converting enzyme and angiotensin I. Angiotensin II results in
  A. decreased secretion of aldosterone from adrenal cells.
  B. hypotension.
  C. increased arterial blood pressure.
  D. release of epinephrine.
  E. decreased arterial blood pressure.

_____196. The duct that carries urine from the bladder to the exterior of the body is the
  A. collecting duct.
  B. Henle duct.
  C. ureter.
  D. urethra.
  E. anus.

_____197. The kidneys are protected relatively well against injury, due to their location in the
  A. chest cavity.
  B. RLQ.
  C. pelvic region.
  D. retroperitoneal space.
  E. LLQ.

_____198. Pain arising in hollow organs such as the ureter and bladder is known as
  A. parietal pain.
  B. referred pain.
  C. somatic pain.
  D. visceral pain.
  E. parenteral pain.

_____199. Pain that occurs when afferent nerve fibers carrying the pain message merge with other pain-carrying fibers at the junction with the spinal cord is
  A. parietal pain.
  B. referred pain.
  C. somatic pain.
  D. visceral pain.
  E. parenteral pain.

_____200. Lloyd's sign, which is an indication of pyelonephritis, is associated with
  A. pain on percussion of the costovertebral angle.
  B. pain on palpation of the anterior costal margin.
  C. periumbilical tenderness.
  D. rebound pain at the level of the umbilicus.
  E. pain on inhalation.

_____ **201.** Hyperkalemia is identified on the ECG by a(n)
- **A.** decrease in QRS duration.
- **B.** depression of the ST segment.
- **C.** erratic U wave.
- **D.** increase in P-R interval.
- **E.** elevation of the T wave.

_____ **202.** Reduced nephron mass can cause all of the following, EXCEPT
- **A.** chronic anemia.
- **B.** hyperkalemia.
- **C.** hyponatremia.
- **D.** loss of glucose.
- **E.** isosthenuria.

_____ **203.** All of the following may be complications related to hemodialysis or peritoneal dialysis, EXCEPT
- **A.** chest pain.
- **B.** dyspnea.
- **C.** hypertension.
- **D.** seizure.
- **E.** infection.

_____ **204.** Which of the following types of renal calculi is found more often in women than in men?
- **A.** Calcium stones
- **B.** Cystine stones
- **C.** Struvite stones
- **D.** Uric acid stones
- **E.** Oxalate stones

_____ **205.** The pathophysiology of urinary tract infections is due primarily to
- **A.** bacterial infections.
- **B.** decreases in sexual intercourse.
- **C.** sexually transmitted disease infections.
- **D.** urinary tract lesions.
- **E.** viral infections.

Chapter 8: Toxicology and Substance Abuse

_____ **206.** The MOST common portal of entry for toxic exposure is
- **A.** absorption.
- **B.** ingestion.
- **C.** inhalation.
- **D.** injection.
- **E.** osmosis.

_____ **207.** For which of the following ingested substances is flumazenil an antidote?
- **A.** Arsenic
- **B.** Benzodiazepines
- **C.** Cyanide
- **D.** Ethylene glycol
- **E.** Methyl alcohol

_____ **208.** All of the following are respiratory signs or symptoms of a toxic inhalation exposure, EXCEPT
- **A.** bradycardia.
- **B.** chest tightness.
- **C.** cough.
- **D.** tachypnea.
- **E.** dyspnea.

_____ **209.** All of the following are signs or symptoms of cyanide toxicity, EXCEPT
- **A.** burning sensation in mouth.
- **B.** confusion.
- **C.** early hypotension and bradycardia.
- **D.** pulmonary edema.
- **E.** tachycardia.

_____ **210.** All of the following are signs or symptoms of carbon monoxide poisoning, EXCEPT
- **A.** arousal.
- **B.** headache.
- **C.** nausea.
- **D.** tachypnea.
- **E.** confusion.

_____ 211. Scenario: A patient has spilled a large quantity of an unknown acid on his skin. Treatment should consist of:
   A. contacting poison control for instructions.
   B. covering the area with activated charcoal.
   C. diluting the acid with bicarbonate.
   D. irrigation with copious amounts of water.
   E. irrigation with copious amounts of milk.

_____ 212. Ingestion of alkalis usually results in
   A. immediate and intense pain.
   B. bradycardia.
   C. local burns to the mouth and throat.
   D. ulceration and perforation of the stomach lining.
   E. liquefaction necrosis.

_____ 213. All of the following procedures are appropriate for hydrofluoric acid exposure, EXCEPT
   A. immersing the injured part in iced water with sodium bicarbonate.
   B. irrigating the affected area with copious amounts of water.
   C. protecting rescue personnel from exposure.
   D. removing exposed clothing.
   E. initiating supportive measures.

_____ 214. All of the following are hydrocarbons, EXCEPT
   A. turpentine.   D. naphtha.
   B. benzene.   E. ammonia.
   C. kerosene.

_____ 215. All of the following are tricyclic antidepressant medications, EXCEPT
   A. doxepin.   D. Zoloft.
   B. Elavil.   E. imipramine.
   C. nortriptyline.

_____ 216. Scenario: A patient has attempted suicide by overdosing on amitriptyline and alcohol. You might expect all of the following signs or symptoms, EXCEPT
   A. hypertension.   D. widened QRS complex.
   B. respiratory depression.   E. hallucinations.
   C. tachycardia.

_____ 217. Which of the following medications can be useful in tricyclic antidepressant overdoses?
   A. Activated charcoal   D. Sodium bicarbonate
   B. Atropine   E. Dextrose
   C. Flumazenil

_____ 218. Monoamine oxidase inhibitors (MAOIs) function by
   A. increasing the availability of norepinephrine and dopamine.
   B. increasing the release of serotonin.
   C. inhibiting the breakdown of norepinephrine and dopamine.
   D. inhibiting the release of serotonin.
   E. releasing endorphins.

_____ 219. All of the following medications are selective serotonin reuptake inhibitors, EXCEPT
   A. Elavil.   D. Zoloft.
   B. Luvox.   E. Paxil.
   C. Prozac.

_____ 220. Signs of lithium toxicity include
   A. hyperactivity.   D. tachycardia.
   B. moist mucous membranes.   E. constipation.
   C. muscle twitching.

©2013 Pearson Education, Inc.
Paramedic Care: Principles & Practice, Vol. 4, 4th Ed.

_____221. An overdose of aspirin at greater than 300 mg/kg results in
- **A.** metabolic acidosis.
- **B.** metabolic alkalosis.
- **C.** respiratory acidosis.
- **D.** respiratory alkalosis.
- **E.** respiratory arrest.

_____222. All of the following are expected signs or symptoms of a salicylate overdose, EXCEPT
- **A.** abdominal pain.
- **B.** cardiac dysrhythmia.
- **C.** hypothermia.
- **D.** pulmonary edema.
- **E.** confusion.

_____223. An overdose of Tylenol at which level is considered toxic?
- **A.** 100 mg/kg
- **B.** 150 mg/kg
- **C.** 200 mg/kg
- **D.** 300 mg/kg
- **E.** 350 mg/kg

_____224. Scenario: A patient has accidentally overdosed on his theophylline medication. He is experiencing PVCs, palpitations, and nausea and vomiting. Which of the following medications can be used to manage the theophylline overdose?
- **A.** Activated charcoal
- **B.** Lidocaine
- **C.** Morphine
- **D.** Phenergan
- **E.** Digoxin

_____225. Chronic ingestion of and exposure to which of the following metals can result in memory disturbances, abdominal pain, confusion, agitation, and tremors?
- **A.** Copper
- **B.** Iron
- **C.** Lead
- **D.** Magnesium
- **E.** Aluminum

_____226. Exposure to contaminated food that has this bacteria, which is the world's most toxic poison, results in respiratory distress or arrest.
- **A.** *Clostridium botulinum*
- **B.** *E. coli*
- **C.** *Salmonella*
- **D.** *Shigella*
- **E.** *Scombroid*

_____227. The pathophysiology of an anaphylactic reaction resulting from a *Hymenoptera* sting involves
- **A.** decreased release of adrenergics.
- **B.** decreased release of endorphins in the body.
- **C.** excessive release of catecholamines.
- **D.** increased production of beta blockers.
- **E.** excessive release of histamine.

_____228. Scenario: Your patient has been bitten by a rattlesnake. He is tachypneic, is nauseated, has vomited once, and has weakness in his extremities. You would also expect all of the following, EXCEPT
- **A.** altered mental status.
- **B.** dyspnea.
- **C.** hypertension.
- **D.** localized pain.
- **E.** thirst.

_____229. Routine emergency care of a pit viper bite includes which of the following?
- **A.** Applying ice to the bite site
- **B.** Encouraging the patient to walk to reduce the concentration of the venom
- **C.** Immobilizing the limb with a splint
- **D.** Using a constricting band to reduce venous circulation
- **E.** Applying a mild electrical shock to reverse the spread of venom

_____230. The condition that occurs when a patient's body reacts severely when deprived of an abused substance is
- **A.** addiction.
- **B.** habituation.
- **C.** tolerance.
- **D.** delirium.
- **E.** withdrawal.

____231. Alcohol is a(n)
    A. depressant.   D. stimulant.
    B. narcotic.   E. oxidant.
    C. opiate.

____232. All of the following are signs of someone who has taken too much Phenobarbital, EXCEPT
    A. coma.   D. respiratory depression.
    B. hypertension.   E. bradycardia.
    C. lethargy.

____233. Scenario: A patient is extremely anxious and complaining of euphoria and a very dry mouth. Your assessment reveals only dilated pupils. The patient states that he smoked "grass" tonight with his friends and this was his first time. Management of this patient should consist of
    A. gentle reassurance.   D. Valium 5 mg.
    B. IV therapy.   E. Decadron.
    C. Phenergan 12.5 mg.

____234. Signs and symptoms associated with amphetamine usage include all of the following, EXCEPT
    A. constricted pupils.   D. psychosis.
    B. exhilaration.   E. tremors.
    C. hypertension.

____235. Which of the following is NOT a sign or symptom of a Xanax overdose?
    A. Altered mental status   D. Respiratory depression
    B. Slurred speech   E. Tachycardia
    C. Hypotension

Chapter 9: Hematology

____236. All of the following organs are part of the hematopoietic system, EXCEPT the
    A. heart.   D. spleen.
    B. kidneys.   E. bone marrow.
    C. liver.

____237. A 75-kg person has approximately how many liters of blood?
    A. 5   D. 8
    B. 6   E. 9
    C. 7

____238. The hormone responsible for red blood cell production is
    A. aldosterone.   D. renin.
    B. cytokine.   E. erythropoietin.
    C. calcitonin.

____239. The phenomenon in which a decrease in PCO_2/acidity causes an increase in the quantity of oxygen that binds with hemoglobin and in which an increase in PCO_2/acidity causes hemoglobin to release oxygen is known as
    A. the Bohr effect.   D. the Frank-Starling law.
    B. Boyle's law.   E. the Clauser principle.
    C. the Fick principle.

____240. Which of the following will REDUCE hemoglobin's affinity for oxygen?
    A. A decrease in 2,3-diphosphoglycerate (2,3-DPG)
    B. Decreased exercise
    C. Increased erythrocyte production
    D. Pyrexia
    E. Mild hypothermia

©2013 Pearson Education, Inc.
Paramedic Care: Principles & Practice, Vol. 4, 4th Ed.

____241. Erythropoietin is secreted when these cells sense hypoxia.
  A. Heart
  B. Liver
  C. Kidney
  D. Spleen
  E. Bone marrow

____242. Hemoglobin is usually expressed as the number of grams per deciliter of whole blood. The normal concentration for men is
  A. 10.5 to 14.0 g/dL.
  B. 12.0 to 15.0 g/dL.
  C. 13.5 to 17.0 g/dL.
  D. 15.0 to 20.0 g/dL.
  E. 20.0 to 22.0 g/dL.

____243. White blood cells originate from which hematopoietic component?
  A. Bone marrow
  B. Kidney
  C. Liver
  D. Spleen
  E. All of the above

____244. All of the following are functions of monocytes, EXCEPT
  A. attacking tumor cells.
  B. repairing tissue.
  C. removing foreign matter.
  D. stimulating the release of cytokine.
  E. secreting growth factors.

____245. Which type of granulocytes mediates an acute allergic response by inactivating chemical mediators?
  A. Basophils
  B. Eosinophils
  C. Neutrophils
  D. Phagocytes
  E. Monocytes

____246. Which white blood cell contains antigen-specific surface receptor sites that can initiate an immune response?
  A. Basophil
  B. Lymphocyte
  C. Eosinophil
  D. Neutrophil
  E. Monocyte

____247. Cellular immunity is mediated through which type of lymphocyte?
  A. A cell
  B. B cell
  C. M cell
  D. T cell
  E. I cell

____248. The normal number of platelets ranges from
  A. 90,000 to 120,000/mcL.
  B. 120,000 to 250,000/mcL.
  C. 150,000 to 450,000/mcL.
  D. 250,000 to 550,000/mcL.
  E. 300,000 to 600,000/mcL.

____249. The primary cell from which thrombocytes are formed is the
  A. lymphocyte.
  B. megakaryocyte.
  C. neutrophil.
  D. thombophil.
  E. leukocyte.

____250. The process of breaking down or dismantling a clot is known as
  A. delamination.
  B. platelet degradation.
  C. prothrombinlysis.
  D. thrombolysis.
  E. fibrinolysis.

____251. The rarest blood type in the United States is
  A. A.
  B. AB.
  C. B.
  D. O.
  E. none of the above.

252. The universal donor blood type is
   A. A.
   B. AB.
   C. B.
   D. O.
   E. none of the above.

253. Lymphatic signs associated with hematological disorders include
   A. enlarged lymph nodes.
   B. hematuria.
   C. petechiae.
   D. shrunken spleen.
   E. jaundice.

254. Which disease may result in slower blood clotting?
   A. AIDS
   B. Cholecystitis
   C. Cirrhosis
   D. Pancreatitis
   E. Malaria

255. Patients who have sickle cell disease typically have complete infarction of the
   A. heart.
   B. liver.
   C. pancreas.
   D. spleen.
   E. gallbladder.

256. The condition in which patients with hemophilia develop swollen, discolored, and painful joints with minimal trauma is
   A. leukotaxis.
   B. dysthralgia.
   C. ecchymotic arthralgia.
   D. hemarthrosis.
   E. arthralgia.

257. A deficiency of _____ is linked to anemia.
   A. calcium
   B. copper
   C. iron
   D. potassium
   E. magnesium

258. Hemophilia is acquired through
   A. defective genetic code.
   B. excessive NSAIDs dosing.
   C. transfusion reaction.
   D. viral infection.
   E. bacterial infection.

259. Patients with hemophilia A are deficient in blood clotting factor
   A. VII.
   B. VIII.
   C. IX.
   D. X.
   E. XII.

260. The disease referred to as consumption coagulation is often caused by any of the following, EXCEPT
   A. hemolytic transfusion reactions.
   B. hypertension.
   C. obstetrical complications.
   D. sepsis.
   E. hypotension.

Chapter 10: Infectious Diseases and Sepsis

261. The individual who first introduced an infectious agent to a population is referred to as the
   A. first incident.
   B. ground zero.
   C. index case.
   D. infectious deliverer.
   E. target case.

262. Which public health agency is responsible for setting standards and guidelines for workplace and worker safety?
   A. CDC
   B. DHHS
   C. FEMA
   D. OSHA
   E. NIHD

©2013 Pearson Education, Inc.
Paramedic Care: Principles & Practice, Vol. 4, 4th Ed.

_____ **263.** Toxic waste products that are produced by living bacteria are
   A. bacterotoxins.
   B. cytotoxins.
   C. endotoxins.
   D. exotoxins.
   E. pathotoxins.

_____ **264.** Which statement about viruses is correct?
   A. A host is susceptible to any particular virus during multiple encounters.
   B. Antibiotic therapy is the only means to treat viral infections.
   C. Viruses cannot be seen under the microscope.
   D. Viruses grow and reproduce only within a host cell.
   E. Viruses are larger than bacteria.

_____ **265.** Which type of organism is yeast?
   A. Bacteria
   B. Fungus
   C. Protozoa
   D. Virus
   E. Endotoxin

_____ **266.** Which of the following diseases is transmitted through an airborne route?
   A. Gonorrhea
   B. Hepatitis B
   C. Lyme disease
   D. Measles
   E. Trichinosis

_____ **267.** _____ is the presence of an agent (pathogen) only on the surface of the host without actual infection.
   A. Communication
   B. Symbiosis
   C. Infection
   D. Virulence
   E. Contamination

_____ **268.** All of the following are factors in disease transmission, EXCEPT
   A. host resistance.
   B. length of exposure.
   C. mode of entry.
   D. virulence.
   E. number of organisms transmitted.

_____ **269.** The time between a host's exposure to an infectious agent and the appearance of symptoms is the
   A. communicable period.
   B. disease period.
   C. incubation period.
   D. latent period.
   E. growth period.

_____ **270.** The marker on the surface of a cell that identifies it as self or nonself is an
   A. antibody.
   B. anticell.
   C. antigen.
   D. antiprion.
   E. antiphon.

_____ **271.** The immunoglobulin that remembers an antigen and recognizes any repeated invasions is
   A. IgA.
   B. IgE.
   C. IgG.
   D. IgM.
   E. IgD.

_____ **272.** The cells in the lymph system that attach to and destroy particulate matter are
   A. killer T-cells.
   B. monocytes.
   C. neutrophils.
   D. reticuloendothelial cells.
   E. chemotactic cells.

_____ **273.** _____ immunity develops after birth as a result of a direct exposure to a pathogen.
   A. Acquired
   B. Age-related
   C. Humoral
   D. Passive
   E. Active

____ **274.** Intermediate-level disinfection is accomplished by using
   A. 1:100 water and bleach solution.   **D.** soap and water.
   B. chemical sterilizing agents.   **E.** an autoclave.
   C. gas sterilization unit.

____ **275.** When should an infectious disease exposure be reported?
   A. At the end of the shift   **D.** Within 24 hours
   B. By the beginning of the next shift   **E.** Within 72 hours
   C. Immediately

____ **276.** Clinical presentation of an HIV-infected person includes all of the following signs or symptoms, EXCEPT
   A. reduced lymph nodes.
   B. general fatigue, fever, lymphadenopathy, and weight loss.
   C. *Pneumocystis carinii* pneumonia.
   D. purplish skin lesions.
   E. enlarged spleen.

____ **277.** Which of the following medications is recommended as part of the triple therapy following HIV exposure?
   A. TCP   **D.** IDG
   B. AZT   **E.** MVC
   C. HBV

____ **278.** The mode of transmission of hepatitis A is
   A. contact with fecal matter to mucous membranes or nonintact skin.
   B. direct blood contact.
   C. saliva.
   D. vaginal secretions.
   E. through the air.

____ **279.** For which of the following diseases is the health care worker at the GREATEST risk of exposure?
   A. Hepatitis B   **D.** Tuberculosis
   B. HIV   **E.** Pneumonia
   C. Meningitis

____ **280.** Hepatitis C is transmitted primarily through
   A. blood transfusions.   **D.** IV drug abuse.
   B. the fecal–oral route.   **E.** contaminated food.
   C. household contact.

____ **281.** The mode of transmission for tuberculosis is
   A. bloodborne.   **D.** respiratory.
   B. cutaneous contact.   **E.** gastrointestinal.
   C. fecal–oral.

____ **282.** Which of the following precautions BEST reduces the emergency responder's risk of tuberculosis exposure?
   A. Administering oxygen via a nasal cannula
   B. A NIOSH-approved respirator
   C. Placing a mask over the patient's face
   D. Opening the ambulance's patient compartment windows
   E. Gloves and standard mask

____ **283.** All of the following significantly increase a patient's risk for developing pneumonia, EXCEPT
   A. a transplanted kidney.   **D.** a splenectomy.
   B. gastroenteritis.   **E.** diabetes mellitus.
   C. sickle cell disease.

_____ **284.** Which virus causes chickenpox?
- **A.** Herpes zoster
- **B.** Influenza zoster
- **C.** Streptococcus zoster
- **D.** Varicella zoster
- **E.** Klebsiella zoster

_____ **285.** A prophylactic postexposure medication for meningitis is
- **A.** Wymox.
- **B.** cyclosporin.
- **C.** erythromycin.
- **D.** Zithromax.
- **E.** Cipro.

_____ **286.** Which patient group is MOST susceptible to influenza?
- **A.** Teenagers
- **B.** Young adults
- **C.** Middle-aged adults
- **D.** The elderly
- **E.** Children

_____ **287.** The most life-threatening sequela of measles in children who are not immunized is
- **A.** encephalitis.
- **B.** eye damage.
- **C.** myocarditis.
- **D.** pneumonia.
- **E.** cardiovascular damage.

_____ **288.** The _____ phase of pertussis is characterized by a deep, high-pitched cough similar to a "whoop."
- **A.** catarrhal
- **B.** convalescent
- **C.** entry
- **D.** paroxysmal
- **E.** virulent

_____ **289.** The MOST common sign of herpes simplex virus type 1 infection is
- **A.** conjunctivitis.
- **B.** Epstein-Barr syndrome.
- **C.** herpetic whitlow.
- **D.** HSV labialis.
- **E.** a rash.

_____ **290.** All of the following are among the "four Ds" associated with epiglottitis, EXCEPT
- **A.** drooling.
- **B.** dyspepsia.
- **C.** dysphagia.
- **D.** dysphonia.
- **E.** distress.

_____ **291.** A viral illness in children characterized by inspiratory and expiratory stridor and seal-bark-like cough is
- **A.** croup.
- **B.** epiglottitis.
- **C.** pertussis.
- **D.** pharyngitis.
- **E.** variola.

_____ **292.** All of the following complications may result from gastroenteritis, EXCEPT
- **A.** dehydration.
- **B.** diarrhea and emesis.
- **C.** dysuria.
- **D.** electrolyte imbalance.
- **E.** hypovolemic shock.

_____ **293.** Urban rabies is transmitted through
- **A.** foxes.
- **B.** raccoons.
- **C.** skunks.
- **D.** unimmunized domestic dogs.
- **E.** rats.

_____ **294.** An acute bacterial infection of the central nervous system that presents with muscle rigidity near the injury site and pain and stiffness of the jaw muscles is
- **A.** meningitis.
- **B.** mumps.
- **C.** rickettsia.
- **D.** tetanus.
- **E.** variola.

_____ **295.** Gonorrhea presentation in men is characterized by
    A. impotence.
    B. priapism.
    C. purulent urethral discharge.
    D. scrotum enlargement.
    E. facial sores.

_____ **296.** The stage of syphilis that is known as the "great imitator" may result in all of the following, EXCEPT
    A. aortic aneurysms.
    B. deep lesions with sharp borders on skin and bones.
    C. increased sensation of pain and temperature.
    D. progressive dementia.
    E. enlargement of the lymph nodes.

_____ **297.** All of the following are transmission routes for chlamydia, EXCEPT
    A. hand-to-hand transfer of eye secretions.
    B. oral intercourse.
    C. sexual intercourse.
    D. respiratory route.
    E. use of infected linens.

_____ **298.** A parasitic infection of the skin, scalp, trunk, or pubic area is
    A. impetigo.
    B. lice.
    C. psoriasis.
    D. scabies.
    E. roundworm.

_____ **299.** Infection of the skin by _staphylococci_ or _streptococci_ is
    A. impetigo.
    B. lice.
    C. psoriasis.
    D. scabies.
    E. roundworm.

_____ **300.** Infections acquired while in the hospital are referred to as
    A. social.
    B. administrative.
    C. nosocomial.
    D. pathological.
    E. opportunistic.

Chapter 11: Psychiatric and Behavioral Disorders

_____ **301.** Normal behavior varies based on culture, ethnic group, and
    A. affective attitude.
    B. interpersonal characteristics.
    C. personal interpretation.
    D. religious beliefs.
    E. financial status.

_____ **302.** Psychological disorders can arise from interactions within society, including all of the following, EXCEPT
    A. economic problems.
    B. dysfunctional families.
    C. social isolation.
    D. witnessing the victimization of another.
    E. clashes of values.

_____ **303.** Psychosocial conditions are related to a patient's personality style and
    A. crisis management methods.
    B. personal values.
    C. social habits.
    D. socioeconomic status.
    E. use of drugs.

_____ **304.** A state of being unclear or unable to make a decision easily is
    A. affect.
    B. ambivalence.
    C. fear.
    D. posture.
    E. confusion.

©2013 Pearson Education, Inc.
Paramedic Care: Principles & Practice, Vol. 4, 4th Ed.

_____ **305.** A feeling of alarm and discontentment in the expectation of danger is
    A. anxiety.
    B. confusion.
    C. depression.
    D. fear.
    E. angst.

_____ **306.** A condition characterized by the rapid onset of widespread disorganized thought is
    A. delirium.
    B. delusions.
    C. dementia.
    D. dysphasia.
    E. dysfunction.

_____ **307.** All of the following conditions typically may cause dementia, EXCEPT
    A. Alzheimer's disease.
    B. Bell's palsy.
    C. head trauma.
    D. Parkinson's disease.
    E. AIDS.

_____ **308.** Impaired ability to recognize objects or stimuli despite intact sensory function is
    A. aphasia.
    B. delirium.
    C. flat affect.
    D. agnosia.
    E. catatonia.

_____ **309.** Scenario: You are called to the scene of a patient threatening suicide. The patient is preoccupied with a sense of persecution, her speech is very disorganized, and she's exhibiting peculiar movements. The best management for this condition is to
    A. tell the patient you hear the same voices that she hears.
    B. present a calm and reassuring demeanor.
    C. reinforce the patient's hallucinations.
    D. restrain the patient.
    E. ignore the patient's speech and just do your job.

_____ **310.** Scenario: A student is preparing to take an exam and suddenly begins to feel palpitations, sweating, shaking, and abdominal distress. These symptoms are BEST characterized as
    A. anxiety.
    B. panic attack.
    C. phobia.
    D. post-traumatic stress.
    E. delirium.

_____ **311.** Displaying hostility or rage to compensate for an underlying feeling of anxiety is
    A. depression.
    B. anger.
    C. paranoia.
    D. phobia.
    E. catatonia.

_____ **312.** A patient who is preoccupied with physical symptoms without physical cause most likely has _____ disorder.
    A. conversion
    B. pain
    C. body dysmorphic
    D. somatization
    E. affective

_____ **313.** In which of the following disorders does the patient avoid stress by separating from his core personality?
    A. Bipolar
    B. Dissociative
    C. Factitious
    D. Somatoform
    E. Affective

_____ **314.** Which of the following disorders is a dissociative disorder?
    A. Anorexia
    B. Conversion
    C. Depersonalization
    D. Factitious
    E. Hypochondriasis

315. A patient with recurrent episodes of binge eating and purging most likely has
    A. fugue state.
    B. bulimia nervosa.
    C. conversion disorder.
    D. anorexia nervosa.
    E. hypochondriasis.

316. _____ behavior involves a pattern of excessive emotions and attention seeking.
    A. Codependent
    B. Histrionic
    C. Narcissistic
    D. Paranoiac
    E. Antisocial

317. Kleptomania, pyromania, trichotillomania, gambling, and intermittent explosive disorder are all types of _____ disorders.
    A. anxiety
    B. impulse control
    C. mood
    D. somatoform
    E. factitious

318. The MOST common method of committing suicide is
    A. cutting.
    B. drowning.
    C. poisoning.
    D. strangulation.
    E. gunshot wound.

319. Which of the following usually would be MOST appropriate when caring for a child experiencing an emotional crisis?
    A. Separate the child from the parent.
    B. Explain in detail what you are doing.
    C. Have the child bring a favorite blanket or toy.
    D. Discourage the child from crying.
    E. Maintain an authoritative distance from the child.

320. Which statement regarding restraining a patient is FALSE?
    A. Preferably five people should restrain the patient, but more may be used if the patient is extremely large or combative.
    B. Combative patients should be hog-tied and placed on the stretcher, then transported to the local hospital.
    C. Restrained patients should be placed supine on the stretcher with one arm extended and restrained above the head and the other arm adducted and restrained next to the body.
    D. The patient's mental status and ABCs should be constantly reevaluated during transport.
    E. Commercial leather restraints, jacket restraints, and soft restraints are optimal.

Chapter 12: Diseases of the Eyes, Ears, Nose, and Throat

321. Movement of the eyes is controlled by the
    A. extraocular muscles.
    B. periorbital muscles.
    C. muscles of the iris.
    D. midclavicular muscles.
    E. pupillary muscles.

322. A membrane that covers and protects the exposed surface of the eye is the
    A. pupil.
    B. iris.
    C. conjunctiva.
    D. optic nerve.
    E. eyebrow.

323. The posterior cavity of the eye behind the lens contains the
    A. iris.
    B. pupil.
    C. oculomotor nerve.
    D. vitreous humor.
    E. aqueous humor.

©2013 Pearson Education, Inc.
Paramedic Care: Principles & Practice, Vol. 4, 4th Ed.

_____ 324. An infection of the eyelid that results from blockage of the oil glands is
   A. an astrocyte.   D. cellulitis.
   B. an ulcer.   E. a sty.
   C. an eye sore.

_____ 325. A conjunctival condition characterized by a raised, wedge-shaped growth of the conjunctiva is called a(n)
   A. sty.   D. pustule.
   B. pterygium.   E. lesion.
   C. eye sore.

_____ 326. A collection of blood in the anterior chamber of the eye is called
   A. lymphoma.   D. cellulitis.
   B. a sty.   E. a hyphema.
   C. glaucoma.

_____ 327. A clouding of the lens of the eye associated with aging is called
   A. diplopia.   D. hyphema.
   B. glaucoma.   E. a neoplasm.
   C. a cataract.

_____ 328. Optic _____ is an inflammation of the optic nerve.
   A. neuritis   D. lesion
   B. necrosis   E. cellulitis
   C. degeneration

_____ 329. A separation of the retina from the supporting structures is called
   A. retinal detachment.   D. retinal abruption.
   B. retinal necrosis.   E. retinal dissection.
   C. retinal shedding.

_____ 330. The membranous labyrinth is filled with a fluid called
   A. endolymph.   D. synoviate.
   B. sebum.   E. CSF.
   C. semen.

_____ 331. A substance that often occludes the external auditory canal is called
   A. concrete sebum.   D. otitis media.
   B. impacted cerumen.   E. obstructed saliva.
   C. viscous mucus.

_____ 332. A common infection of the middle ear is
   A. otitis interna.   D. malignant otitis.
   B. otitis intima.   E. otitis media.
   C. otitis externa.

_____ 333. Swelling and irritation of the inner ear is
   A. nystagmitis.   D. mastoiditis.
   B. urethritis.   E. labyrinthitis.
   C. cellulitis.

_____ 334. An area of the nose made up of four arteries, making it highly vascular, is called
   A. the choroid plexus   D. the nasal-septal cyst.
   B. Kisselbach's plexus.   E. the cribriform cavity.
   C. the nasal plexus.

_____ 335. Inflammation of the nose resulting in a "runny nose" often seen with seasonal allergies is called
   A. cholecystitis.   D. rhinitis.
   B. cystitis.   E. endometritis.
   C. cellulitis.

_____ **336.** Group A *Streptococcus* (strep throat) is often associated with a red and swollen throat and is commonly referred to as

A. pharyngitis.
B. cellulitis.
C. cystitis.
D. cholecystitis.
E. otitis.

_____ **337.** A collection of infected material (pus) in the area around the tonsils is called

A. periorbital cellulitis.
B. a peritonsillar abscess.
C. a palate lesion.
D. a dental rupture.
E. a salivary ulcer.

_____ **338.** A type of oral bacterial cellulitis that involves the floor of the mouth under the tongue is called

A. Ludwig's angina.
B. Prinzmittle's angina.
C. Mittelschmerz angina.
D. a ruptured oral cyst
E. a sublingual blastoma.

_____ **339.** An infection of the trachea characterized by deep cough, dyspnea, and fever is

A. tracheitis.
B. bronchitis.
C. laryngitis.
D. tonsillitis.
E. pharyngitis.

_____ **340.** A disorder that results from problems with the joint between the temporal bones and mandible is called

A. articular joint disorder.
B. temporomandibular joint syndrome.
C. degenerative jaw disorder.
D. mandibular degenerative disease.
E. maxilla framework disorder.

Chapter 13: Nontraumatic Musculoskeletal Disorders

_____ **341.** Physicians who specialize in the treatment of nontraumatic musculoskeletal disorders are

A. gerontologists.
B. cardiologists.
C. endocrinologists.
D. proctologists.
E. rheumatologists.

_____ **342.** Many nontraumatic musculoskeletal disorders are caused by inflammatory or

A. autoimmune disorders.
B. endocrine disorders.
C. immune disorders.
D. hematological disorders.
E. gastrointestinal disorders.

_____ **343.** Other body systems, such as the _____ system, also play a major role in nontraumatic medical conditions.

A. cardiovascular
B. integumentary
C. pulmonary
D. nervous
E. gastrointestinal

_____ **344.** The type of joints that are found in the forearm allowing for pronation and supination are called _____ joints.

A. hinge
B. ball-and-socket
C. ellipsoidal
D. saddle
E. pivot

©2013 Pearson Education, Inc.
Paramedic Care: Principles & Practice, Vol. 4, 4th Ed.

_____ 345. Joints contain a lubricant referred to as _____ fluid.
   A. synovial
   B. gliding
   C. ellipsoid
   D. skeletal
   E. hyaline

_____ 346. Most patients with nontraumatic musculoskeletal disorders will present with
   A. deformity or bleeding.
   B. ecchymosis or swelling.
   C. pain or tenderness.
   D. swelling or deformity.
   E. crepitation or deformity.

_____ 347. A form of trauma caused by chronic repeated events such as using a computer keyboard is called a
   A. chronic work disorder.
   B. persistent-motion disorder.
   C. repetitive-motion disorder.
   D. repetitive-action disorder.
   E. persistent-movement disorder.

_____ 348. The condition known as tennis elbow is clinically referred to as
   A. myalgia.
   B. cellulitis.
   C. herniation.
   D. epicondylitis.
   E. phyarngitis.

_____ 349. Inflammation of the joints that affects the knee, elbow, and hip is called
   A. bursitis.
   B. tendonitis.
   C. myalgia.
   D. epicondylitis.
   E. herniation.

_____ 350. A condition caused by pressure on the median nerve in the wrist often caused by repetitive motion is called
   A. osteoarthritis.
   B. carpal tunnel syndrome.
   C. osteoporosis.
   D. degenerative nerve disorder.
   E. bursitis.

_____ 351. Wear and tear on the joints may cause
   A. osteoarthritis.
   B. osteoporosis.
   C. nucleus pulposus.
   D. joint stenosis.
   E. gout.

_____ 352. Rheumatoid arthritis is a chronic disease that leads to inflammation and injury to the joints and surrounding tissues and is considered a(n)
   A. infectious disease.
   B. environmental disease.
   C. multiple-trauma disease.
   D. autoimmune disease.
   E. gastrointestinal disease.

_____ 353. A form of inflammatory arthritis that primarily affects the spine is called
   A. ankylosing spondylitis.
   B. osteoarthritis.
   C. osteoporosis.
   D. degenerative epicondylitis.
   E. systemic lupus erythematosus.

_____ 354. Gout results from an abnormal elevation of the amount of _____ acid in the body.
   A. lactic
   B. uric
   C. pyruvic
   D. gastric
   E. ketonic

_____ 355. The treatment of cellulitis includes pain medication and
   A. emetics.
   B. cathartics.
   C. antibiotics.
   D. mycolytics.
   E. proton-pump inhibitors.

____ **356.** An infectious condition characterized by the death of soft tissue is called
    A. peripheral neuropathy.   **D.** osteomyelitis.
    B. peripheral necrosis.   **E.** gangrene.
    C. diabetic foot.

____ **357.** Skin ulcers that are commonly seen in bedridden patients as a result of pressure and friction are called
    A. infectious neoplasms.   **D.** decubitus ulcers.
    B. bone spurs.   **E.** skin lesions.
    C. septic spots.

____ **358.** A condition characterized by widespread pain in the muscles and soft tissues throughout the body is
    A. fibromyalgia.   **D.** sympathetic pain dystrophy.
    B. central pain syndrome.   **E.** somatrophic disorder.
    C. psychotic pain disorder.

©2013 Pearson Education, Inc.
Paramedic Care: Principles & Practice, Vol. 4, 4th Ed.

WORKBOOK ANSWER KEY

Note: Throughout Answer Key, textbook page references are shown in italic.

Chapter 1: Pulmonology

Part 1

CONTENT SELF-EVALUATION

MATCHING TERMS—SECTION A *pp. 3–40*

1. acute respiratory distress syndrome (ARDS)   L
2. apnea   D
3. asphyxia   T
4. bradypnea   O
5. carina   J
6. carbaminohemoglobin   S
7. chronic obstructive pulmonary disease (COPD)   A
8. cor pulmonale   P
9. crepitus   W
10. cyanosis   N
11. deoxyhemoglobin   B
12. diaphoresis   V
13. diffusion   C
14. dyspnea   M
15. flail chest   I
16. reactive oxygen species (ROS)   E
17. free radicals   X
18. hemoglobin   F
19. hemoptysis   Q
20. hemothorax   Y
21. hypoxia   K
22. hyperoxia   G
23. nasal flaring   R
24. normoxia   H
25. orthopnea   U

MATCHING TERMS—SECTION B *pp. 3–40*

1. oxyhemoglobin   F
2. oxidative stress   P
3. pallor   H
4. paroxysmal nocturnal dyspnea   A
5. perfusion   J
6. pH   N
7. pleuritic   K
8. pneumothorax   B
9. polycythemia   G
10. positive end-expiratory pressure (PEEP)   T
11. respiration   E
12. spontaneous pneumothorax   Q
13. subcutaneous emphysema   C
14. surfactant   I
15. tachycardia   S
16. tachypnea   M
17. tactile fremitus   L
18. tracheal deviation   O
19. tracheal tugging   D
20. ventilation   R

MULTIPLE CHOICE

1.	C	*p. 3*	13.	E	*p. 14*	25.	D	*p. 16*
2.	D	*p. 5*	14.	B	*p. 14*	26.	D	*p. 16*
3.	E	*p. 6*	15.	A	*p. 14*	27.	D	*p. 17*
4.	E	*p. 7*	16.	C	*p. 14*	28.	B	*p. 17*
5.	A	*p. 7*	17.	B	*p. 14*	29.	E	*p. 18*
6.	A	*p. 7*	18.	A	*p. 14*	30.	B	*p. 18*
7.	D	*p. 10*	19.	B	*p. 15*	31.	E	*p. 18*
8.	E	*p. 10*	20.	A	*p. 25*	32.	D	*p. 18*
9.	C	*p. 12*	21.	C	*p. 31*	33.	C	*p. 18*
10.	D	*p. 13*	22.	A	*p. 16*	34.	A	*p. 18*
11.	B	*p. 13*	23.	A	*p. 16*	35.	C	*p. 20*
12.	B	*p. 25*	24.	E	*p. 16*			

MATCHING

pp. 7–14

36.	D
37.	V
38.	V
39.	V
40.	D
41.	D
42.	P
43.	V
44.	V
45.	P
46.	P

LABEL THE DIAGRAMS *pp. 4–12*

47.	J	55.	D	63.	D
48.	H	56.	I	64.	D
49.	G	57.	M	65.	C
50.	C	58.	N	66.	A
51.	E	59.	O		
52.	F	60.	K		
53.	B	61.	B		
54.	A	62.	E		

SPECIAL PROJECT: Evaluating Abnormal Breathing Patterns

SUGGESTED RESPONSES TO SCENARIOS

pp. 12–18

Scenario 1: *Breathing pattern:* Cheyne-Stokes; *Probable cause:* terminal illness

Scenario 2: *Breathing pattern:* ataxic (Biot's); *Probable cause:* hemorrhagic stroke. (The ataxic breathing is a clue that the stroke is hemorrhagic rather than obstructive because ataxic breathing typically results from a buildup of intracranial pressure as would be caused by bleeding into the brain.) Other possibilities include intracranial bleeding caused by a blow to the head when the patient fell. A brain infection or tumor could also cause increased intracranial pressure and ataxic breathing, but the sudden onset and severe headache are more indicative of a stroke.

Scenario 3: *Breathing pattern:* Kussmaul's; *Probable cause:* diabetic ketoacidosis. (A variety of medical emergencies can result from diabetes. The clue to acidosis is the deep, rapid breathing, which is a compensatory mechanism that rids the body of excess CO_2 to alleviate the acidic condition. The cause in this case is that the patient has not been taking her insulin. Insulin is necessary to help glucose enter the body cells. When insulin is absent, the cells turn to metabolism of fats instead of the normal glucose metabolism. A by-product of fat metabolism is ketones, resulting in acidosis.)

Part 2

CONTENT SELF-EVALUATION

MULTIPLE CHOICE

1.	E	*p. 29*	11.	B	*p. 35*	21.	A	*p. 42*
2.	C	*p. 25*	12.	A	*p. 36*	22.	A	*p. 42*
3.	A	*p. 28*	13.	B	*p. 37*	23.	C	*p. 40*
4.	A	*p. 28*	14.	A	*p. 39*	24.	B	*p. 38*
5.	B	*p. 29*	15.	B	*p. 40*	25.	D	*p. 438*
6.	B	*p. 30*	16.	A	*p. 40*	26.	D	*p. 42*
7.	B	*p. 32*	17.	A	*p. 40*	27.	B	*p. 42*
8.	D	*p. 32*	18.	D	*p. 40*	28.	A	*p. 38*
9.	D	*p. 32*	19.	C	*p. 40*	29.	B	*p. 42*
10.	B	*p. 34*	20.	A	*p. 41*	30.	B	*p. 38*

MATCHING

31.	C	*p. 25*	34.	E	*p. 35*	37.	D	*p. 539*
32.	F	*p. 28*	35.	G	*p. 36*			
33.	A	*p. 30*	36.	B	*p. 37*			

SPECIAL PROJECT: Assessing Respiratory Emergencies

pp. 25–40

Scenario 1: *Probable cause:* asthma

Scenario 2: *Probable cause:* pneumonia; *Underlying probable cause:* emphysema (COPD)

Scenario 3: *Probable cause:* pulmonary embolism

Chapter 2: Cardiology

Part 1

CONTENT SELF-EVALUATION

MULTIPLE CHOICE

1.	C	*p. 48*	14.	B	*p. 62*	27.	A	*p. 80*
2.	E	*p. 49*	15.	A	*p. 62*	28.	B	*p. 80*
3.	C	*p. 50*	16.	E	*p. 62*	29.	B	*p. 82*
4.	B	*p. 49*	17.	B	*p. 63*	30.	A	*p. 83*
5.	B	*p. 51*	18.	A	*p. 63*	31.	D	*p. 83*
6.	E	*p. 51*	19.	C	*p. 64*	32.	E	*p. 85*
7.	A	*p. 52*	20.	B	*p. 66*	33.	A	*p. 86*
8.	C	*p. 53*	21.	D	*p. 68*	34.	C	*p. 86*
9.	D	*p. 54*	22.	C	*p. 69*	35.	C	*p. 88*
10.	D	*p. 54*	23.	E	*p. 69*	36.	A	*p. 88*
11.	E	*p. 57*	24.	C	*p. 71*	37.	B	*p. 90*
12.	A	*p. 58*	25.	C	*p. 71*	38.	B	*p. 71*
13.	E	*p. 57*	26.	D	*p. 77*	39.	B	*p. 90*

40.	C	*p. 92*	44.	D	*p. 97*	48.	D	*p. 101*
41.	E	*p. 95*	45.	A	*p. 96*	49.	A	*p. 101*
42.	A	*p. 95*	46.	E	*p. 99*	50.	E	*p. 102*
43.	B	*p. 94*	47.	B	*p. 101*			

MATCHING

51.	B	*p. 53*	55.	H	*p. 54*	59.	B	*p. 61*
52.	I, G	*p. 54*	56.	C	*p. 54*	60.	C	*p. 61*
53.	D	*p. 54*	57.	F	*p. 54*	61.	A	*p. 61*
54.	A	*p. 54*	58.	E	*p. 54*			

LABEL THE DIAGRAMS *pp. 49–68*

Figure 1 *p. 50* (fig. 2–3)

62.	D	65.	C	68.	C
63.	A	66.	F	69.	D
64.	B	67.	E		

Figure 2 *p. 61* (fig. 2–16)

70.	F	72.	E	74.	A
71.	G	73.	B		

Figure 3 *p. 64* (fig. 2–20)

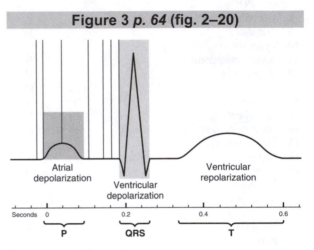

SPECIAL PROJECT: ECG Interpretation

pp. 68–99

ECG 1

Rate: P wave 72, QRS 72

Rhythm: P wave regular, QRS regular

P waves: upright, smooth and rounded

P-R interval: regular at 0.12 sec

QRS complexes: normal at 0.08

Overall rhythm (or dysrhythmia): normal sinus rhythm

ECG 2

Rate: P wave 75, QRS ~ 55

Rhythm: P wave regular, QRS irregular due to skipped beats

P waves: upright, smooth and rounded

P-R interval: increasing until dropped beat (4 P waves to 3 QRS complexes)

QRS complexes: normal at 0.08 sec.

Overall rhythm (or dysrhythmia): second-degree heart block, type I (Wenckebach)

©2013 Pearson Education, Inc.
Paramedic Care: Principles & Practice, Vol. 4, 4th Ed.

ECG 3

Rate: P wave 70, QRS 70—except for extra beat

Rhythm: P wave and QRS regular except for extra beat

P waves: upright, smooth and rounded, none preceding extra beat

P-R interval: 0.12 and regular, none before extra beat

QRS complexes: normal at 0.08 except extra beat, then 0.12 and bizarre morphology

Overall rhythm (or dysrhythmia): sinus rhythm with a premature ventricular contraction (PVC)

ECG 4

Rate: P wave 68, QRS 68

Rhythm: P wave and QRS regular

P waves: upright, smooth and rounded

P-R interval: 0.22, prolonged but regular

QRS complexes: normal at 0.08

Overall rhythm (or dysrhythmia): first-degree heart block

ECG 5

Rate: P wave 72, QRS 72

Rhythm: P wave and QRS regular except for extra beats

P waves: upright, smooth and rounded, extra beats—abnormal (biphasic)

P-R interval: normal at 0.128, shorter with extra beats

QRS complexes: normal at 0.08

Overall rhythm (or dysrhythmia): sinus rhythm with premature junctional contractions (PJCs)

ECG 6

Rate: P wave 145, QRS 145

Rhythm: P wave and QRS regular

P waves: indiscernible (probably biphasic—atrial)

P-R interval: between 0.08 and 0.12

QRS complexes: normal at 0.08

Overall rhythm (or dysrhythmia): supraventricular tachycardia (probably atrial)

ECG 7

Rate: P wave 92, QRS 44

Rhythm: P wave and QRS regular but different rates

P waves: upright, smooth and rounded

P-R interval: varies (unrelated)

QRS complexes: greater than 0.20, bizarre, uniform

Overall rhythm (or dysrhythmia): third-degree heart block

ECG 8

Rate: no discernible P waves or QRS complexes

Rhythm: chaotic

P waves: no discernible P waves

P-R interval: no discernible P-R interval

QRS complexes: no discernible QRS complexes

Overall rhythm (or dysrhythmia): ventricular fibrillation

ECG 9

Rate: P wave 106, QRS 38

Rhythm: P wave and QRS regular, but different rates (3 P waves/QRS)

P waves: upright, smooth and round

P-R interval: 0.12 for every 3rd beat, other two not related

QRS complexes: normal at 0.08

Overall rhythm (or dysrhythmia): second-degree heart block type II

ECG 10

Rate: P wave indiscernible, QRS 152

Rhythm: P wave indiscernible, QRS regular

P waves: none discernible

P-R interval: none discernible

QRS complexes: 0.12+ and bizarre

Overall rhythm (or dysrhythmia): ventricular tachycardia

ECG 11

Rate: P wave 280, QRS 70

Rhythm: P wave and QRS regular, but different

P waves: sawtooth

P-R interval: regular at 0.12 for conducted beats (every 4th beat)

QRS complexes: normal at 0.06

Overall rhythm (or dysrhythmia): atrial flutter (4:1)

ECG 12

Rate: P wave 0, QRS 0

Rhythm: no rhythm present

P waves: none present

P-R interval: none

QRS complexes: none

Overall rhythm (or dysrhythmia): asystole

ECG 13

Rate: P wave 34, QRS 34

Rhythm: P wave and QRS regular

P waves: upright, smooth and rounded

P-R interval: normal at 0.12

QRS complexes: normal at 0.6

Overall rhythm (or dysrhythmia): sinus bradycardia

ECG 14

Rate: P wave indiscernible, QRS 40

Rhythm: QRS regular

P waves: indiscernible

P-R interval: indiscernible

QRS complexes: normal at 0.06

Overall rhythm (or dysrhythmia): junctional rhythm

ECG 15

Rate: P wave indiscernible, QRS 148

Rhythm: QRS regular

P waves: indiscernible

P-R interval: indiscernible

QRS complexes: normal at 0.06

Overall rhythm (or dysrhythmia): supraventricular tachycardia

ECG 16

Rate: P wave indiscernible, QRS about 90

Rhythm: QRS irregularly irregular

P waves: indiscernible

P-R interval: indiscernible

QRS complexes: normal at 0.06

Overall rhythm (or dysrhythmia): atrial fibrillation

ECG 17

Rate: P wave 74, QRS 74 except for extra beats

Rhythm: P wave and QRS regular except for extra beats

P waves: upright, smooth and regular, no P wave preceding extra beats

P-R interval: normal at 0.12 except with extra beats

QRS complexes: normal at 0.06 except extra beats at 0.18+ and bizarre, extra beats are different in morphology

Overall rhythm (or dysrhythmia): sinus rhythm with multifocal premature ventricular contractions (PVCs)

ECG 18

Rate: P wave 60, QRS 70

Rhythm: P wave and QRS regular except with extra beat

P waves: upright, smooth and rounded, except with extra beat (possibly biphasic)

P-R interval: normal at 0.12, except with extra beat (0.04)

QRS complexes: normal at 0.06

Overall rhythm (or dysrhythmia): sinus rhythm with a premature atrial contraction

ECG 19

Rate: P wave 75, QRS 65

Rhythm: P wave regular, QRS irregular due to skipped beats

P waves: upright, smooth and rounded

P-R interval: increasing until QRS is dropped (4 P-waves to 3 QRS)

QRS complexes: normal at 0.06

Overall rhythm (or dysrhythmia): second-degree heart block type I (Wenckebach)

ECG 20

Rate: P wave indiscernible, QRS 90

Rhythm: irregularly irregular

P waves: indiscernible

P-R interval: indiscernible

QRS complexes: normal at 0.06

Overall rhythm (or dysrhythmia): atrial fibrillation

Part 2

CONTENT SELF-EVALUATION

MULTIPLE CHOICE

1.	A	*p. 103*	**10.**	C	*p. 112*	**19.**	D	*p. 123*
2.	B	*p. 103*	**11.**	B	*p. 70*	**20.**	B	*p. 123*
3.	D	*p. 103*	**12.**	B	*p. 96*	**21.**	E	*p. 131*
4.	B	*p. 105*	**13.**	B	*p. 99*	**22.**	A	*p. 135*
5.	C	*p. 106*	**14.**	B	*p. 107*	**23.**	A	*p. 141*
6.	E	*p. 109*	**15.**	A	*p. 115*	**24.**	D	*p. 141*
7.	D	*p. 110*	**16.**	C	*p. 115*	**25.**	C	*p. 142*
8.	E	*p. 111*	**17.**	B	*p. 118*			
9.	B	*p. 112*	**18.**	A	*p. 120*			

MATCHING

26.	B	*p. 104*	**33.**	E	*p. 107*	**40.**	B	*p. 128*
27.	F	*p. 106*	**34.**	D	*p. 115*	**41.**	F	*p. 136*
28.	E	*p. 115*	**35.**	A	*p. 110*	**42.**	E	*p. 124*
29.	G	*p. 130*	**36.**	B	*p. 112*	**43.**	G	*p. 131*
30.	C	*p. 130*	**37.**	C	*p. 118*	**44.**	D	*p. 128*
31.	D	*p. 141*	**38.**	C	*p. 120*	**45.**	H	*p. 133*
32.	A	*p. 142*	**39.**	A	*p. 128*			

Part 3

CONTENT SELF-EVALUATION

MULTIPLE CHOICE

1.	A	*p. 144*	**6.**	D	*p. 148*	**11**	A	*p. 158*
2.	B	*p. 144*	**7.**	C	*p. 152*	**12.**	A	*p. 159*
3.	A	*p. 144*	**8.**	D	*p. 154*	**13.**	E	*p. 167*
4.	D	*p. 148*	**9.**	E	*p. 158*	**14.**	B	*p. 149*
5.	A	*p. 148*	**10.**	A	*p. 158*	**15.**	E	*p. 149*

MATCHING

16.	C	*p. 144*	**22.**	C	*p. 155*	**28.**	D	*p. 166*
17.	A	*p. 145*	**23.**	B	*p. 155*	**29.**	G	*p. 166*
18.	B	*p. 149*	**24.**	D	*p. 155*	**30.**	E	*p. 166*
19.	A	*p. 155*	**25.**	E	*p. 155*	**31.**	B	*p. 166*
20.	G	*p. 155*	**26.**	C	*p. 164*	**32.**	F	*p. 166*
21.	F	*p. 155*	**27.**	A	*p. 164*			

SPECIAL PROJECT: Interpreting an ECG

pp. 103–107

1. The QRS complexes are widened and have a notched appearance that is readily apparent in leads I, II, aVL, V5, III, aVF, and V6. In addition, there are deep S waves in leads V1, V2, and V3 and relatively tall R waves in leads I, aVL, V5, and V6. This strongly suggests left bundle branch block.

2. The tracing shows significant ST segment depression and inverted T waves in leads aVL, V5, and V6, which suggests myocardial ischemia in the anterolateral part of the heart. However, you know that left bundle branch block can produce these changes in the absence of any ischemia, so the ECG is not useful in detecting or localizing ischemia or an acute MI.

   Note: Although the ECG is not useful in this instance, the presence of left bundle branch block in no way negates the possibility of myocardial ischemia or infarction in the patient, and you should treat and transport accordingly.

You should give the tracing to the emergency team when you deliver Mr. Benon so they can compare the tracing with previous ECGs and any ECGs that may be taken while he is at the hospital.

Chapter 3: Neurology

CONTENT SELF-EVALUATION

MULTIPLE CHOICE

1.	A	*p. 186*	6.	A	*p. 197*	11.	B	*p. 205*
2.	C	*p. 189*	7.	C	*p. 201*	12.	A	*p. 205*
3.	B	*p. 190*	8.	E	*p. 201*	13.	C	*p. 206*
4.	E	*p. 194*	9.	B	*p. 202*	14.	E	*p. 213*
5.	C	*p. 194*	10.	B	*p. 202*			

FILL IN THE BLANKS

15. heart rate, bronchioles, pupils *p. 188*
16. temporal, cerebrum *p. 184*
17. involuntary *p. 187*
18. smooth, cardiac *p. 188*
19. thalamus, hypothalamus, limbic *p. 184*
20. dendrites *p. 181*
21. somatic nervous system, autonomic nervous system *p. 182*
22. central nervous system, peripheral nervous system *p. 181*
23. meninges *p. 184*
24. axon *p. 182*
25. heart rate, bronchioles, pupils *p. 188*
26. mesencephalon, pons, medulla oblongata *p. 184*
27. cerebrospinal fluid (CSF) *p. 184*
28. consciousness, stimuli *p. 186*
29. occipital, cerebrum *p. 184*
30. frontal, cerebrum *p. 186*
31. voluntary, conscious *p. 0187*
32. synapse, neurotransmitter *p. 182*
33. brain, spinal cord *p. 181*

LABEL THE DIAGRAM

pp. 183–186

34. Thalamus, H
35. Hypothalamus, E
36. Pituitary gland, G
37. Midbrain, B
38. Pons, D
39. Medulla oblongata, C
40. Cerebrum, F
41. Cerebellum, A

MATCHING

42.	B, G	*p. 192*	47.	A, D	*p. 198*
43.	E, H	*p. 192*	48.	C, E	*p. 199*
44.	A, D	*p. 192*	49.	C, F	*p. 198*
45.	C, I	*p. 192*	50.	B, C	*p. 199*
46.	F, J	*p. 192*			

LISTING

51. A, alert and oriented to surroundings; V, responsive to verbal stimuli; P, responsive to painful stimuli; U, unresponsive to all *p. 191*
52. M, mood; T, thought processes; P, perception of surroundings; J, judgment in context of situation; MA, memory and attention *p. 151*

53. Increased blood pressure, decreased pulse, decreased respirations, increased temperature *p. 194*
54. A, acidosis or alcohol; E, epilepsy; I, infection; O, overdose; U, uremia; T, trauma, toxin, or tumor; I, insulin (either hypoglycemia or ketoacidosis); P, psychosis or poison; S, stroke or seizure *p. 196*
55. Thrombotic, embolic *p. 198*
56. Intracerebral, subarachnoid *p. 199*
57. Tremor, rigidity, bradykinesia, postural instability *p. 211*
58. Occulta, meningocele, myelomeningocele *p. 212* (*order DOES matter for this question*)
59. Migraine, cluster *p. 206*

SPECIAL PROJECT: Distinguishing Different Conditions in the Field

Scenario 1 *pp. 194–196*

Vital Signs	Shock	Increased ICP
Blood pressure	Decreased	Increased
Pulse	Increased	Decreased
Respirations	Increased	Decreased
Level of consciousness	Decreased	Decreased

Scenario 2 *pp. 202–206*

Trait	Syncope	Tonic-Clonic Seizure
Starting position	Usually begins in standing position	May begin in any position
Warning	Patient usually remembers warning of fainting	May or may not have warning; may be preceded by aura
Jerking motions	Jerking motions usually not present	Jerking motions present while unconscious
Return of consciousness	Consciousness returns almost immediately on becoming supine	Patient unconscious during seizure and drowsy during postictal period

Chapter 4: Endocrinology

CONTENT SELF-EVALUATION

MULTIPLE CHOICE

1.	C	*p. 220*	11.	E	*p. 225*	21.	E	*p. 230*
2.	C	*p. 228*	12.	C	*p. 225*	22.	A	*p. 230*
3.	B	*p. 221*	13.	B	*p. 226*	23.	C	*p. 235*
4.	B	*p. 224*	14.	C	*p. 226*	24.	E	*p. 232*
5.	A	*p. 224*	15.	A	*p. 226*	25.	A	*p. 235*
6.	B	*p. 224*	16.	A	*p. 226*	26.	B	*p. 236*
7.	B	*p. 225*	17.	A	*p. 226*	27.	A	*p. 237*
8.	D	*p. 225*	18.	E	*p. 227*	28.	E	*p. 237*
9.	B	*p. 225*	19.	B	*p. 229*	29.	A	*p. 237*
10.	B	*p. 225*	20.	D	*p. 229*	30.	B	*p. 237*

MATCHING

31.	J	*p. 238*	35.	G	*p. 225*	39.	B	*p. 220*
32.	C	*p. 228*	36.	D	*p. 228*	40.	A	*p. 220*
33.	E	*p. 224*	37.	F	*p. 224*			
34.	H	*p. 226*	38.	I	*p. 226*			

SPECIAL PROJECT: Label the Diagram

pp. 221–223

A. Pineal gland: melatonin
B. Hypothalamus: growth-hormone-releasing hormone, growth-hormone-inhibiting hormone, corticotropin-releasing hormone, thyrotropin-releasing hormone, gonadotropin-releasing hormone, prolactin-releasing hormone, prolactin-inhibiting hormone
C. Pituitary gland: antidiuretic hormone, oxytocin, growth hormone, adrenocorticotropic hormone, thyroid-stimulating hormone, follicle-stimulating hormone, luteinizing hormone, prolactin
D. Thyroid gland: thyroxine, triiodothyronine, calcitonin
E. Parathyroid gland: parathyroid hormone
F. Thymus: thymosin
G. Pancreas: glucagon, insulin, somatostatin
H. Adrenal glands: epinephrine, norepinephrine, glucocorticoids (cortisol), mineralocorticoids (aldosterone), androgenic hormones (estrogen, progesterone, testosterone)
I. Gonads (ovaries): estrogen, progesterone, testosterone from testes

Chapter 5: Immunology

CONTENT SELF-EVALUATION

MULTIPLE CHOICE

1.	B	*p. 224*	6.	A	*p. 242*	11.	A	*p. 246*
2.	D	*p. 243*	7.	C	*p. 245*	12.	B	*p. 248*
3.	B	*p. 243*	8.	C	*p. 242*	13.	C	*p. 248*
4.	C	*p. 243*	9.	C	*p. 244*	14.	D	*p. 248*
5.	D	*p. 244*	10.	B	*p. 244*	15.	D	*p. 246*

MATCHING

16.	E	*p. 250*	18.	D	*p. 250*	20.	A	*p. 250*
17.	C	*p. 250*	19.	B	*p. 250*			

SPECIAL PROJECT: Completing Tables

Part A *p. 251*

Skin: flushing, itching, hives, swelling, cyanosis

Respiratory: respiratory difficulty, sneezing, coughing, wheezing, stridor, laryngeal edema, laryngospasm, bronchospasm

Cardiovascular: vasodilation, increased heart rate, decreased blood pressure

Gastrointestinal: nausea and vomiting, abdominal cramping, diarrhea

Nervous system: dizziness, headache, convulsions, tearing

Part B *p. 250*

Albuterol: beta agonist, reverses bronchospasm and laryngeal edema

Diphenhydramine: blocks histamine receptors

Dopamine: potent vasopressor to support blood pressure (vasoconstrictors)

Epinephrine: sympathetic agonist that increases heart rate, increases cardiac contractile force, increases peripheral vasoconstriction, and reverses much of the capillary permeability caused by histamine

Methylprednisolone: suppresses the inflammatory response

Chapter 6: Gastroenterology

CONTENT SELF-EVALUATION

MULTIPLE CHOICE

1.	D	*p. 256*	9.	A	*p. 262*
2.	A	*p. 257*	10.	E	*p. 273*
3.	B	*p. 257*	11.	B	*p. 263*
4.	E	*p. 256*	12.	A	*p. 260*
5.	A	*p. 256*	13.	C	*p. 264*
6.	C	*p. 258*	14.	D	*p. 268*
7.	D	*p. 258*	15.	B	*p. 272*
8.	B	*p. 260*			

MATCHING

16.	C	*p. 256*	20.	A	*p. 256*	24.	D	*p. 267*
17.	E	*p. 256*	21.	E	*p. 259*	25.	A	*p. 273*
18.	A	*p. 256*	22.	A	*p. 256*	26.	B	*p. 267*
19.	B	*p. 256*	23.	D	*p. 258*	27.	C	*p. 272*

FILL IN THE BLANKS

28. Symptoms; Allergies; Medications; Past medical history; Last oral intake; Events *p. 258*
29. Six hours *p. 258*
30. ligament of Treitz *p. 260*

SPECIAL PROJECT: History Taking

Question types (in sequence) are Severity, Associated Symptoms, Time, Quality, Region, Onset, Provocation/Palliation, Pertinent Negatives *p. 258*

Probable field diagnosis: Appendicitis (probably ruptured, with peritonitis) *p. 270*

Chapter 7: Urology and Nephrology

CONTENT SELF-EVALUATION

MULTIPLE CHOICE

1.	B	*p. 278*	6.	E	*p. 284*	11.	D	*p. 289*
2.	A	*p. 281*	7.	B	*p. 284*	12.	A	*p. 289*
3.	D	*p. 281*	8.	A	*p. 278*	13.	E	*p. 278*
4.	B	*p. 282*	9.	A	*p. 286*	14.	B	*p. 278*
5.	C	*p. 282*	10.	C	*p. 289*	15.	C	*p. 294*

MATCHING

16.	A	*p. 278*	19.	C	*p. 287*	22.	D	*p. 295*
17.	B	*p. 278*	20.	A	*p. 278*	23.	A	*p. 295*
18.	B	*p. 286*	21.	C	*p. 295*	24.	B	*p. 295*

FILL IN THE BLANKS

25. proximal tubule, descending loop of Henle, ascending loop of Henle, distal tubule *p. 279*
26. Bowman's capsule, filtrate *p. 280*
27. water, sodium and chloride ions *p. 281*
28. secretion *p. 280*
29. Onset, Provocation/Palliation, Quality, Region, Severity, Time *p. 284*
30. semipermeable membrane, dialysate *p. 291*
31. semipermeable membrane *p. 291*
32. artificial graft connecting an artery and vein, arteriovenous fistula *p. 291*
33. Infection *p. 292*

p. 279

34.	D	**38.**	D	**42.**	G
35.	C	**39.**	A	**43.**	E
36.	B	**40.**	C	**44.**	F
37.	A	**41.**	B		

SPECIAL PROJECT: Making a Call

1. The external portion of the indwelling catheter is visible above the skin. Beneath the skin, the catheter tunnels through the abdominal wall and into the peritoneal cavity. *p. 292*
2. Infection *p. 292*
3. The skin and subcutaneous tissues, the muscle of the abdominal wall, and the peritoneal membrane itself. Peritonitis is unlikely given history of pain, so infection probably has not spread as far as the peritoneal membrane. *p. 292*
4. You already know that the patient has had either vascular (shift in blood pressure?) or neurological (because of change in chemical milieu for the brain) complications because of the fainting episode. You should be prepared for rapid evolution of physiological instability (as in all patients with chronic renal failure/end-stage renal failure), with treatment during transport including close monitoring and support of ABCs with high-flow oxygen, constant monitoring of ECG, and establishment of IV access. The risks/benefits of peritoneal lavage may be discussed with medical direction. Talking quietly with the patient helps to monitor mental status. Monitoring of BP may note development of hypotension. *p. 292*

Chapter 8: Toxicology and Substance Abuse

CONTENT SELF-EVALUATION

MULTIPLE CHOICE

1.	C	*p. 300*	**15.**	A	*p. 306*
2.	A	*p. 302*	**16.**	B	*p. 317*
3.	D	*p. 301*	**17.**	A	*p. 317*
4.	B	*p. 302*	**18.**	C	*p. 319*
5.	A	*p. 302*	**19.**	E	*p. 322*
6.	B	*p. 303*	**20.**	A	*p. 335*
7.	E	*p. 303*	**21.**	B	*p. 320*
8.	B	*p. 301*	**22.**	D	*p. 324*
9.	B	*p. 303*	**23.**	E	*p. 319*
10.	C	*p. 303*	**24.**	A	*p. 324*
11.	A	*p. 302*	**25.**	A	*p. 325*
12.	D	*p. 301*	**26.**	C	*p. 332*
13.	B	*p. 301*	**27.**	B	*p. 337*
14.	E	*p. 306*			

MATCHING

28.	E	*p. 302*	**34.**	G	*p. 319*	**40.**	D	*p. 331*
29.	A	*p. 302*	**35.**	B	*p. 331*	**41.**	C	*p. 300*
30.	O	*p. 331*	**36.**	K	*p. 302*	**42.**	F	*p. 331*
31.	N	*p. 306*	**37.**	L	*p. 301*	**43.**	H	*p. 301*
32.	P	*p. 331*	**38.**	M	*p. 332*			
33.	I	*p. 337*	**39.**	J	*p. 324*			

44. ingestion, inhalation, surface absorption, injection *p. 300*
45. organophosphates *p. 301*

SPECIAL PROJECT: Analyzing an Emergency Scene

p. 301–306

1. This probably represents an accidental ingestion overdose involving multiple medications of unknown type(s). This is not an uncommon call; you will see this kind of situation.
2. As in all other cases involving a potentially unstable patient, the first priority is support of the ABCs: After checking that the airway is clear, high-flow oxygen should be started and attention paid on an ongoing basis that the airway remains clear (suspect possible vomiting and aspiration; intubate if necessary). Ventilation does not appear to need support at the moment, but you are aware that ventilation can decompensate quickly. Circulation clearly is impaired based on the peripheral pulses. Prepare for ECG monitoring and for pulse oximetry. If it looks like IV access can be established easily, it may be done at this point.
3. Transport of this unstable, elderly man with unclear toxic ingestion and underlying medical conditions is the first priority. Contact with medical direction can be made en route as the focused physical is done and evaluation of vitals and patient condition continues. The poison control center is not useful until you have some idea of the medications involved in the ingestion.
4. Take the pill case. If there are any empty or partially full glasses/cups around, check for signs of alcohol or coffee or tea (which might contain caffeine). Look for opened bottles of over-the-counter medications such as aspirin. If one team partner has time while en route, he can inspect the medications to see if any are definitely recognizable.

Chapter 9: Hematology

CONTENT SELF-EVALUATION

MULTIPLE CHOICE

1.	C	*p. 342*	**8.**	B	*p. 346*	**15.**	D	*p. 351*
2.	B	*p. 342*	**9.**	A	*p. 346*	**16.**	E	*p. 352*
3.	C	*p. 343*	**10.**	B	*p. 346*	**17.**	A	*p. 352*
4.	A	*p. 344*	**11.**	E	*p. 346*	**18.**	C	*p. 353*
5.	D	*p. 354*	**12.**	D	*p. 347*	**19.**	E	*p. 357*
6.	A	*p. 344*	**13.**	B	*p. 349*	**20.**	D	*p. 357*
7.	E	*p. 345*	**14.**	C	*p. 344*			

MATCHING

21.	C	*p. 344*	**26.**	G	*p. 354*	**31.**	B	*p. 345*
22.	J	*p. 348*	**27.**	I	*p. 352*	**32.**	H	*p. 348*
23.	L	*p. 349*	**28.**	E	*p. 353*	**33.**	M	*p. 357*
24.	N	*p. 351*	**29.**	A	*p. 342*	**34.**	O	*p. 358*
25.	D	*p. 353*	**30.**	K	*p. 356*	**35.**	F	*p. 347*

pp. 353–357

Hematological	Common Signs and Symptoms	Prehospital Disorder Management
Anemia	Dyspnea, tachycardia, fatigue, syncope, diaphoresis, pallor, hypotension	Oxygen, control bleeding, volume replacement, expedite transport
Hemophilia	Bleeding	Oxygen, control bleeding, volume replacement, analgesia, expedite transport
Leukemia	Bleeding, fever, weakness, anorexia, weight loss, abdominal pain, fatigue	Oxygen, control bleeding, volume replacement, analgesia, expedite transport
Lymphoma	Fatigue, night sweats, anorexia and weight loss, pruritus	Oxygen, control bleeding, volume replacement, analgesia, expedite transport
Sickle cell anemia	Abdominal or joint pain, pulmonary problems, renal infarction, priapism	Oxygen, control bleeding, volume replacement, analgesia, expedite transport

Chapter 10: Infectious Disease and Sepsis

CONTENT SELF-EVALUATION

MULTIPLE CHOICE

1.	B	*p. 365*	16.	C	*p. 370*
2.	E	*p. 366*	17.	E	*p. 371*
3.	B	*p. 363*	18.	D	*p. 370*
4.	C	*p. 365*	19.	A	*p. 372*
5.	D	*p. 367*	20.	A	*p. 378*
6.	A	*p. 368*	21.	B	*p. 380*
7.	E	*p. 368*	22.	D	*p. 382*
8.	C	*p. 368*	23.	C	*p. 383*
9.	B	*p. 365*	24.	D	*p. 384*
10.	E	*p. 368*	25.	E	*p. 399*
11.	A	*p. 369*	26.	A	*p. 399*
12.	D	*p. 369*	27.	E	*p. 386*
13.	C	*p. 369*	28.	B	*p. 391*
14.	B	*p. 370*	29.	A	*p. 392*
15.	B	*p. 374*	30.	C	*p. 395*

pp. 373–375

Low-level disinfection

Agent: EPA-registered disinfectant

Indication: Routine housekeeping/cleaning and removing visible body fluids

Effectiveness: Destroys most bacteria and some viruses and fungi

Intermediate-level disinfection

Agent: 1:10 to 1:100 dilution of water and chlorine bleach, hard-surface germicide, EPA-registered disinfectant/chemical germicide

Indication: All equipment that has been in contact with intact skin

Effectiveness: Destroys *Mycobacterium tuberculosis,* most viruses, fungi

High-level disinfection

Agent: EPA-approved chemical sterilizing agent, hot water (176°F to 212°F) immersion

Indication: Reusable devices that have been in contact with mucous membranes

Effectiveness: Destroys all forms of microorganisms except certain bacterial spores

Sterilization

Agent: Autoclave (pressurized steam or ethylene-oxide gas), EPA-approved chemical sterilizing agent (prolonged immersion)

Indication: Contaminated invasive instruments

Effectiveness: Destroys all microorganisms

Chapter 11: Psychiatric and Behavioral Disorders

CONTENT SELF-EVALUATION

MULTIPLE CHOICE

1.	B	*p. 408*	6.	D	*p. 420*	11.	C	*p. 411*
2.	B	*p. 407*	7.	E	*p. 411*	12.	A	*p. 411*
3.	C	*p. 409*	8.	C	*p. 412*	13.	A	*p. 414*
4.	C	*p. 409*	9.	C	*p. 412*	14.	E	*p. 419*
5.	B	*p. 410*	10.	A	*p. 410*	15.	B	*p. 420*

MATCHING

16.	J	*p. 415*	20.	E	*p. 411*	24.	G	*p. 411*
17.	A	*p. 411*	21.	H	*p. 413*	25.	B	*p. 411*
18.	D	*p. 411*	22.	F	*p. 411*			
19.	I	*p. 415*	23.	C	*p. 411*			

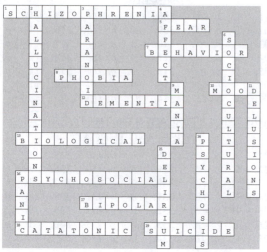

Chapter 12: Diseases of the Eyes, Ears, Nose, and Throat

CONTENT SELF-EVALUATION

MULTIPLE CHOICE

1.	D	*p. 426*	6.	A	*p. 430*	11.	E	*p. 436*
2.	A	*p. 428*	7.	E	*p. 431*	12.	A	*p. 437*
3.	C	*p. 428*	8.	B	*p. 432*	13.	C	*p. 437*
4.	A	*p. 429*	9.	D	*p. 434*	14.	E	*p. 439*
5.	C	*p. 430*	10.	A	*p. 434*	15.	A	*p. 440*

Chapter 13: Nontraumatic Musculoskeletal Disorders

CONTENT SELF-EVALUATION

MULTIPLE CHOICE

1.	A	*p. 445*	6.	A	*p. 449*	11.	A	*p. 453*
2.	B	*p. 446*	7.	D	*p. 449*	12.	C	*p. 453*
3.	D	*p. 446*	8.	B	*p. 450*	13.	B	*p. 453*
4.	B	*p. 442*	9.	C	*p. 452*	14.	E	*p. 454*
5.	E	*p. 449*	10.	D	*p. 451*	15.	C	*p. 455*

Medicine: Content Review

ANSWER KEY

CHAPTER 1: PULMONOLOGY

1.	D	*p. 4*	13.	D	*p. 9*	25.	E	*p. 13*
2.	A	*p. 5*	14.	B	*p. 9*	26.	C	*p. 13*
3.	E	*p. 5*	15.	C	*p. 9*	27.	B	*p. 13*
4.	A	*p. 5*	16.	C	*p. 10*	28.	C	*p. 13*
5.	B	*p. 5*	17.	B	*p. 10*	29.	D	*p. 14*
6.	E	*p. 7*	18.	C	*p. 11*	30.	D	*p. 17*
7.	C	*p. 7*	19.	A	*p. 11*	31.	A	*p. 17*
8.	C	*p. 7*	20.	C	*p. 11*	32.	C	*p. 17*
9.	C	*p. 7*	21.	A	*p. 11*	33.	D	*p. 18*
10.	E	*p. 8*	22.	A	*p. 11*	34.	E	*p. 18*
11.	A	*p. 9*	23.	A	*p. 11*	35.	C	*p. 18*
12.	B	*p. 9*	24.	B	*p. 13*	36.	D	*p. 18*

37.	A	*p. 19*	42.	A	*p. 30*	47.	A	*p. 32*
38.	A	*p. 20*	43.	C	*p. 28*	48.	A	*p. 34*
39.	A	*p. 25*	44.	B	*p. 29*	49.	A	*p. 38*
40.	D	*p. 25*	45.	A	*p. 30*	50.	A	*p. 39*
41.	C	*p. 28*	46.	B	*p. 14*			

CHAPTER 2: CARDIOLOGY

51.	C	*p. 48*	68.	C	*p. 60*	85.	D	*p. 79*
52.	A	*p. 49*	69.	D	*p. 59*	86.	C	*p. 79*
53.	B	*p. 50*	70.	C	*p. 61*	87.	C	*p. 80*
54.	A	*p. 50*	71.	C	*p. 62*	88.	A	*p. 81*
55.	A	*p. 52*	72.	A	*p. 63*	89.	E	*p. 87*
56.	C	*p. 52*	73.	C	*p. 64*	90.	D	*p. 92*
57.	D	*p. 57*	74.	B	*p. 64*	91.	C	*p. 94*
58.	D	*p. 53*	75.	E	*p. 65*	92.	D	*p. 111*
59.	A	*p. 128*	76.	C	*p. 66*	93.	C	*p. 111*
60.	C	*p. 128*	77.	D	*p. 66*	94.	B	*p. 111*
61.	E	*p. 129*	78.	A	*p. 65*	95.	C	*p. 111*
62.	B	*p. 54*	79.	A	*p. 67*	96.	D	*p. 125*
63.	D	*p. 58*	80.	B	*p. 68*	97.	D	*p. 79*
64.	E	*p. 58*	81.	D	*p. 68*	98.	E	*p. 103*
65.	B	*p. 58*	82.	C	*p. 69*	99.	B	*p. 128*
66.	D	*p. 59*	83.	A	*p. 70*	100.	C	*p. 128*
67.	D	*p. 59*	84.	A	*p. 76*			

CHAPTER 3: NEUROLOGY

101.	C	*p. 181*	108.	E	*p. 184*	115.	D	*p. 196*
102.	D	*p. 181*	109.	D	*p. 184*	116.	B	*p. 197*
103.	C	*p. 182*	110.	D	*p. 186*	117.	D	*p. 197*
104.	C	*p. 184*	111.	A	*p. 186*	118.	B	*p. 203*
105.	C	*p. 184*	112.	E	*p. 189*	119.	C	*p. 203*
106.	A	*p. 185*	113.	D	*p. 189*	120.	C	*p. 210*
107.	D	*p. 185*	114.	C	*p. 189*			

CHAPTER 4: ENDOCRINOLOGY

121.	C	*p. 220*	128.	D	*p. 235*	135.	C	*p. 229*
122.	A	*p. 220*	129.	B	*p. 225*	136.	E	*p. 230*
123.	D	*p. 220*	130.	B	*p. 225*	137.	A	*p. 230*
124.	A	*p. 220*	131.	B	*p. 226*	138.	A	*p. 232*
125.	C	*p. 221*	132.	E	*p. 227*	139.	B	*p. 237*
126.	B	*p. 223*	133.	C	*p. 228*	140.	A	*p. 237*
127.	A	*p. 226*	134.	C	*p. 229*			

CHAPTER 5: IMMUNOLOGY

141.	C	*p. 243*	146.	E	*p. 244*	151.	A	*p. 246*
142.	B	*p. 243*	147.	C	*p. 245*	152.	D	*p. 247*
143.	B	*p. 243*	148.	B	*p. 245*	153.	C	*p. 248*
144.	B	*p. 244*	149.	C	*p. 243*	154.	B	*p. 250*
145.	C	*p. 243*	150.	D	*p. 245*	155.	B	*p. 250*

CHAPTER 6: GASTROENTEROLOGY

156.	D	*p. 256*	165.	E	*p. 260*	174.	D	*p. 270*
157.	B	*p. 256*	166.	B	*p. 260*	175.	C	*p. 270*
158.	C	*p. 256*	167.	B	*p. 260*	176.	E	*p. 271*
159.	B	*p. 258*	168.	A	*p. 262*	177.	D	*p. 271*
160.	C	*p. 258*	169.	D	*p. 262*	178.	A	*p. 272*
161.	A	*p. 259*	170.	C	*p. 262*	179.	A	*p. 273*
162.	A	*p. 264*	171.	A	*p. 264*	180.	A	*p. 273*
163.	C	*p. 264*	172.	B	*p. 262*			
164.	D	*p. 263*	173.	C	*p. 270*			

CHAPTER 7: UROLOGY AND NEPHROLOGY

181.	C *p. 278*	190.	A *p. 280*	199.	B *p. 283*
182.	D *p. 278*	191.	E *p. 280*	200.	A *p. 296*
183.	D *p. 278*	192.	C *p. 280*	201.	E *p. 288*
184.	D *p. 278*	193.	C *p. 281*	202.	C *p. 289*
185.	D *p. 278*	194.	A *p. 281*	203.	C *p. 291*
186.	C *p. 279*	195.	C *p. 281*	204.	C *p. 278*
187.	B *p. 280*	196.	D *p. 282*	205.	A *p. 294*
188.	A *p. 280*	197.	D *p. 279*		
189.	D *p. 280*	198.	D *p. 283*		

CHAPTER 8: TOXICOLOGY AND SUBSTANCE ABUSE

206.	B *p. 301*	216.	A *p. 319*	226.	A *p. 324*
207.	B *p. 304*	217.	D *p. 319*	227.	E *p. 326*
208.	A *p. 301*	218.	C *p. 320*	228.	C *p. 329*
209.	C *p. 315*	219.	A *p. 320*	229.	C *p. 329*
210.	A *p. 315*	220.	C *p. 322*	230.	E *p. 331*
211.	D *p. 317*	221.	A *p. 322*	231.	A *p. 335*
212.	E *p. 317*	222.	C *p. 322*	232.	B *p. 334*
213.	A *p. 318*	223.	B *p. 322*	233.	A *p. 334*
214.	E *p. 319*	224.	A *p. 323*	234.	A *p. 334*
215.	D *p. 319*	225.	C *p. 324*	235.	E *p. 334*

CHAPTER 9: HEMATOLOGY

236.	A *p. 342*	245.	B *p. 346*	254.	C *p. 252*
237.	B *p. 342*	246.	B *p. 346*	255.	D *p. 253*
238.	E *p. 342*	247.	D *p. 346*	256.	D *p. 257*
239.	A *p. 344*	248.	C *p. 347*	257.	C *p. 354*
240.	D *p. 343*	249.	B *p. 347*	258.	A *p. 257*
241.	C *p. 342*	250.	E *p. 348*	259.	B *p. 257*
242.	B *p. 343*	251.	B *p. 349*	260.	B *p. 353*
243.	A *p. 344*	252.	D *p. 349*		
244.	D *p. 346*	253.	A *p. 351*		

CHAPTER 10: INFECTIOUS DISEASE AND SEPSIS

261.	C *p. 364*	275.	C *p. 374*	289.	D *p. 389*
262.	D *p. 364*	276.	A *p. 376*	290.	B *p. 390*
263.	D *p. 365*	277.	B *p. 376*	291.	A *p. 390*
264.	D *p. 365*	278.	A *p. 378*	292.	C *p. 391*
265.	B *p. 366*	279.	A *p. 378*	293.	D *p. 392*
266.	D *p. 387*	280.	D *p. 378*	294.	D *p. 393*
267.	E *p. 368*	281.	D *p. 380*	295.	C *p. 395*
268.	B *p. 368*	282.	B *p. 380*	296.	C *p. 395*
269.	C *p. 368*	283.	B *p. 382*	297.	D *p. 397*
270.	C *p. 368*	284.	D *p. 383*	298.	B *p. 398*
271.	C *p. 369*	285.	E *p. 384*	299.	A *p. 398*
272.	D *p. 369*	286.	D *p. 385*	300.	C *p. 399*
273.	E *p. 370*	287.	A *p. 392*		
274.	A *p. 373*	288.	D *p. 388*		

CHAPTER 11: PSYCHIATRIC AND BEHAVIORAL DISORDERS

301.	C *p. 407*	308.	D *p. 311*	315.	B *p. 415*
302.	B *p. 407*	309.	B *p. 416*	316.	B *p. 415*
303.	A *p. 408*	310.	B *p. 411*	317.	B *p. 415*
304.	E *p. 409*	311.	B *p. 412*	318.	E *p. 416*
305.	D *p. 409*	312.	D *p. 414*	319.	C *p. 417*
306.	A *p. 411*	313.	B *p. 414*	320.	B *p. 419*
307.	B *p. 411*	314.	C *p. 415*		

CHAPTER 12: DISEASES OF THE EYES, EARS, NOSE, AND THROAT

321.	A *p. 426*	328.	A *p. 430*	335.	D *p. 435*
322.	C *p. 427*	329.	A *p. 430*	336.	A *p. 437*
323.	D *p. 426*	330.	A *p. 431*	337.	B *p. 437*
324.	E *p. 427*	331.	B *p. 432*	338.	A *p. 439*
325.	B *p. 428*	332.	E *p. 432*	339.	A *p. 440*
326.	E *p. 429*	333.	E *p. 433*	340.	B *p. 440*
327.	C *p. 429*	334.	B *p. 434*		

CHAPTER 13: NONTRAUMATIC MUSCULOSKELETAL DISORDERS

341.	E *p. 445*	348.	D *p. 449*	355.	C *p. 453*
342.	A *p. 445*	349.	A *p. 450*	356.	E *p. 454*
343.	D *p. 448*	350.	B *p. 450*	357.	D *p. 454*
344.	E *p. 445*	351.	A *p. 450*	358.	A *p. 456*
345.	A *p. 450*	352.	D *p. 452*		
346.	C *p. 449*	353.	A *p. 452*		
347.	C *p. 449*	354.	B *p. 453*		

©2013 Pearson Education, Inc.
Paramedic Care: Principles & Practice, Vol. 4, 4th Ed.

PATIENT SCENARIO FLASH CARDS

The following pages contain prepared 3" × 5" index cards. Each card presents a patient scenario with the appropriate signs and symptoms. On the reverse side are the appropriate field diagnosis and the care steps you should consider providing for your patient.

Detach the pages, cut out the cards, and review each of them in detail. If there are any discrepancies with what you have been taught in class, please review these with your instructor and medical director and employ what is appropriate for your EMS system. Record any changes directly on the cards.

Once your cards are prepared and you have reviewed them carefully, shuffle them and then read the scenario and signs and symptoms. Try to identify the patient's problem and the treatment you would employ. Compare your diagnosis and care steps with those on the reverse side of your flash card. This exercise will help you recognize and remember the common serious medical emergencies, their presentation, and the appropriate care. Remember that Standard Precautions should always be taken in any scenario.

SCENARIO 1:   You find a 68-year-old female inside her car, which has slid off into a slight ditch along the interstate.

S/S: Unilateral pupil dilation
Breathing with cheeks puffing on expiration
Snoring respirations
Paralysis on right side
Reduced LOC, responds to verbal stimuli only
Hypertension
Bradycardia

SCENARIO 2:   Your patient is a 43-year-old male complaining of a sudden onset of acute abdominal pain while working.

S/S: Temp of 103°F
RLQ pain, not relieved by position
No significant previous medical history
Ate a normal breakfast 3 hours ago

SCENARIO 1:

Field Diagnosis: Cerebrovascular accident (CVA) resulting in motor vehicle collision

Management:
Scene size-up—Determine nature of illness/mechanism of injury/index of suspicion.
  Standard Precautions—gloves
Initial Assessment
  Spinal precautions—manual immobilization and cervical collar.
  Calm and reassure patient.
  Airway—Maintain a patent airway; keep suction available.
  Breathing—Administer oxygen to keep $SaO_2 \geq 94\%$.
  Circulation—Establish an IV of NS or LR at 25 mL/hr rate.
Rapid Trauma Assessment
  Fully immobilize patient based on MOI.
  Determine blood glucose level; consider administration of 50% dextrose if hypoglycemia is present.
  Monitor ECG rhythm.
Provide ongoing assessment(s).
Protect paralyzed extremities and transport rapidly to accredited trauma center. Notify receiving facility to activate trauma team.

SCENARIO 2:

Field Diagnosis: Appendicitis

Management:
Scene size-up—Determine nature of illness, rule out traumatic injury.
  Standard Precaution—gloves
Initial Assessment
  Airway—Maintain a patent airway; keep suction available.
  Breathing—Administer oxygen to keep $SaO_2 \geq 94\%$.
  Circulation—Establish an IV w/large-bore catheter. Monitor ECG and vital signs.
Focused History and Physical Exam
  Calm and reassure patient.
  Monitor ECG rhythm.
Provide ongoing assessment(s). Treat signs of shock as indicated.
Transport. Alert receiving hospital.

SCENARIO 3: Your patient is a 47-year-old female who was pulling weeds in her garden when she suddenly collapsed with respiratory distress.

S/S: Sudden onset, less than minute
Anxious, scared
Difficulty breathing
Hypoxia
Blood pressure 88/64
Peripheral edema
Urticaria
Tachycardia
Small bite found on L arm

SCENARIO 4: Your patient is a 63-year-old male with increased dyspnea on exertion.

S/S: Recent weight loss
Barrel chest
Prolonged expirations
Rapid resting expirations
30-pack/year smoking history
Purses lips to breathe
Clubbed fingers
Wheezes
JVD
Peripheral edema

SCENARIO 5: You find an 18-year-old female lying on the sidewalk outside a warehouse known to house frequent "raves." The patient became unconscious and was brought outside by a friend. Unknown drugs were frequently available at the party. The patient is unresponsive to painful stimuli and is breathing 12 times per minute.

S/S: CNS depression
Constricted pupils
Blood pressure 90/52
Cool skin
Bradycardia
Pulmonary edema

SCENARIO 3:

Field Diagnosis: Anaphylaxis

Management: Scene size-up—Determine nature of illness.
    Standard Precautions—gloves
Initial Assessment
    Airway—Protect the airway. Consider early endotracheal intubation.
    Be prepared to establish surgical airway if necessary.
Breathing—Administer oxygen to keep $SaO_2 \geq 94\%$. Assist ventilations if indicated.
    Circulation—Establish one or two IVs w/large-bore catheters.
    Monitor ECG
Focused History and Physical Exam
    SAMPLE history
    Consider administering medications—epinephrine (0.3–0.5 mg 1:1,000 solution SQ/IM)
    may repeat if needed, diphenhydramine (25–50 mg IV), corticosteroids, and beta agonists
    per protocol.
Provide ongoing assessment(s). Treat hypotension with volume replacement; consider use of
vasopressors to maintain BP per protocol.
Transport rapidly. Alert receiving facility.

SCENARIO 4:

Field Diagnosis: Emphysema

Management: Scene Size-up—Determine nature of illness.
    Standard Precautions—gloves
Initial Assessment
    Airway—Maintain a patent airway.
Breathing—Place patient in position of comfort. Administer oxygen to keep $SaO_2 \geq 94\%$.
Prepare to assist ventilations of intubate if respiratory depression develops.
Circulation—Establish an IV of NS or LR at TKO rate. Monitor ECG.
Focused History and Physical Exam
    SAMPLE history
    Consider medication administration—bronchodilators, corticosteroids per protocol.
Provide ongoing assessment(s).
Transport. Alert receiving facility.

SCENARIO 5:

Field Diagnosis: Narcotic overdose

Management: Scene size-up—Determine nature of illness.
    Standard Precautions—gloves
Initial Assessment
    Airway—Maintain a patent airway; keep suction ready.
Breathing—Administer oxygen to keep $SaO_2 \geq 94\%$.
    Assist ventilations as indicated.
    Circulation—Establish an IV of NS or LR at 25ml/hr rate. Monitor ECG.
Focused History and Physical Exam
    SAMPLE history
    Consider medication administration—naloxone (0.4–2 mg IV prn titrated to improvement
    in respiratory status).
Provide ongoing assessment(s).
Transport. Alert receiving facility.

SCENARIO 6:   Your patient is a 92-year-old cancer case who is being cared for at home in a wealthy part of town. Examination reveals blunt trauma to the right arm.

S/S: Uncleaned sheets and room
Previous incontinence still evident
Senile dementia
Inconsistent story of how trauma occurred

SCENARIO 7:   Your patient is a 23-year-old sexually active female who has "pain on walking."

S/S: Lower abdominal pain
Pain with intercourse
Yellow vaginal discharge
Rebound tenderness
Fever

SCENARIO 8:   Your patient is a 42-year-old male taxi driver who experiences colicky pain.

S/S: Acute onset of back and flank pain
Pain appears to migrate downward as episode continues
Pain described as worst patient ever experienced
History of difficulty/painful urination for last 12 hours

SCENARIO 6:

Field Diagnosis: Geriatric neglect/abuse

Management: Scene size-up—Determine nature of illness/mechanism of injury.
    Standard Precautions—gloves
Initial Assessment
    Airway—Maintain a patent airway.
    Breathing—Administer oxygen to keep $SaO_2 \geq 94\%$.
    Circulation—Assess circulatory status. Monitor ECG.
Focused History and Physical Exam
    Document patient history, sources of information, and inconsistencies.
    Avoid confrontational situations.
Provide ongoing assessment(s).
Transport. Alert receiving facility. Report suspicions to appropriate authorities per protocol.

SCENARIO 7:

Field Diagnosis: Pelvic inflammatory disease

Management: Scene size-up—Determine nature of illness.
    Standard Precautions—gloves
Initial Assessment
    Airway—Maintain a patent airway.
    Breathing—Administer oxygen to keep $SaO_2 \geq 94\%$.
    Circulation—Assess circulatory status. Establish IV access if signs of sepsis.
Focused History and Physical Exam
    SAMPLE history
    Provide supportive care. Avoid walking the patient and allow her to remain in a position of comfort.
Provide ongoing assessment(s).
Transport. Notify receiving facility.

SCENARIO 8:

Field Diagnosis: Renal calculi (kidney stones)

Management: Scene size-up—Determine nature of illness.
    Standard Precautions—gloves
Initial Assessment
    Airway—Maintain a patent airway.
    Breathing—Administer oxygen to keep $SaO_2 \geq 94\%$.
    Circulation—Establish an IV of NS or LR at 100 mL/hr rate.
Focused History and Physical Exam
    SAMPLE history
    Provide supportive care; coach the patient through pain episodes; place the patient in a position of comfort.
    Consider medication administration—Toradol, narcotic analgesics and antiemetics per protocol.
Provide ongoing assessment(s).
Transport. Notify receiving facility.

SCENARIO 9:   Your patient is a 55-year-old female who just returned home from recent hip fracture surgery.

S/S: Sudden onset of unexplained dyspnea
Chest pain
Tachypnea with labored breathing
Tachycardia
JVD
Progressive hypertension

SCENARIO 10:   Your patient is an 18-year-old female distraught over the breakup with her boyfriend.

S/S: Tachycardia
Dilated pupils
Respiratory depression
Slurred speech
Twitching and jerking
Seizures
ST and T wave changes on ECG
Blood pressure 84/52

SCENARIO 11:   Your patient is a 52-year-old office executive who has had a stressful day and about 2 hours ago started having chest pains.

S/S: Diaphoresis
Anxiety
Apprehension
Dyspnea
Pallor
Irregular pulse
Bradycardia
Pain radiating down left arm and into the back
"Crushing pain in my chest"

SCENARIO 9:

Field Diagnosis: Pulmonary embolism

Management:
Scene size-up—Determine nature of illness.
    Standard Precautions—gloves
Initial Assessment
    Airway—Maintain a patent airway.
    Breathing—Administer oxygen to keep $SaO_2 \geq 94\%$. Assist ventilations as necessary.
    Perform endotracheal intubation if indicated.
    Circulation—Establish an IV of NS or LR at 25 mL/hr rate. Monitor ECG and vital signs.
    Use waveform capnography to monitor $EtCO_2$ and ventilatory function.
Focused History and Physical Exam
    SAMPLE history
Provide ongoing assessment(s).
Transport rapidly. Alert receiving facility.

SCENARIO 10:

Field Diagnosis: Tricyclic antidepressant overdose

Management:
Scene size-up—Determine nature of illness.
    Standard Precautions—gloves
Initial Assessment
    Airway—Maintain a patent airway.
    Breathing—Administer oxygen to keep $SaO_2 \geq 94\%$. Assist ventilations as necessary.
    Perform endotracheal intubation if indicated. Use waveform capnography to monitor
    $EtCO_2$ and ventilatory function.
    Circulation—Establish an IV of NS or LR at 25 mL/hr rate. Monitor ECG and vital signs.
    Treat dysrhythmias per protocol.
Focused History and Physical Exam
    SAMPLE history
    Contact poison control.
    Consider placement of nasogastric tube and gastric lavage or administration of activated
    charcoal to reduce absorption if ingestion occurred less than 1 hour ago. Contact local
    poison control center.
Provide ongoing assessment(s).
Transport rapidly. Alert receiving facility.

SCENARIO 11:

Field Diagnosis: Myocardial infarction/Acute coronary syndrome (ACS)

Management:
Scene size-up—Determine nature of illness.
    Standard Precautions—gloves
Initial Assessment
    Airway—Maintain a patent airway.
    Breathing—Administer oxygen to keep $SaO_2 \geq 94\%$.
    Assist ventilations as necessary. Perform endotracheal intubation if indicated.
    Circulation—Establish 2 large-bore IVs of NS or LR at 25 mL/hr rate if possible. Monitor
    ECG and vital signs. Use waveform capnography to monitor $EtCO_2$ and ventilatory func-
    tion. Treat specific dysrhythmias per protocol.
Focused History and Physical Exam
    SAMPLE history
    Place patient in position of comfort.
    Obtain 12-lead or 15-lead ECG and transmit to medical control. Consider transport to
    closest cardiac catheterization facility. Repeat 12-lead or 15-lead ECG en route.
    Consider medication administration—aspirin, narcotic analgesics, antiemetics, nitroglyc-
    erin (SL or IV) per protocol.
Provide ongoing assessment(s).
Transport rapidly. Alert receiving facility.